Handbook of
and Gynaecology

Handbook of Obstetrics and Gynaecology

THIRD EDITION

Edited by

Barry G. Wren

Director
Centre for the Management of the Menopause
Royal Hospital for Women, Paddington, Sydney

and

Rogerio A. Lobo

Professor
Department of Obstetrics and Gynecology
University of Southern California
Los Angeles, California

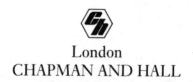

London
CHAPMAN AND HALL

First published in 1979 by Cassell Australia Ltd
Second edition 1985 published by Chapman and Hall Ltd
11 New Fetter Lane, London EC4P 4EE
Third edition 1989

© 1989 Barry G. Wren and Rogerio A. Lobo

Typeset in 10/12 Ehrhardt by
Best-Set Typesetter Limited, Hong Kong
Printed in Hong Kong

ISBN 0 412 31060 0

British Library Cataloguing in Publication Data

Handbook of obstetrics and gynaecology.—
3rd ed.
1. Gynaecology & obstetrics
I. Wren, Barry G. II. Lobo, Rogerio A.
618

ISBN 0-412-31060-0

Contents

Contents

Preface to the third edition

When the *Handbook of Obstetrics and Gynaecology* was first written as internal course material in 1974, it was designed to assist students in understanding the core of knowledge required for the curriculum at the University of New South Wales in Sydney. The *Handbook* was to contain only that information which was essential to the undergraduate course, and it was published with a specific size in mind — it had to slip easily into a ward coat pocket.

Since then, there have been two further publications of this book and it is now bought by students in many parts of the English-speaking world. The original concepts have been maintained in all publications, but new ideas and changing technology have meant a continual need for updating.

In this, the third edition, the *Handbook* has become international, with Professor Rogerio Lobo accepting our invitation not only to write a chapter, but also to co-edit the content.

Because the original staff of the University of New South Wales have now all retired, their replacements have been invited to assist with this most recent review. Some of the chapters have been re-written, in which case the original authors have been deleted from the list of contributors, whilst in other cases, the chapter has been revised and brought up to date, with only a few changes to the text. In these latter cases, both the original and the new authors are accredited with the contribution.

We hope the new edition of the *Handbook of Obstetrics and Gynaecology* remains as popular as the early versions. It must be regarded as a guide to undergraduates and not as a major resource manual. However, it has a logical, easy-to-understand text, simple diagrams and, most important, it is highly relevant to those common obstetric and gynaecological activities which are faced by students, interns and nurses. Those who use the book will find it of great practical value, and we hope that students continue to find it useful both before and after graduation.

Barry G. Wren, *Sydney*
Rogerio A. Lobo, *Los Angeles*
1988

Contributors

Michael J. Bennett MD, ChB(UCT), FCOG(SA), FRACOG, DDU.
Professor and Head, School of Obstetrics and Gynaecology, University of New South Wales, Sydney, Australia

C. R. Climie MB ChB, FFARCS, FFARACS
Former Staff Anaesthetist, Royal Hospital for Women, Paddington, Syndey, Australia

C. Fisher MB BS, MRACGP, MRCOG, FRACOG
Staff Obstetrician and Gynaecologist, Royal Hospital for Women, Paddington, Sydney, Australia

Stephen P. Gatt MD, LRCP, MRCS, FFARACS, FFA Intensive Care
Director of Anaesthesia, Royal Hospital for Women, Paddington, Syndey, Australia

J. M. Gupta MB BS, MD, DCH, MRCP, MRACP
Associate Professor, School of Paediatrics, University of New South Wales, Sydney, Australia

Graeme Hughes MB BS, MRCOG, FRACOG
Senior Lecturer, School of Obstetrics and Gynaecology, University of New South Wales, Sydney, Australia

Leo R. Leader FRACOG
Senior Lecturer, School of Obstetrics and Gynaecology, University of New South Wales, Sydney, Australia

Rogerio A. Lobo MD
Professor and Chief of Division of Reproductive Endocrinology and Infertility, Department of Obstetrics and Gynecology, University of Southern California, The Women's Hospital, Los Angeles

Rosalind Robertson MA
Psychologist in Departments of Gynaecological Endocrinology and Oncology, Royal Hospital for Women, Paddington, Sydney, Australia

Debbie Wass MRCOG, FRACOG
Lecturer, School of Obstetrics and Gynaecology, University of New South Wales, Sydney, Australia

Michael Webster MB BS, MRCOG, FRACOG
Lecturer, School of Obstetrics and Gynaecology, University of New South Wales, Sydney, Australia

Barry G. Wren MD, MB BS, MHPeD, FRACOG, FRCOG
Director, Centre for the Management of the Menopause, Royal Hospital for Women, Paddington, Sydney, Australia

History taking and physical examination

Barry G. Wren

1.1 GENERAL INSTRUCTIONAL OBJECTIVE

The students are expected to develop competence in taking a history and performing a physical examination so that obstetric or gynaecological abnormalities can be recognized and appropriate management initiated.

1.2 SPECIFIC BEHAVIOURAL OBJECTIVES

1. Elicit a relevant history from a patient with an obstetric or gynaecological problem.
2. Examine the pelvis and abdomen of a patient with an obstetric or gynaecological problem.
3. Discuss the history, physical findings and possible diagnoses of a patient with obstetric and gynaecological problems.
4. Demonstrate care, consideration, tact and kindness when taking a history, examining or managing a patient who presents with an obstetric or gynaecological problem.

1.3 REASONS FOR LEARNING TO TAKE A RELEVANT HISTORY AND PERFORMING A SPECIFIC OBSTETRIC AND GYNAECOLOGICAL EXAMINATION

Most medical students are taught to take a good general history and to perform an adequate physical examination, but at first they tend to ask too many questions, to ask far too many irrelevant time- and space-filling questions, or to fail to obtain sufficient information on an important symptom. It is, however, necessary to focus on only the more relevant facts and to ask for some very specific information. Without knowledge regarding the relevance of material or the knowledge of the pathophysiology of the disease, it becomes very difficult for students to sort out the important from the unimportant facts that a patient may offer to a doctor. Specific and leading questions may never be asked unless the student knows that a certain symptom may be the key to opening the diagnosis. Symptoms that the patient may regard as irrelevant may hold the answer to the diagnosis. It is important that the student is aware not only of some of these specialized symptoms, but also how to obtain a history from a female patient.

There is often a reluctance on the part of the patient to state what actually is the problem. Female patients may feel embarrassed to talk to strangers about vaginal discharge, sexual problems or other personal gynaecological symptoms. Students should be aware of the problem and be able to show sympathy. Questions should be open-ended, beginning with such queries as 'How did you feel?', 'What happened then?', 'Tell me about it'. Students must avoid the use of any questions implying a judgement, such as 'Why did you do that?'. The justification necessary to answer such questions may make the patient defensive, tense and anxious, so that a correct easily expressed history is not obtained.

If possible, students should avoid writing answers immediately to all the questions. It is more natural and comforting to a patient for the doctor to appear to be having a chat or a pleasant talk than to be conducting a staccato interview. Students would of course obtain the necessary coding information early. Facts such as age, parity and marital state should be obtained and recorded early — then the doctor must relax and let the patient tell her story. It is important only to interrupt in order to clarify a certain point. When she has finished, the doctor will have a sound idea of what is wrong and can then ask the specific, probing and detailed questions that allow a diagnosis to be made.

Without the ability to take a good history and to perform an adequate examination, no medical practitioner can assist women who attend complaining of obstetric or gynaecological problems.

The specific questions that it may be necessary to ask include the following:

1.4 OBSTETRIC HISTORY

1. Name and address.
2. It is best to obtain the actual date of birth. People age from year to year but the birth date remains constant.

3. Gravidity and parity. Gravidity refers to the number of times a woman has conceived, whilst parity refers to the number of pregnancies, of more than 20 weeks of amenorrhoea, she has delivered. Parity is often noted as P2 + 3, meaning the woman has delivered two babies and also had three pregnancies that have terminated prior to 20 weeks of amenorrhoea.

4. Last normal menstrual period (LNMP). This should be recorded from the first day of the last normal period. Ask about its duration, the volume of flow, any associated pain or other symptoms. Did it appear normal or was it merely 'spotting'? If the latter was the case, then the second-last menstrual period should also be recorded, and, if that was also abnormal, keep going back until the last normal menstrual period can be ascertained. Abnormalities of 'menstrual flow' are frequently found in such conditions as dysfunctional uterine haemorrhage, fibromyoma, threatened abortion, implantation bleed and ectopic pregnancy.

5. Menstrual cycle. This usually varies from 3 to 5 per 21–35 days. It may become grossly irregular in a variety of states, particularly dysfunctional uterine haemorrhage and certain infertility problems. A regular pattern generally suggests a normal hypothalamic–pituitary –ovarian function.

6. Period of amenorrhoea should be calculated accurately by counting from the first day of the last normal period. The length of time should *always* be recorded accurately in weeks and days (a month is *not* a scientific measure of time!).

7. Expected date of confinement (EDC). A rough guide for doctor and patient is achieved by the knowledge that most infants will deliver 283 (±14) days after the first day of the last normal period. An easy ready reckoner is achieved by adding 9 months and ~~10~~ 7 days to the date of the LNMP to determine the EDC. *Neagle's rule*

	Days	Months	Year
e.g. If LNMP was 8 April 1983, then add 10 days and 9 months	8	4	1983
	~~10~~ 7	9	
and the EDC is approximately	~~18~~ 15	1	1984

8. Nationality may be important, as Mediterranean peoples have a higher incidence of thalassaemia, tuberculosis and other locally acquired diseases.

9. Does the patient smoke, drink or take drugs? All of these may have

a deleterious effect on a pregnancy and the medical officer should warn patients accordingly.

10. Obstetric record.

Preg. No.	Year	Complications of pregnancy	Length of labour	Type of delivery	Weight	Sex	A SB NND

A = alive; SB = still birth; NND = neonatal death.

11. Medical history. Some medical diseases are particularly relevant to pregnancy and care must be taken to enquire about these, such as heart disease, rheumatic fever, hypertension, tuberculosis, asthma, bronchitis, urinary tract infection or 'fits'.
12. Surgical history. Take particular care to record such previous operations as dilatation and curettage, abdominal operations or accidents, as well as blood transfusions.
13. Family history. Enquire about illness in close relatives, such as tuberculosis, diabetes, hypertension, multiple pregnancy or congenital abnormalities.
14. Social history. Enquire about marital status, financial support, smoking and drinking habits, work or occupation, and knowledge regarding social benefits, reproductive education, baby care, contraception, sexual attitudes and community child-care centres.
15. Gynaecological history regarding her menstrual life, contraception and sexual intercourse. Difficulty, pain or ignorance in any of these areas would suggest that either counselling or further investigation may be necessary.

1.5 HISTORY OF THE PRESENT PREGNANCY

1. Ask about the common symptoms of pregnancy, such as:
   (a) Nausea or vomiting
   (b) Breast tenderness or swelling
   (c) Frequency of micturition
   (d) Fainting
   (e) Vaginal discharge

2. Determine when fetal movements are first felt. In primigravid women they are usually first detected at about 18–20 weeks of amenorrhoea. In multigravida, because of prior experience, they are usually first detected at about 17–19 weeks. Movements are usually felt as faint 'bubbles' or 'like a butterfly'. Note carefully and record the exact date that fetal movements are first felt.
3. Abnormal symptoms may be pain, vaginal bleeding and an abnormal discharge. Specific questions should be asked, and further enquiries made if the response is affirmative.
4. If there is any response that indicates the presence of an abnormality, it is wise to investigate all the associated factors by careful enquiry or by physical examination.

Always check at each obstetric visit that the patient is taking her iron and folic acid, and has enough to last until the next visit. Then, make an appointment for the next visit.

1.6 OBSTETRIC EXAMINATION

General impression

Note anything obvious such as height, weight, accent, configuration and gait.

General examination

1. Blood pressure, pulse, hands, nails.
2. Feet, varicose veins, oedema.
3. Mouth, tongue and teeth.
4. Neck, thyroid.
5. Thorax and breasts (observe the nipples, areola, Montgomery tubercles, veins and breast secretions).
6. Listen to heart and lungs for abnormal sounds.

Abdominal examination

1. Inspect the abdomen for the presence of striae, scars or bruises.
2. Palpate for the liver, spleen, kidneys and uterus.

Uterine palpation

The uterus grows from a small organ, 8 cm long, in the pelvis to a large mass, 30–35 cm long, which reaches to the subcostal margins by the 36th week of a normal pregnancy. The regular palpation and observation of changes in parameters of the growing uterus allow an attendant to determine normal and abnormal growth patterns, and to modify the antenatal care as necessary. The parameters that should be closely examined as often as necessary and recorded on a chart are as follows:

1. Uterine fundus (Fig. 1.1). This is just palpable above the symphysis pubis by the 12th week of pregnancy, reaches approximately to the umbilicus by the 24th week, and finally ceases to ascend at about the 36th week. When the uterine fundus is about halfway from the symphysis pubis to the umbilicus, the gestational age is about 16 weeks (soon after, the fetal movements may be first felt). From the umbilicus to the subcostal margins, the uterine fundus grows at a rate equivalent to one finger's breadth (2 cm) every 2 weeks. (Note that the umbilicus becomes flattened after 24 weeks due to the intra-abdominal distension.) The fundus of the uterus generally remains at about the level of the xiphisternum (or the subcostal margins) from the 36th week until the time of delivery (38–42 weeks), unless the head actually engages in the pelvis — in which case, as the head and body descend, so will the fundus appear to decrease in height (to the 32 or 34 weeks fundal height).

2. Fetal lie (Fig. 1.2). The fetal lie is the relationship of the long axis

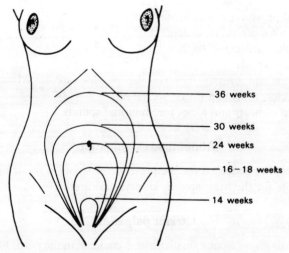

Fig. 1.1 Estimated gestational age from equivalent fundal heights.

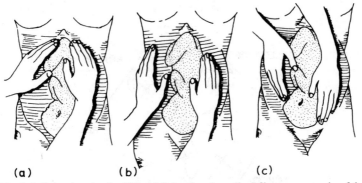

Fig. 1.2 Palpating the fetal lie. (a) Palpating the soft, diffuse, upper pole of the fetal breech; (b) Palpating the broad, firm back of the fetus. Note that there is little resistance at the convex front of the fetus; (c) Palpating the firm, round, mobile head of the fetus.

of the fetus to the long axis of the uterus. As the uterus generally lies longitudinally to the mother, the lie is often referred to as being the relationship of the fetal axis to the maternal axis. The fetal axis can generally be detected easily by finding the two ends (poles) of the fetus. The head is usually harder and rounder than the large, diffuse, soft bottom of the fetus. A line drawn between these two poles is the fetal axis. To confirm the lie, the fetal back can also be palpated parallel to the axis. An oblique or transverse lie usually indicates some abnormality.

3. Fetal position is the relationship of the denominator of the presenting part of the fetus to the mother's pelvis. When the head is presenting with one of the usual degrees of flexion, then the occiput is the denominator. The position is stated as being occipito-anterior (OA), occipito-lateral (OL) or occipito-posterior (OP) in relationship to the maternal pelvic brim. The common positions before the onset of labour are: left occipito-lateral (LOL), 50%; and right occipito-lateral (ROL), 25% (Fig. 1.3). However, at the end of labour, 60% of positions are found to be left occipito-anterior (LOA) and 30% are right occipito-anterior (ROA), indicating that internal rotation to an anterior position is the commonest outcome during labour. Other positions relate to the mentum (face) and sacrum (breech).

4. Fetal presentation. Over 95% of all babies present by the fetal head and less that 5% are found to have a breech, shoulder or other form of presentation. The head is generally easily palpated lying in the

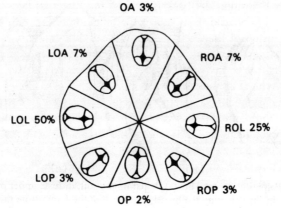

Fig. 1.3 Frequency of distribution of positions of the occiput at the onset of labour.

lower segment as a firm, round, mobile mass, but if doubt exists an ultrasound examination should be taken after the 34th week to confirm the presence of breech or other abnormal presentation.
5. Fetal attitude. The fetal head is normally universally flexed so that the fetal head presents the smallest diameters (9.5 cm) to the maternal pelvic brim. However, when the fetus is in the occipito-

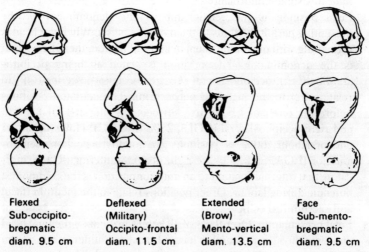

Flexed	Deflexed	Extended	Face
Sub-occipito-bregmatic	(Military)	(Brow)	Sub-mento-bregmatic
	Occipito-frontal	Mento-vertical	
diam. 9.5 cm	diam. 11.5 cm	diam. 13.5 cm	diam. 9.5 cm

Fig. 1.4 Fetal attitude.

posterior position, its back is against the maternal back and the maternal lumbar lordosis causes the fetus to present with a degree of extension of the back, neck and head (the 'military' attitude). This extension means that a larger diameter — occipito-frontal (11.5 cm) or vertico-mental (13.5 cm) — presents at the maternal pelvic brim (Fig. 1.4).

6. Fetal engagement is the term used when the largest diameter of the presenting diameters has passed through the pelvic brim. With a well-flexed fetal head, the suboccipito-bregmatic diameter and the biparietal diameter are both about 9.5 cm and will easily pass through a pelvis that has dimensions of average size. However, a fetal head that is extended due to an occipito-lateral or occipito-posterior position may not engage until strong labour contractions cause flexion and then descent of the head. Engagement may be detected either by abdominal palpation or by vaginal examination.

7. Fetal heart rate is usually between 120 and 160 per minute and is detected over the portion of the fetal chest that lies closest to the uterine wall.

DETERMINING THE FETAL POSITION

1. First determine the presentation. If the head presents, the denominator will almost always be the occiput.

2. The occiput always lies on the same side of the fetal body as the back, so palpate for the back. Palpate across the abdomen at the level of the umbilicus. The back is detected as a broad band of resistance on one side. Palpate along the back to the breech, and then down to the shoulder and the head. The portion of the fetal head that is first palpated after the fetal back is the occiput.

3. Having determined the side on which the occiput lies, it is relatively easy to determine whether the occiput is anterior, lateral or posterior. The fetal head is an oval shape, with the occiput at one end and the sinciput at the other. A line drawn through the occiput and sinciput passes along the sagittal suture, and a line drawn at right angles to the sagittal suture will pass through the tips of both fetal shoulders (Fig. 1.5). Knowing this simple geometry allows one to palpate not only the back but the shoulder, occiput and the sinciput, and so by spatial imagery to determine the fetal position. Final confirmation can be obtained at a vaginal examination to feel the sagittal suture, the anterior and posterior fontanelles or the fetal ear.

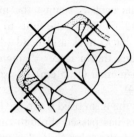

Fig. 1.5 Showing that a line drawn through the two shoulders will be at right angles to a line drawn through the sagittal suture. This piece of geometry is helpful when determining the position of the fetus during labour.

ABDOMINAL PALPATION TO DETERMINE FETAL LIE, PRESENTATION, POSITION AND ENGAGEMENT

It is essential in obstetrics that from the 30th week of pregnancy medical practitioners can palpate accurately the lie, presentation, position and engagement of a fetus, as it is by mastering these skills that they can diagnose such conditions as breech, transverse lie, twins, disproportion, occipito-posterior position, polyhydramnios and may suspect other conditions such as placenta praevia, hydrocephalus or failure of fetal growth.

Medical practitioners who do not have these skills in palpation will be seriously handicapped in management of normal pregnancy and will fail to diagnose problems that might be present. Students who fail to master the steps and techniques of fetal palpation will be unable to assist in antenatal clinics or in the labour ward.

STEPS IN PALPATION OF UTERUS AT MORE THAN 30 WEEKS

1. Ensure that the patient is lying comfortably in a bed (or on an examination couch), on her back and with her abdominal muscles completely relaxed.
2. Expose the whole abdomen from the symphysis pubis to the xip-histernum. Make sure that underclothes are pulled below the level of the hips and the symphysis.
3. Observe the configuration of the uterus. It is generally oval in shape with the long axis parallel to the long axis of the mother. Abnormal shapes to the uterus may be due to transverse lie, subseptate uterus, multiple pregnancy, polyhydramnios or disproportion.

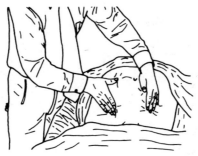

Fig. 1.6 Demonstrating that to palpate an abdomen satisfactorily, the position of the body must allow the flat of the hands to press against the fetus.

4. Palpate the uterine outline. Stand in a position so that you face either the head or the feet of your patient — in this way you can place a hand easily on either side of the uterus without undue effort. Use the flat of the hand and fingers when palpating, as it causes less discomfort than when one or two fingers are pressed into the abdominal wall (Fig. 1.6). Run your hands gently over the uterus to feel its configuration. This gentle palpation helps in two ways. First, you can determine the general outline of the uterus and can confirm that it is indeed of an oval (or an uneven) shape; secondly, by being gentle with your initial palpation you can assist in relaxing the patient for the next steps in palpation.
5. Now determine the lie of the fetus. Using both hands on either side of the uterus and approximately at the same level, palpate the fetus as it lies within the uterus. Usually it will be lying longitudinally, it is then easy to feel the fetal back as a broad, firm and resistant mass on one side. Having found the back, move both hands up and down (on either side of the utrus), following the back to the two ends (poles) of the fetus. Determine very carefully the size and consistency of the two poles. A line drawn between the midpoint of each pole is the axis of the fetus. To obtain the lie, relate the axis of the fetus to the axis of the uterus. An oblique lie will have the lower pole lying in one iliac fossa, whilst a transverse lie will have both poles lying in the flanks (Fig. 1.7).
6. The presentation is usually the head, which is felt as a firm, round mass. A breech is usually soft, diffuse and often feels larger than the head. Again, palpation should be with both hands working opposite each other on either side of the uterus. Be gentle but firm with all palpation and avoid 'playing the piano' when palpating.

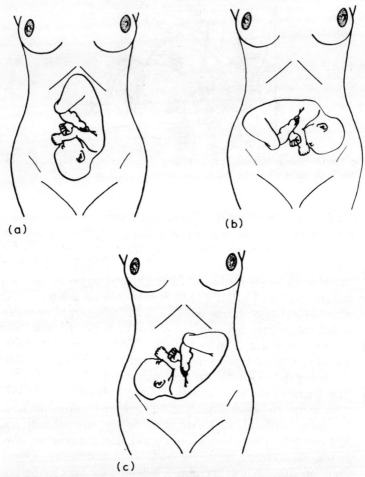

Fig. 1.7 Fetal lie. (a) Longitudinal; (b) Transverse; (c) Oblique.

Irregular movement in palpation is more likely to produce a uterine contraction or cause pain so that further palpation is difficult.

7. Finding the position can be difficult, but remember that the occiput and the sacrum both lie on the same side as the fetal back. If you can palpate the firm, resistant back at the level of the umbilicus and can follow this down to the lower pole, then the denominator is easily detected. As the head usually presents, the first part of the head that is palpated after moving off the back must be the occiput (Fig. 1.8). Mostly the fetus will be in the occipito-lateral position,

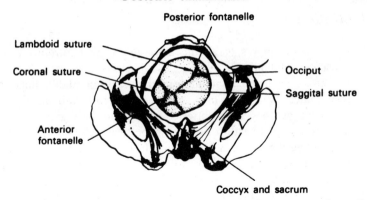

Posterior fontanelle

Lambdoid suture

Coronal suture

Occiput

Saggital suture

**Anterior
fontanelle**

Coccyx and sacrum

Fig. 1.8 Fetal skull within the bony pelvis. The skull sutures can be easily palpated to determine the fetal position. In this case it is left occipito-anterior.

and this can be confirmed by pressing down on the fetal occiput and the synciput to ascertain that both lie approximately equidistant from the skin over the anterior abdominal wall.

8. It is sometimes difficult to be sure whether a head is engaged in the pelvis, but it is easy to decide when it is high above the brim. If your fingers can be made to pass around in front of the head above the symphysis pubis, then it is clearly not engaged. When you cannot get your fingers in front of the head then the head is obviously fitting into the brim. The point of decision between engagement and non-engagement in these cases is a fine one, and probably not important unless you are considering applying forceps prior to delivery. In this case, a vaginal examination must become the final arbiter.

+ Pawlock's manoeuvre

Vaginal examination in labour

A digital vaginal examination is usually performed to determine: .

1. The cervical dilatation and effacement.
2. The descent of the fetal head in the pelvis.
3. The presence of caput succedaneum or of fetal skull moulding.
4. The shape of the maternal bony pelvis.
5. Whether a prolapsed cord is present following rupture of membranes.

Never perform a digital vaginal examination in the presence of an antepartum haemorrhage unless full preparations have been made for an urgent delivery (placenta praevia may be present).

TECHNIQUE

1. Using sterile gloves, swab the labia and vaginal introitus with antiseptic solution.
2. Use an antiseptic cream to lubricate the index and middle fingers, then under *direct observation*, separate the labia with one hand whilst the two fingers are inserted gently into the vagina.
3. Feel for the fetal head. It can usually be easily felt as a bony hard mass filling the pelvis. A breech may feel firm and is occasionally mistaken for the head, unless care and thought are involved during the procedure.
4. The cervix is usually easily detected, unless effacement is almost complete. Pass the fingers inside the cervix and feel for the extent of dilatation. Try to estimate the diameter of the cervical dilatation and express it in centimetres. The cervix may be thick when only slightly dilated, but becomes thinner (or effaced) as the cervix dilates beyond 5 cm.
5. When performing a vaginal examination in labour, it is important to determine how far down the pelvis the presenting part has advanced. The leading part of the head is usually the vertex and this point is related to the ischial spines. The distance of the vertex above or below the ischial spines is assessed in centimetres and expressed as -3, -2, -1, 0, $+1$, $+2$, $+3$, etc. to indicate the degree of descent.
6. The skull of the fetus is carefully palpated. Early in labour, before caput formation has occurred, the sagittal suture and the fontanelles can be easily felt, and from this the position is usually determined. Later in labour, the degree of moulding and skull bone overlap may be extreme; the fontanelles are difficult to feel and when the head has been pressing against the dilating cervix for some hours, oedematous thickening of the scalp can be felt (caput succedaneum). The more moulding and caput occurring, the more likely it is that a long difficult labour is taking place. When difficulty is experienced in determining the position (because of caput formation), then a hand slipped over the side of the fetal skull will easily feel the fetal ear. When this is moved backwards and forwards, it is easy to determine the direction of the pinna. The pinna of the ear always points backwards towards the occiput.
7. Maternal pelvic findings (Fig. 1.9). Generally it is difficult to assess a pelvis from the point of view of obstetric outcome. However, a rough guide can be established:

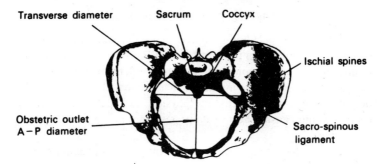

Transverse diameter   **Sacrum**   **Coccyx**

Ischial spines

**Obstetric outlet
A – P diameter**

**Sacro-spinous
ligament**

Fig. 1.9 Landmarks of bony pelvis showing well-rounded features of a gynaecoid brim shape.

(a) Feel for the sacral promontory (Fig. 1.10). Generally it cannot be palpated unless the true conjugate diameter is less than 10.5 cm.

(b) Feel for the sacral curve. Generally the sacrum cannot be felt, but in a narrow funnel-shaped pelvis (associated with an android-shaped brim) the first four segments may appear flat.

(c) The sacro-spinous ligament is generally 4 cm or more in length, but a reduction in distance may indicate an increased 'funnelling' of the pelvis.

(d) Feel for the forepart of the pelvic brim. It is usually rounded, but may have straight rami and a narrow angle at the back of the symphysis pubis — this would indicate an android-shape to the brim.

(e) The subpubic angle may be narrow and less than 80° in arc. This would force the fetal head farther posteriorly in an attempt to pass out of the pelvis, and is obviously an additional problem if associated with an android-shaped pelvic brim.

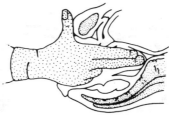

Fig. 1.10 Feel for the sacral promontory and then palpate the sacral curve.

Vaginal speculum examination

Passing a vaginal speculum is an essential skill required by all medical students to enable them to identify and diagnose problems presenting in obstetric and gynaecological patients. Students will be required to pass a vaginal speculum in such a manner that they will be able to display, identify and describe the physical findings of the vagina and cervix without causing hurt or embarrassment to the patients they are examining.

Many females attend a medical practitioner complaining of symptoms that suggest that a vaginal or cervical problem exists. When the patient complains of symptoms referable to the bladder (stress incontinence, dysuria or frequency), or of dyspareunia, a lump in the vagina or bleeding in late pregnancy, then it is important that the speculum used is of a single-blade type (Sims' speculum) (Fig. 1.11). However, when the symptoms are of vaginal discharge, postcoital bleeding or bleeding due to problems in early pregnancy (abortion, ectopic pregnancy, hydatidiform mole), or if a Papanicolaou smear is to be obtained, then a bivalve speculum is the more convenient instrument. The better types of bivalve instrument will come apart (Grave's speculum) (Fig. 1.12), allowing the anterior blade of the speculum to be removed — the posterior blade can then be used as a Sims' speculum.

Whichever speculum is used, several steps should be taken before actually attempting to pass the speculum.

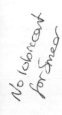

1. Make sure the speculum is at an acceptable temperature. Warm the speculum in a bowl of water at about 40–45°C.
2. Apply a thin smear of lubricant to the surface of the speculum. Make sure that no lubricant is on the inner (concave) surfaces as it may be mistaken for a discharge, and may also mix with a cervical smear and ruin a cytological examination.
3. Choose all your equipment before the examination and have it

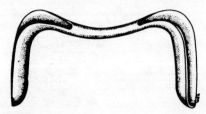

Fig. 1.11 Sims' speculum.

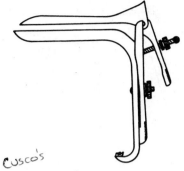

Cusco's

Fig. 1.12 Bivalve (Grave's) speculum.

ready to hand. You may need Ayre's spatula, sponge-holding forceps, cotton-wool swabs, swab-sticks, culture media or transport
media.

PASSING THE SPECULUM (Figs 1. 13–1.22)

Several techniques are employed, and all are satisfactory if the condition is displayed adequately without causing hurt or embarrassment
to the patient. A common method for passing a Grave's speculum is
described:

1. Position the patient on her back so that the buttocks are over the
   end of the couch or table and the feet are supported on a ledge or
   in stirrups.
2. Drape the sheet over the lower abdomen, and the legs so that the
   thighs and abdomen are covered but the vulva is easily seen.
3. Explain to the patient that you are about to pass a metal speculum
   into the vagina.

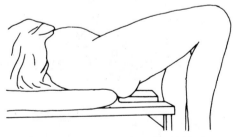

Fig. 1.13 Demonstrating that to obtain the best position to examine a patient
using a speculum, the buttocks must be over the end of the couch.

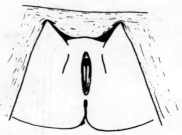

Fig. 1.14 Demonstrating that when a patient is draped and lying comfortably on a couch, the labia are apposed and examination is difficult.

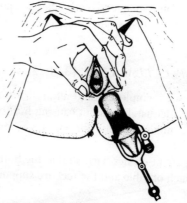

Fig. 1.15 Demonstrating that when the labia are widely separated the speculum may be more easily inserted into the vagina.

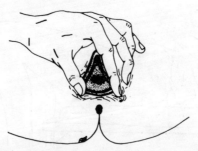

Fig. 1.16 Showing that if the index finger and thumb are inserted between the labia and then separated, the vaginal introitus is clearly seen, a speculum can be passed easily and sometimes even the cervix can be visualized.

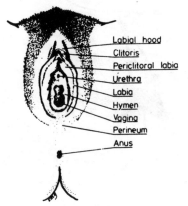

Fig. 1.17 Illustrating the anatomy of the labia and vaginal introitus, which should be carefully inspected when the labia are separated.

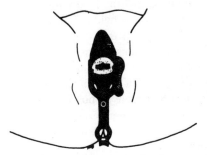

Fig. 1.18 Visualization of cervix through the bivalve speculum.

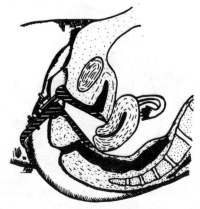

Fig. 1.19 Open the speculum to visualize the cervix.

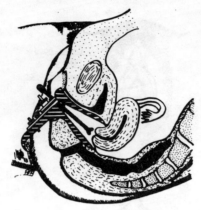

Fig. 1.20 To show how a cancer smear is taken using a bivalve speculum.

4. Hold the speculum so that the blades are between the index and middle finger, the handle is held comfortably in the hand and the thumb is resting lightly on the lever of the anterior blade.
5. Inspect the labia for any signs of masses, inflammation or discharge.
6. Insert the forefinger and thumb of the other hand between the labia towards the posterior third of the vaginal introitus and then separate the labia as widely as possible. This manoeuvre transforms the introitus from an antero-posterior slit into a triangular shape with the base stretched to a width of about 5 cm between the finger and thumb.

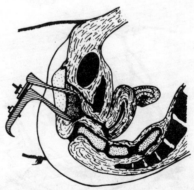

Fig. 1.21 Illustrating that if a bivalve speculum is opened before it is fully inserted into the vagina, the walls of the vagina only are seen.

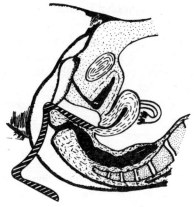

Fig. 1.22 Use a Sims' speculum or the posterior blade of a bivalve speculum to visualize the anterior wall of the vagina.

7. Press the speculum against the straight line made by the stretching of the fourchette and then gently insert the speculum so that it enters the vagina in an upward (towards the patient's head) and backward inclination. It should slide easily to the full length of the vagina, but if resistance is felt do not exert force, just change direction a little until the resistance is overcome.
8. When the speculum is fully inserted into the vagina, open the blades by pressing with the thumb on the lever of the anterior blade. If the speculum has been correctly inserted, the cervix should become clearly visible. (If the speculum is opened when only part way in the vagina, the vaginal walls beyond the speculum will be found to be in apposition and, to the novice, may appear to be the cervix.)
9. Describe first the cervix, then the os and finally the type of vaginal discharge. When the cervix has been completely inspected, the anterior blade may be removed to disclose the anterior wall of the vagina.
10. Observe the anterior wall of the vagina for any epithelial changes such as neoplasm, atrophic changes or other abnormalities. Note whether the bladder bulges down and if there is a cystocoele, whether it is related to a urethrocoele or if stress incontinence can be elicited.
11. Finally, note the level of the cervix as the speculum is withdrawn. There may be a prolapse of the uterus or bladder. If a prolapse is

noted, then it may be graded by degrees depending on its relationship to the vaginal introitus. If the uterus is prolapsed but the cervix is still within the vaginal introitus, it is termed a first-degree prolapse. A second-degree prolapse is found when the cervix passes through the introitus but the body of the uterus is still within the vagina. A third-degree prolapse (or procidentia) occurs when the cervix and the uterus are completely outside the vaginal introitus.

Description of the cervix

When describing the cervix it is best to develop a routine observational check-list which can be used in all written histories and which acts as a base for future reference.

The significant features that should be noted on all cervices are:

1. The condition of the epithelium. Normally the cervix is covered by flat squamous epithelium which meets the endocervical columnar epithelium at the margin of the external cervical os. However, under the influence of excessive oestrogen (at menarche, in pregnancy, certain contraceptive pills, post-menopausal oestrogen), the columnar epithelium of the endocervix proliferates and grows out over the ectocervix. This ectopic columnar epithelium (ECE) is identified as an orange or red, velvety, irregular-looking epithelium. (It was formerly called an 'erosion' but because there is no loss of epithelium this term is a misnomer.) It produces a clear mucous discharge which frequently becomes white when normal vaginal desquamation is mixed with the mucus. If the ectopic columnar epithelium becomes infected (as a result of trichomonas vaginalis, coliform infection, gonorrhoea, etc.), it produces a yellowish or brownish pus-like discharge — and if traumatized may bleed easily. Following stabilization of oestrogen levels, the ectopic columnar epithelium will undergo metaplasia to squamous epithelium. This process often leads to blockage of mucous crypts, so producing retention cysts (Nabothian follicles). In this metaplastic area, neoplasia may occur, so the squamo–columnar junction is sampled when taking a smear for cytological analysis.

2. The colour of the epithelium. Normal non-pregnant squamous epithelium in a young woman is of a mid-pink colour, but may range from a pale-pink to bright-pink shade. The darker colour is associated with an increase in blood supply to the cervix (such as in pregnancy, neoplasia, infection) — and if the blood flow is very

much increased, the epithelium may even be mauve or plum-coloured. In fact a dark-plum colour is regarded as a diagnostic sign of pregnancy.

In post-menopausal women the epithelium is often very pale, or may be mottled orange or red. The mottled colour is due to the extremely thin atrophic epithelium allowing the blood vessels below the epithelium to be easily seen. Sometimes, the vaginal epithelium is so thin and fragile that any trauma such as intercourse or passage of a speculum will cause a loss of, or a tear of the epithelium, producing minute haematomas or haemorrhages.

In women who have vaginal infection due to trichomonas, the epithelium may show a diffuse red discoloration or may present with punctate red spots ('strawberry' cervix). Monilia results in a bright-pink or red discoloration, with typical white plaques covering patches of the epithelium.

3. Cervical os. The cervical os is usually round or oval in shape in a nulliparous woman and the squamo–columnar junction is seen at the ectocervical opening. In multiparas, the cervix often discloses evidence of tears and lacerations so that the os has a distorted appearance. Tears usually take place at the lateral (3 o'clock and 9 o'clock) positions, so that the os has a transverse appearance. The cervix will appear to gape open like two lips pouting and a large area of columnar epithelium is then seen. This is not ectopic epithelium, for once the speculum is allowed to close, the cervical 'lips' close and normal cervical epithelium is seen. The condition where mucous epithelium is seen in association with cervical tears is called an ectropion.

4. Vaginal discharges. Physiological vaginal discharge may be clear and thin due to transudation across the vaginal epithelium, of a mucousy nature from columnar epithelium, or milky in colour due to the normal desquamation of cells and admixture with other cellular debris.

Pathological discharges may be difficulty to differentiate, but two in particular are relatively easy to identify. Infection with *Trichomonas vaginalis* results in a thin, yellowish discharge (sometimes grey, and at other times greenish in colour), which has a few frothy bubbles present (due to the low surface tension) and has a distinct odour. Monilial infection results in a white, flaky discharge (like thin cottage cheese), which is intensely itchy. If a secondary bacterial infection occurs in the vagina, the discharge may have a yellowish appearance and appear to be the result of trichomonal infection. Bacterial invasion of columnar epithelium produces a pus-like mucous discharge from the cervix.

5. Neoplastic conditions of the cervix. These may include polyps of endocervical or endometrial aetiology and appear as tear-shaped lesions protruding through the external os. They are covered by mucous epithelium in most cases, are usually a bright-red colour, and vary from several millimetres to a few centimetres in size.

   Carcinoma may present as ulcers or as sessile or polypoid lesions. It is usually identified by the presence of haemorrhage, increase in blood vessels, abnormal epithelium (leukoplakia, dysplasia), loss of epithelium and distortion of the normal features of the cervix.

6. Papanicolaou smears. These are usually obtained using an Ayre's spatula which should be so applied to the cervix that the spatula, when rotated through 360° around the squamo–columnar junction, scrapes off the superficial cells from this region.

   Smears obtained in this manner are usually classified as:
   Negative — no malignant cells seen.
   Doubtful — abnormal cells of doubtful significance — repeat.
   Suspicious — suspicion of malignancy.
   Positive — cancer cells seen.

   Suspicious or positive smears must have a biopsy performed to obtain a histological diagnosis before any definitive therapy can be initiated. It is usual to perform a curettage at the same time as the cervical biopsy to exclude the possibility that the abnormal smear is arising from the endometrial cavity.

SUMMARY

When passing a vaginal speculum to examine a patient, take the following steps:

1. Choose an appropriate speculum.
2. Position the patient correctly.
3. Lubricate the speculum and make sure it is warmed.
4. Inspect the labia.
5. Separate the labia and inspect the introitus.
6. Pass the speculum in an upward, backward direction for the full length of the vagina.
7. Open the speculum to disclose the cervix.
8. Describe the cervix (epithelium, colour, cervical os, vaginal discharges, any neoplastic lesions).

Digital vaginal examination

Performing a digital vaginal examination is also an important part of
gynaecological examination, but often is difficult to perform or the
findings are incorrectly interpreted. Unless a medical practitioner
knows what to feel and how to examine a pelvis, then many pathological conditions may be missed. A subitable technique is described:

1. Wear a glove of suitable size and lightly lubricate the middle and
   index fingers.
2. Separate the labia and under direct vision insert the two fingers
   gently into the vagina.
3. Pass the fingers in an upward, backward direction to the full
   length of the vagina. Normally the thumb will be found to rest
   firmly on the symphysis pubis and further pressure becomes
   difficult.
4. The cervix. Feel for the cervix. It is usually easily felt as a firm
   rounded mass about 3 cm in diameter. The os is felt as a dimple
   or pit in the surface of the cervix, and an imaginary rod passing
   out of the cervical canal through the os would normally point
   in a downward and backward direction if the uterus was anteverted. When the cervix is felt to point directly downward or in a
   downward and forward direction, then the uterus is usually in a
   retroverted position.
5. Determine the consistency of the cervix. Non-pregnant women
   will have a firm well-defined cervix, whereas pregnancy usually
   produces a softening and enlargement of the tissue.
6. When a patient is pregnant it is important that extreme gentleness
   be employed when feeling for the cervical os. It may be dilated
   or patulous and the finger can then be accidentally inserted
   into the canal, introducing infection or precipitating a rupture of
   membranes (such as in cervical incompetence or late pregnancy).
   When the cervix is dilated in early pregnancy, it usually indicates
   cervical incompetence (when no uterine contractions have occurred previously), or inevitable or incomplete abortion (when
   uterine contractions have been present).
7. Determine the mobility of the cervix. It will normally move up or
   laterally by 1–2 cm when pushed by the examining fingers. There
   may be complete or partial immobility, indicating induration (due
   to infection or neoplasia) in the surrounding tissue.
8. Pain on moving the cervix is usually minimal, but conditions producing blood, pus or chemical irritation of the pelvic

peritoneum will be accompanied by extreme discomfort when the cervix is moved. This occurs because the cervix is like one end of a lever that has the uterine fundus (and its covering peritoneum) at the other end, and both can then move around the fulcrum of the lateral cervical ligaments. Lateral movement of the cervix produces a marked movement of the uterine fundus and consequently extreme peritonism in association with ectopic pregnancy, salpingitis and pelvic peritonitis.

9. The uterus. A bimanual examination of the uterus is now performed. The uterus is normally about 8–9 cm long from the cervix to the fundus, and is normally found in an anteverted position with the cervix pointing downwards and backwards (Figs 1.23–1.25). Determine the size (relate it to common household goods with which you are familiar — a large hen's egg is about 6–7 cm long, an average-size lemon is about 8–9 cm, an orange about 10 cm, a grapefruit about 12 cm). Try to develop the skill of spatial imagery when performing bimanual examinations. Skill and accuracy come after many examinations, but will always be difficult for the beginner to achieve.

10. Determine the size of the uterus, its consistency (normally it is firm, but in pregnancy it becomes softer), its outline or shape (normally a regular pyriform shape, but pathological states produce irregularity), its mobility and any tenderness that may be present.

11. Feel for the adnexae. This consists of the parametria, the ovaries

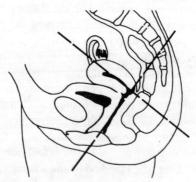

Fig. 1.23 Illustrating the axis of various anatomical organs in the pelvis, using the cervix as a fulcrum and a point of reference. The uterus is normally upwards and forwards while the cervix points downwards and backwards. The vagina passes into the pelvis in an upward and backward direction.

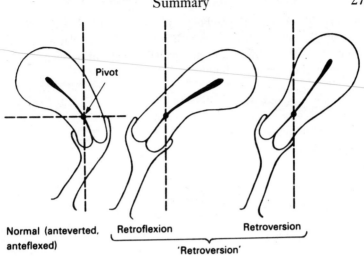

Fig. 1.24 When the cervix points downwards and backwards, the uterine fundus is upwards and forwards (anteverted).

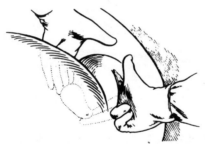

Fig. 1.25 Showing vaginal examination using the bimanual digital technique.

and the tubes. Normally the anatomical detail cannot be palpated. However, if a mass is present, it can be felt by passing the examining vaginal fingers into the lateral fornices and then pressing upwards, backwards and laterally towards the abdominal fingers which press down from the pelvic brim towards the vaginal fingers. Determine the size, mobility, consistency (solid or cystic, soft or hard) and tenderness of the mass.

1.7 SUMMARY

Obstetric and gynaecological history-taking and examination are relatively easy, but do require thought and expertise to be conducted adequately. To learn the techniques it is important that some logical and simple steps be taken. This chapter attempts to clarify the basic concepts in these procedures and explain what can be seen and felt, and how to describe the findings.

Adverse factors affecting embryo or fetus

Debbie Wass

2.1 GENERAL INSTRUCTIONAL OBJECTIVE

The students should appreciate the pre-conceptual, antenatal and intrapartum factors that may adversely affect an embryo or fetus so that they can initiate the management of related problems.

2.2 SPECIFIC BEHAVIOURAL OBJECTIVES

1. Take a relevant history to reveal congenital and hereditary factors that may affect the fetus.
2. Discuss the adverse effects of exogenous hormones, drugs, irradiation and infectious conditions that may alter the physiological processes or cause abnormal development in a fetus or child.
3. Discuss the maternal factors that may be associated with inadequate fetal nutrition.
4. Discuss oxygen transfer to the fetus, those factors that may impair or interrupt it, and the effects of hypoxia on the fetus.
5. Discuss the examination, relevant investigations and findings, and their significance in relation to detecting abnormalities of fetal growth.
6. Discuss the initial management when either hypoxia or intra-uterine growth retardation is identified by symptoms, signs or by investigations.
7. Explain how induction of labour, vaginal delivery or Caesarean section may adversely affect the fetus.

8. Discuss those factors that contribute to cerebral damage and birth trauma.
9. Discuss the effects on the fetus of analgesics and anaesthetic agents used in labour.
10. Discuss those signs during pregnancy that may indicate fetal malformation.
11. Discuss perinatal mortality and identify the major factors contributing to perinatal mortality and morbidity.
12. Describe how a fetus may become infected *in utero*.
13. Discuss the effect of maternal trauma on the fetus.
14. Discuss the formation, constitution and significance of amniotic fluid.

2.3 REASONS FOR LEARNING TO APPRECIATE THE PRE-CONCEPTUAL, ANTENATAL AND INTRAPARTUM FACTORS THAT MAY ADVERSELY AFFECT AN EMBRYO OR FETUS *IN UTERO*

This chapter discusses the major reasons why the medical and paramedical professions should be involved in the care of couples who are either planning or expecting a further addition to their family unit.

A fetus may succumb to noxious influences *in utero* resulting in miscarriage or stillbirth, or a potentially healthy infant may die in labour or suffer significant morbidity which may affect the whole of his or her often shortened life.

Fortunately many of the causes of antenatal and postnatal morbidity and mortality can be predicted, or at least identified early, so that detrimental effects on the future child can be eliminated or alleviated by appropriate antenatal management. However, medical care itself is not without hazard: iatrogenic damage to the embryo, fetus or newborn must also be guarded against, as many of the procedures commonly used with the aim of improving the outcome of pregnancy may lead to increased perinatal mortality and morbidity if used inappropriately or on the basis of misleading information.

As most parents enter a pregnancy in good health, obstetrics is one medical speciality where prophylaxis should be the main aim. This, or course, is not possible unless the medical practitioner appreciates those factors that may adversely affect the fetus, knows how to investigate and identify those problems when they occur, and how to initiate the appropriate management of any such problem.

Perinatal deaths are regrettable, but perinatal morbidity may in many ways disrupt a family unit to a greater extent and produce untold suffering for the child. There is also great cost to the community in the form of special educational facilities or the establishment of total care institutions for the more severely handicapped.

Adverse factors can begin their influence prior to conception, during the antenatal course, or during labour and delivery. The problems can be broadly divided into two groups: genetic and environmental. Environmental factors include the mother's external environment, the mother's general health and also intrauterine factors. The fetus can be likened to a goldfish in a fish tank, in that it is dependent for survival on the purity of its environment (the water), which in turn is in part dependent on the purity of the environment outisde the tank (poisons in the air entering the water), as well as the addition of appropriate nutrients and oxygen and competition from other inhabitants of the tank for the nutrients.

Only about 2% of ongoing pregnancies after the first trimester result in a child with a significant congenital abnormality. Minor malformations are recognized in a further 5%. The proportion of these abnormalities resulting from drug usage is probably less than 1 in 20. This factor albeit small is largely avoidable.

2.4 EXOGENOUS FACTORS THAT MAY ADVERSELY AFFECT THE FETUS

Hormones

1. Progestogens of the 19-nortestosterone group may produce pseudo-hermaphroditism in female infants.
2. Cortisone may produce a minimal increase in the incidence of cleft palates among neonates.
3. Oestrogens administered to the mother may rarely produce changes leading to carcinoma of the vagina in adolescent girls. They may also affect normal development of the genital tract in both male and female offspring.

Anaesthetic agents

Female operating theatre personnel form a high-risk group for both abortion and fetal abnormality. No specific anaesthetic agent has been named.

Analgesics

1. Aspirin may rarely cause impaired platelet aggregation.
2. Prostaglandin synthetase inhibitors may delay the onset of spontaneous labour. There are reports of premature closure of the ductus arteriosus *in utero* associated with these drugs when used for the suppression of pre-term labour.
3. Narcotic analgesics, sedatives and tranquillizers may cause depression of the fetal respiratory centre.

Antibiotics

1. Tetracycline may produce mottling and staining of neonatal teeth.
2. Sulphonamides may interfere with bilirubin conjugation leading to neontal jaundice.

Anticoagulants

Warfarin if used in the first trimester may cause an embryopathy. In the third trimester there is a risk of haemorrhagic complications.

Anticonvulsants

Phenytoin and other anticonvulsants can cause fetal abnormality in up to 6% of exposed fetuses. It is associated with congenital heart abnormalities and cleft lip or palate. Sodium valproate may be associated with neural tube defects.

Antithyroid drugs

Carbimazole and radioactive ^{131}I may lead to neonatal goitre or disturbed thyroid function in 2–5% of infants.

Cytotoxic drugs

Alkylating agents and antimetabolites may lead to abortion and fetal abnormality.

Irradiation

X-rays during pregnancy should be avoided but with modern equipment there appears to be no increase in fetal abnormality rates if X-rays are inadvertently taken or necessary during pregnancy.

2.5 GENETIC AND SOCIAL FACTORS

These are best detected by a careful history and examination when the patient attends for her first visit. Socio-economic and environmental factors should be noted and modified, if possible, to achieve the optimum results.

The history should include:

- Age and parity
- Height and weight
- Occupation and domestic circumstances
- Smoking habits
- Drug and alcohol intake
- Previous obstetric history
- Past medical history
- Family history of inherited disorders
- Immunity or otherwise to rubella, exposure to animals.

The importance of these individual factors varies. All the factors should be weighed together in an attempt to determine whether the present or planned pregnancy is one with a high risk of morbidity or mortality. Approximately 10–20% of women fall into the high-risk category and account for greater than 50% of the fetal and neonatal deaths. Some of the important maternal characteristics that are associated with the high-risk group include the following:

1. Maternal age and parity. The risk is least between 20 and 29 years of age and between the second and fourth pregnancies. Thus a woman older than 35 years who has more than four children falls into the high-risk category. The nulliparous teenager is also at increased risk.
2. Maternal height. Height has a negative linear correlation to perinatal mortality. Women under 152 cm (5 ft) have smaller babies. This may be due to familial trends; however, it may also be due to a poor environment which limited the mother's growth potential. Perinatal mortality is increased for mothers of shorter height and lower socio-economic class. There is also a greater incidence of pre-eclampsia and Caesarean section in this group of women.
3. Socio-economic class. The socio-economic class of the father has a less direct relationship with perinatal mortality than that of the mother, but the lower the class the higher the risk. Where the mother is unsupported and the pregnancy unplanned, the incidence of small for gestational age infants and of perinatal mortality is

double that found for those married women between 25 and 30 years of age. This group of patients also commonly have several other high-risk social factors, the effects of which are cumulative.

4. Social habits. Smoking more than ten cigarettes a day, significant alcohol intake and/or drug addiction increases the risk of perinatal mortality.

5. Nutrition. Weight gain during pregnancy and pre-pregnancy weight are all relevant to the outcome of the pregnancy. Specific associations include the following:

   (a) Iron or vitamin deficiencies are associated with anaemias and infection.

   (b) Poor nutrition is associated with small for gestational age babies.

   (c) Severe nutritional lack in pregnancy can cause impairment of the development of the fetal central nervous system.

   (d) Women with a pre-pregnant weight of less than 50 kg and a pregnancy weight gain of less than 5 kg tend to have low birth weight babies.

6. Trauma. Mothers who are exposed to trauma, especially severe mental trauma, have an increased incidence of pre-term labour and a higher perinatal mortality. Abdominal trauma may rarely cause premature separation of the placenta (accidental haemorrhage) or rupture of the uterus. Massive blood loss leading to shock and decreased placental blood flow can cause an acute hypoxic insult to the fetus. Mothers who are exposed to repeated violence in the home are frequently without emotional or sufficient financial support, all of which may adversely affect the pregnancy and all of which may be aggravated further by the anticipated addition to the family unit.

7. Obstetric history. The patient's previous obstetric history can give a good indication of possible problems in the present pregnancy, and provides a good summary of any high-risk factors that remained or have become worse since the previous pregnancy. Those previous obstetric complications that may indicate a problem in the present pregnancy include:

   (a) Previous stillbirth or neonatal death

   (b) Small for gestational age baby

   (c) Pre-term labour

   (d) Cervical incompetence and/or uterine abnormality

   (e) Previous fetal abnormality

   (f) Antepartum haemorrhage

(g) Rhesus disease
(h) Diabetes
(i) Cardiovascular problems, including congenital heart conditions and hypertension
(j) Anaemia
(k) Prolonged labour or difficult delivery
(l) Caesarean section
(m) Significant postpartum haemorrhage
(n) Postpartum depression

A women who delivered a pre-term infant in a previous pregnancy has at least a two-fold increased risk of delivering another pre-term infant. A previous perinatal loss is associated with a threefold increased risk of another such outcome, particularly if the first loss was associated with a low birth weight infant. It has been found that patients who have previously delivered a low birth weight infant face more than a threefold increased risk of doing so in a subsequent pregnancy.

8. Past medical history. The taking of a medical history is an important method of detecting chronic and continuing problems in the health of the mother which may affect the outcome of her pregnancy, as well as any maternal problems that may be aggravated by the pregnancy such as:

(a) Diabetes mellitus, even with the best of care, can result in 10% fetal mortality.
(b) Hypertension may through alterations in placental vasculature lead to growth retardation or intrauterine asphyxia due to placental separation.
(c) Cardiac disease in pregnancy is usually the result of a congenital heart defect or rheumatic fever, and may result in the mother not being able to increase her cardiac output or cope with the increased cardiac work required during pregnancy. Cardiac failure or arrhythmias may develop and increase the risk of venous and arterial thrombosis, embolism and maternal death. The severity of the disease will determine the mother's antenatal admission and modify her care in labour.
(d) Renal disease may complicate a pregnancy and produce problems related to filtration, renal blood flow and hypertension. Patients who have had renal transplants, however, can be guided through a successful pregnancy with care.
(e) Anaemia and other medical problems in the mother can increase the risk to both the mother and fetus.

(f) Ulcerative colitis, which may be exacerbated by pregnancy, if severe can interfere with the absorption of important nutrients.

(g) Surgical problems, especially those that result in or have caused bony deformities in the spine, pelvis, lower limbs and chest can give rise to problems of discomfort during pregnancy and may interfere with the normal birth mechanisms. Abdominal or pelvic soft-tissue tumours, or abnormalities such as uterine fibroids or a vaginal septum, can also cause problems during pregnancy and labour.

9. Family history. The family history of the potential parents, especially that of the mother's immediate family, may also provide definite indications as to whether the pregnancy is at risk or not. A history of diabetes mellitus in a first-degree relative would be an indication to screen the mother during pregnancy for this disorder. Where there is a family history of a chromosomal or genetic abnormality antenatal diagnosis may be indicated.

Physical examination

A thorough physical examination is the next logical step after eliciting from the history the presence or absence of any of the risk factors mentioned. It is important to determine the size of the uterus early in the pregnancy and thus confirm the estimated gestation as accurately as possible. This may involve the use of an ultrasound scan. The timing of any management of a high-risk patient may depend on an accurate estimate of fetal maturity.

2.6 RETARDED INTRAUTERINE GROWTH OF THE FETUS

Retarded intrauterine growth may occur because of abnormalities in the mother, the placenta or the fetus leading to defective nutrient transfer or a decrease in nutrients. Examples are as follows:

1. The mother
   (a) Medical conditions such as hypertension, renal disease, endocrine disease or advanced cardiovascular disease.
   (b) Toxins such as cigarette smoke.
   (c) Nutritional problems associated with poor intake (dieting, food fads and vegans) or severe malabsorption syndrome.
2. The placenta

(a) Impaired placental transport associated with antepartum hae-morrhage, placental infarction and poor implantation (such as that which results in a circumvallate placenta).

(b) Transplacental circulation in twins.

3. The fetus

(a) Congenital abnormalities.

(b) Infection.

(c) Twins.

Signs of retarded intrauterine growth

There is a small group of neonates who are born small for gestational age when there has been no detectable reason during the pregnancy. Thus, while it is important to be vigilant for the risk factors associated with small for gestational age infants, it is also important to observe the growth of both the uterus and the fetus so as to detect at the earliest possible opportunity any sign of fetal growth retardation.

The signs of retarded intrauterine growth include the following:

1. Uterine size smaller than expected for the period of amenorrhoea as judged by:
   (a) Symphyseal–fundal height measurement, which is in part dependent on the lie and engagement of the fetus, and
   (b) Uterine volume.
2. Fetal size. If there is any question about intrauterine growth an attempt should be made to estimate the weight of the fetus.
3. The volume of amniotic fluid. Oligohydramnios tends to be a poor sign when associated with intrauterine growth retardation and should lead to further investigations.
4. Decreased number of fetal movements may be reported by the mother.
5. Maternal weight loss or lack of weight gain during the third trimester.
6. A maternal girth measurement that remains the same or decreases.
7. Abnormal fetal development. Asymetrical growth or the presence of fetal abnormality.

Investigation of suspected retarded intrauterine growth

This should be directed towards confirming its presence, attempting to estimate the severity, and eliciting the cause. Growth retardation can be confirmed and its severity estimated by:

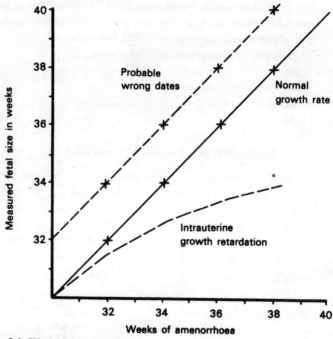

Fig. 2.1 Weeks of amenorrhoea.

1. Repeated clinical observation, including:
   (a) Abdominal palpation.
   (b) Symphyseal–fundal height and girth measurements.
   (c) Maternal weight.
   These repeated observations should be made by the same observer.
2. Ancillary tests
   (a) Ultrasound examination. Many pregnant women, having been identified as of high risk, may have had an ultrasound examination performed before 24 weeks to aid the confirmation of their dates. Repeated echograms will then give information as to whether the growth rate is normal, decreased or ceased. The ultrasound examination in addition will give information about the presence or absence of some fetal structural abnormalities. It can also give a more accurate estimation of the amount of liquor present than can clinical examination alone. Research is being carried out to determine if a prognostic value can be placed upon signs of placental ageing and fetal blood flow measurements.

(b) Tests on amniotic fluid. Amniotic fluid is formed by transudation across the placenta and membranes, facilitated by an active transport system. The fetus also contributes some of its waste products, particularly urine, to the amniotic fluid. Sampling of the amniotic fluid by amniocentesis can give some clues as to the well-being of the fetus. The osmolality of liquor decreases in the second half of pregnancy and any increase may indicate fetal jeopardy. Liquor creatinine should increase near term, whilst the pH value of the liquor is reduced and the pCO_2 rises.

None of the above measurements correlate well with the fetal condition or outcome, and at the present time the risks of the invasive test (amniocentesis) outweigh any benefit that may be obtained. The exceptions to this statement are related to those special situations where bilirubin estimations may predict the severity of Rhesus disease, where the lecithin/sphingomyelin ratio or presence of phosphatidyl glycerol may predict fetal lung maturity and where chromosome studies or alpha-fetoprotein levels may detect fetal abnormality.

(c) Activity of the fetus.

(i) Fetal movements can be used to evaluate the status of the fetus at risk. Normally a fetus moves at frequent intervals and these movements can be easily felt by the mother and counted. If movements are counted for four segments of half hour each during the day, greater than 10 movements is reasurring. Less than 10 detected movements over the same 2 hours indicates the need for closer observation and further testing.

(ii) Cardiotocography involves a continuous recording of the fetal heart rate. The machine calculates the rate from a series of fetal heart beats and graphs the result in relationship to any uterine activity that may be occurring. A normal trace shows a short-term variation of greater than 5 beats, a rate between 120 and 160 beats per minute, and no slowing of the fetal heart rate in relation to contractions, movements or maternal activity. Spontaneous accelerations of the fetal heart rate with movements or contractions is a good sign. A normal cardiotocograph trace is reassuring, as the fetus is very unlikely to die in the ensuing 4–6 days in the absence of any acute insults such as an accidental haemorrhage. An abnormal result may mean the presence of fetal hypoxia and may indicate the need to deliver the fetus if the cause of the heart rate abnormality is not reversible.

2.7 SMALL FOR GESTATIONAL AGE BABIES

Babies who are small for gestational age may show symmetrical or asymmetrical growth retardation.

Symmetrical growth retardation (appropriate head to body ratio) occurs from an early period of gestation and is more commonly associated with primary fetal pathology such as chromosomal abnormality or fetal infection.

Babies who demonstrate asymmetrical growth appear long and thin with relatively large heads. They lack subcutaneous fat and organs such as the liver, lungs and heart are smaller relative to total body weight than those of a normal infant. Neurological development is mature and brain weight is relatively greater in relation to birth weight. These changes usually result from an abnormality of placental function which may be due to reduced placental circulation, fibrin deposition or thrombotic occlusion of the arterioles in the deciduo–placental circulation. Separation of a portion of the placenta and infarction of the separated placenta (as occurs with accidental haemorrhage) reduces the functioning placenta. A circumvallate placenta is often associated with a restricted area of implantation, which may be severe enough to compromise placental function. Chronic poor placental function leads to a reduced oxygen supply, resulting in a greater demand on the less efficient anaerobic metabolic pathways. Also there is a reduction in placental transfer of nutrients, including amino acids and carbohydrates. The combination of hypoxia and nutritional deprivation results in a rapid depletion of glycogen and fat stores, and the commencement of acidosis and further hypoxia.

2.8 MANAGEMENT OF GROWTH RETARDATION

The decision that must be made whenever fetal growth retardation is detected is when to deliver the fetus. In other words, is the fetus safer in the uterus or in the nursery? As knowledge of antenatal fetal medicine advances, it may be possible in some cases to correct the problem causing retarded intrauterine growth. At the present time, most of the explored avenues have proved fruitless. These have included the use of heparin to prevent intravascular coagulation and intravenous feeding of the mother with hyperosmolar dextrose. The main aims at present are to limit the effect of placental inadequacy in pregnancy and to improve placental blood flow by resting the patient in bed with precautions to prevent postural hypotension.

If clinical evidence and investigations indicate that the fetus is compromised and growth has ceased then delivery needs to be considered and expedited if the fetus is mature. The fetal maturity depends upon gestational age and the severity of the growth retardation. The number of infants who die from the effects of pre-term delivery decrease markedly after 34 weeks of amenorrhoea.

However, prior to 34 weeks of amenorrhoea, each week of maturity gained produces a significant increase in the likelihood of the fetus surviving neonatally. Thus accurate knowledge of the last normal menstrual period, and the length of the cycle, is most important. If this information is available it should have been correlated with the size of the uterus at the first visit and the onset of fetal movements. If there is any discrepancy between the clinical signs, ultrasound examination can give an accurate guide to gestational age if it is performed before 24 weeks of amenorrhoea.

Regular clinical assessment of symphyseal–fundal height measurements, biophysical parameters of fetal well-being (fetal movements, fetal breathing and cardiotocography) and ultrasound assessment of fetal size, growth and liquor volume are invaluable in deciding how long to keep the pre-term growth retarded infant *in utero*. Ultrasound assessement of fetal subcutaneous fat and measurements of fetal blood flow appear at the moment to be a useful adjuvant.

It is important to individualize each case rather than make strict guidelines as to when fetuses should be delivered or remain *in utero*. Biochemical assessment of fetal lung maturity generally is not particularly helpful. If the fetus is considered to be sufficiently compromised *in utero* then delivery will be indicated independent of fetal lung maturity. There are, however, cases where delivery may be, in part, elective either to make sure the patient is delivered in a large hospital or where fetal surgery may be indicated. Assessment of fetal lung maturity in these cases may well help with the timing of delivery.

2.9 DELIVERY

The type and timing of delivery can affect the perinatal morbidity and mortality. Providing there are no complicating factors, the spontaneous onset of labour at term (38–40 weeks of amenorrhoea), with a vaginal delivery occurring after 2 hours but before 12 hours of labour, is the ideal aim.

Pre-term delivery carries a higher risk of respiratory distress, intracranial haemorrhage, neonatal death, jaundice, infection, low birth weight and hypoglycaemia. Prolonged stay in the intensive care nursery for the baby may lead to increased parent anxiety and problems with parent–child handling and bonding.

Pre-term delivery may be essential in the presence of marked intrauterine growth retardation. However, elective induction or induction of convenience, together with over-interpretation of signs of fetal jeopardy and incorrect or misleading estimates of gestational age, have all been implicated as causes of unnecessary preterm deliveries.

Postmaturity (pregnancy prolonged more than 42 weeks of amenorrhoea) is not synonymous with post-dates. Postmaturity is present when the pregnancy is prolonged so far beyond term that a risk to the fetus exists. The fetus has all the features of a growth-retarded baby, except it has signs consistent with a term infant (long finger nails, skin creases on heels and feet, joint movements, cartilage in the ears), but has almost no subcutaneous fat and no glycogen stores. The postmature baby frequently develops hypoglycaemia, and meconium is often present in the liquor.

2.10 INDUCTION OF LABOUR

Labour may be induced because of the following reasons:

1. Fetal
   (a) Signs of fetal hypoxia
   (b) Intrauterine growth retardation
   (c) Diabetes
   (d) Rhesus incompatibility
   (e) Infection
2. Maternal
   (a) Pre-eclampsia, eclampsia or hypertension
   (b) Dead or grossly abnormal fetus
   (c) Antepartum haemorrhage
3. Social

In most cases, induction involves an oxytocin (Syntocinon) infusion and the surgical rupture of the membranes.

1. Surgical rupture of membranes. Fetal problems may arise from the following:

(a) Prolapse of the cord. This results in cord compression and rapid onset of fetal distress, leading to death if immediate delivery (usually by Caesarean section) is not accomplished. The membranes should not be ruptured if the cord is presenting, or the presenting part is not well applied to the lower segment of the uterus.

(b) Intrauterine infection. This usually only occurs when aseptic techniques are not adhered to. Membranes that have been ruptured for more than 12 hours during a labour predispose to intrauterine infection. The risk is greatly magnified after 24 hours or if the membranes have been ruptured for some time prior to the onset of labour.

Repeated vaginal or rectal examinations markedly increase the risk of infection.

Fetal infection may result in pneumonia, septicaemia and meningitis. The haemolytic streptococcus group B is particularly virulent, and an intrauterine infection with these organisms results in a high risk of neonatal mortality.

In order to shorten any delay in the onset of labour, it is now common to combine Syntocinon with the surgical rupture of the membranes.

2. Oxytocin infusion. This may cause the following problems:

(a) Abnormally strong or prolonged contractions. These reduce the placental blood flow below that required by the fetus to maintain an aerobic form of metabolism, resulting in acidosis, fetal distress and, if prolonged and severe, fetal death. Thus it is important to monitor both the fetal heart rate and the contractions closely.

(b) Rupture of the uterus. This is usually associated with a uterus weakened by a scar, grand multiparity, or obstructed labour. Rupture of the uterus commonly results in maternal haemorrhage, hypotension, greatly reduced or absent placental circulation, death of the fetus and a threat to the life of the mother.

Failure to achieve induction of labour

Once the membranes have been ruptured for the purpose of inducing labour, the fetus should be delivered within 24 hours. Thus a Caesarean section may be the end result of an induction of labour.

Caesarean section may adversely affect the baby in the following ways:

1. There may be an increased risk to the baby of respiratory distress due to hyaline membrane disease. The risk must be foremost in the mind of the obstetrician planning an elective Caesarean section.
2. 'Wet lung syndrome' may be present where the baby has inhaled copious quantities of liquor. This is very irritating, especially if the liquor contains meconium. This may result in a syndrome that is similar to hyaline membrane disease, but is usually less severe and prolonged. In a delivery by Caesarean section, 'wet lung syndrome' is more difficult to prevent.
3. Accidental incision of the fetus when the uterus is being opened.
4. Anaesthetic complications:
   (a) Postural hypotension is more prone to develop in the anaesthetized patient. Her muscles are paralysed, and the uterus presses on the inferior vena cava and the iliac veins. This reduces the venous return to the heart, impairs cardiac output, lowers the blood pressure and reduces uterine blood flow. The reduction in uterine blood flow often may be sufficient to cause severe distress or death to an already compromised fetus. The incidence and effect of postural hypotension may be reduced by shortening the time between induction of the anaesthetic and the delivery of the baby, and by tilting the patient, using a wedge under one side of her back.
   (b) Effects of the anaesthetic agents on the fetus. If time between the induction of anaesthesia and the delivery of the fetus is prolonged, then anaesthetic agents may depress the fetus, in particular its respiration. If a narcotic has been given prior to the anaesthetic or cyclopropane is used for maintenance of the anaesthetic, this effect is aggravated.
   (c) Complications occurring to the mother. In particular, the inhalation of gastric contents (Mendelson's syndrome), may result in severe hypotension and poor oxygenation.

2.11 ANAESTHESIA

General anaesthesia within the labour ward increases the risks to both the mother and child, as the anaesthetic is frequently associated with an emergency procedure and is performed in a room primarily designed for the delivery of the patient rather than the routine administration of general anaesthesia.

Epidural anaesthesia has replaced general anaesthesia for many procedures within the labour ward, because the mother is provided with pain relief and is still able to witness and cooperate in the birth of her child. Epidural anaesthesia may result in vasodilatation which is followed by hypotension; thus the position and hydration of the patient must be watched carefully to prevent reduced placental blood flow.

Local anaesthetic agents, sedatives and narcotic agents may reduce the short-term variation of the fetal heart rate. This is one of the parameters observed when monitoring an at-risk fetus in labour. Narcotic analgesics may also cause neonatal respiratory depression when they are given between 1 and 4 hours prior to the delivery.

2.12 VAGINAL DELIVERY

Vaginal delivery is not without its risks of trauma to the fetus. Intracranial haemorrhage may occur in association with a traumatic delivery, and is particularly predisposed to by hypoxia. Situations in which the fetus is particularly at risk are:

1. Breech delivery.
2. Pre-term infants, as the moulding of the head may be marked or occur over a short period of time. (With a rapid delivery, the cranial bones may spring apart when the vaginal pressure is released, resulting in the tearing of an intracranial vein.)
3. Forceful forceps delivery, where a great deal of traction is required to bring the head through the pelvis, may fracture the fetal skull. The difficult forceps delivery should be abandoned in favour of a Caesarean section, which would result in a lower morbidity and mortality.
4. Fractures of the fetal leg or arm can occasionally occur from incorrect manipulation during a breech delivery or excessive traction.
5. Internal version and breech extraction of a fetus is associated with a high perinatal morbidity and mortality and should only be performed for the management of the second twin.

2.13 SUMMARY

1. Be aware of problems that may occur.
2. Seek problems out with appropriate history, examination and investigation.
3. Assess both the patients (mother and fetus) before instituting treatment.
4. Ensure that any treatment used will improve the outcome for the family.

Normal pregnancy

Colin Fisher
Revised by *Michael Bennett*

3.1 GENERAL INSTRUCTIONAL OBJECTIVE

The students should understand the anatomical, physiological and psychological changes consequent upon conception, so that they can diagnose and manage a normal pregnancy.

3.2 SPECIFIC BEHAVIOURAL OBJECTIVES

1. Discuss the physiological changes associated with normal implantation of a fertilized ovum.
2. Discuss the changes in female anatomy occurring during a normal pregnancy.
3. Discuss the symptoms that are presumptive of early pregnancy.
4. Perform a vaginal examination on a patient who is less than 14 weeks pregnant and describe the findings.
5. Correlate the uterine size with the period of gestation.
6. Specify the problems in determining the time of conception in relation to the date of the last menstrual period.
7. Discuss the origin and the effects of the endogenous hormones (oestrogen, progesterone, human placental lactogen, oxytocin, prostaglandins and chorionic gonadotrophin) in relation to the materno-fetal unit.
8. Discuss investigations and tests that are used to assess fetal well-being.
9. Palpate the abdomen of a patient after 28 weeks of gestation and accurately describe the lie, presentation, position and engagement of the fetus.
10. Discuss the relevance of specific antenatal investigations.
11. Take a history, examine a pregnant patient attending for a routine visit to the antenatal clinic, and discuss the findings.

12. Discuss physiological and emotional changes that may occur in pregnancy.
13. Discuss the relevance of nutrition and supplements during pregnancy.
14. Discuss counselling of patients on breast care, posture, diet, smoking, exercise, intercourse and drugs during pregnancy.
15. Identify and demonstrate an ability to manage the minor discomforts in pregnancy.
16. Discuss the counselling of a woman about her normal pregnancy.

3.3 REASONS FOR UNDERSTANDING THE NORMAL PREGNANCY

The most important concepts to be understood about the management of a normal pregnancy are the following:

1. It is a process that involves normal people who undergo numerous physical, physiological and psychological changes.
2. Medically speaking, the management of such a pregnancy is an exercise in preventive medicine.

Each piece of information gained during the pregnancy, either voluntarily offered by the patient or by specific interrogation or physical examination, should be evaluated with these concepts in mind. There may not be an immediate use for this information; however, it may be invaluable later in pregnancy when a complication may arise or when labour commences (Fig. 3.1).

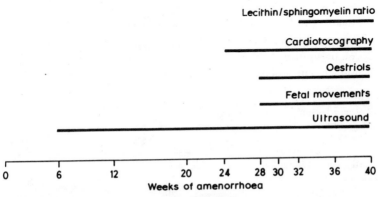

Fig. 3.1 Ideal times to perform placental function tests.

Failure to grasp these concepts can lead to uncertainty in the mind of the practitioner and in some instances, decisions may be made that will have adverse effects on the mother and her child.

The material in this chapter will provide information about the changes that occur in a woman during the course of her pregnancy and how this information can be applied to the advantage of all concerned.

3.4 PHYSIOLOGICAL CHANGES IN THE MOTHER

Blood and its components

In the course of a pregnancy there is an increase in the total blood volume, the plasma volume and red cell mass (Table 3.1). The total blood volume increases by 30–40% by about 34 weeks. This is largely due to an increase in plasma volume (45%), whilst the red cell mass increases by 18%. This results in haemodilution, often incorrectly called a physiological anaemia (Fig. 3.2).

The white cell count increases from approximately $7000/mm^3$ before pregnancy to $10\,000-15\,000/mm^3$. This is due to an increase in neutrophils — the other cells do not increase. Platelets rise considerably from $180\,000/mm^3$ to over $300\,000/mm^3$, and this rise is doubled again in the puerperium.

The erythrocyte sedimentation rate (ESR) rises due to increased fibrinogen and globulin levels. The plasma protein changes are shown in Table 3.2.

All lipid fractions increase, whilst there is a fall in the levels of all electrolytes associated with haemodilution.

Cardiovascular system

The main changes relate to increased cardiac output, which is produced by an increase in both heart rate and stroke volume. Peripheral resistance falls and as a result blood pressure usually remains steady

Table 3.1 Blood volume changes

	Non-pregnant	34 weeks
Total blood volume (ml)	4000	5500
Plasma volume (ml)	2500	3750
Red cell volume (ml)	1500	1750
Haemoglobin (g)	492	597

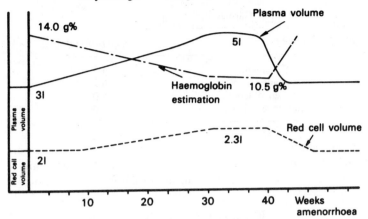

Fig. 3.2 Showing that as the pregnancy advances both the ciculating red cell mass and the plasma volume increase, but as the plasma volume increases by up to 50%, the haemoglobin concentration appears to fall.

throughout pregnancy, or frequently it may fall below pre-pregnancy levels during midpregnancy.

The cardiac output increases by 30–60% during pregnancy. Most of this increase occurs by the end of the first trimester, then slowly rising to 28 weeks, and is maintained to term. Further increases in cardiac output occur during labour (Table 3.3). During the first stage, a 30% increase occurs, whilst in the second stage an even greater output can be measured during bearing down.

Supine hypotension

During late pregnancy, a fall in blood pressure and a feeling of faintness occurs in some women who lie supine. This is due to vena caval

Table 3.2 Plasma protein alterations during pregnancy

Protein	Change
Total protein	Rises
Total protein concentration	Falls (due to haemodilution)
Albumin: globulin ratio	Falls
Albumin: α, α2 and β	Falls
Globulins: α, α2 and β	Rise (transport globulins)
Gamma globulins	No change
Fibrinogen	Rises (25–50% increases)
Clotting factors 1, 2, 5, 7, 8, 9, 10, 12	Rise

Table 3.3 Cardiac blood output

Condition	Output (l/min)
Non-pregnant	4.5
Pregnant	6.7
1st stage of labour	8.0
2nd stage of labour	9.0

compression by the enlarging uterus in the presence of a poor para-vertebral collateral circulation. The resultant fall in venous return reduces the cardiac output, and thus also a fall in blood pressure.

Regional blood flow changes

The regional blood flow to the liver and brain does not significantly alter during pregnancy, but the uterine blood flow increases ten-fold: from 50 ml/min in early pregnancy to 500 ml/min at term. The renal blood flow increases by 30%, renal plasma flow by 45% and glomerular filtration rate by up to 50%. However, because tubular reabsorption is unaltered, the clearance of many solutes (for example, urea, uric acid and glucose) is increased.

Metabolic changes in pregnancy are complex, and currently under much investigation. There is a general increase in the metabolic rate, largerly due to fetal demands. Oxygen consumption rises by 20%, and the thyroid gland hypertrophies in perhaps 70% of patients.

Carbohydrate metabolism is affected by human placental lactogen during pregnancy. This hormone antagonizes the action of insulin, breaks down body fat, and thus acts towards the elevation of blood glucose levels. As a result, insulin rises to even higher levels, so increasing glucose utilization but restricting any abnormal blood levels (Fig. 3.3). The increased demand on the pancreas may at this stage uncover a latent diabetic.

Protein metabolism shows an overall positive nitrogen balance, and about 500 g of protein are retained by term. Thus a high protein diet is required during pregnancy.

Fat is the main form of maternal energy store during pregnancy, mostly in the form of depot fat. Blood lipid also increases significantly. It is important to note that because glycogen stores are low, any major stress will draw quickly on fat for energy and so ketosis may occur.

The average total weight gain should be about 12.5 kg (28 lb), the main increase being in the second half of the pregnancy.

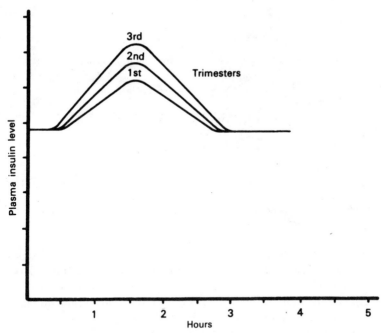

Fig. 3.3 Plasma insulin level to a glucose test meal. Pancreatic stimulation by glucose during the third trimester is maximal due to the inhibiting effect of placental lactogen.

3.5 FERTILIZATION

Pregnancy occurs following the fertilization of an ovum by a sperm. The sperm and the ovum usually survive for no longer than 24 hours, thus conception is unlikely to occur unless coitus occurs 1–2 days before or after ovulation.

The sex of the child is determined at fertilization, and depends on whether the ovum is fertilized by an X sperm or a Y sperm. Some workers believe that the sex of the child can be predetermined by the timing of coitus: X sperms live longer than Y sperms, and it is said that intercourse prior to ovulation is likely to produce a female, whilst intercourse at the time of ovulation favours a male.

Following fertilization, cell division ensues within 24 hours. Each daughter cell contains genetic material from both parents. By the 3rd or 4th day the morula is formed, which then becomes partly cystic. By the 7th day a single layered fluid-filled cyst, with a solid collection of cells in one area of its wall, is formed. This is the blastocyst. The solid

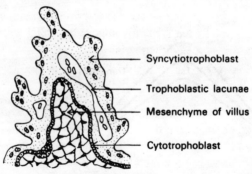

Fig. 3.4 Early stage of development of chorionic villus. The trophoblast has separated into two cellular layers — the syncytiotrophoblast and the cytotrophoblast. There is a coalescence of lacunae which contain a few red cells. A mesenchymal core is beginning to form.

area (the inner cell mass) forms the fetus, whilst the cyst wall becomes the trophoblast. This trophoblast differentiates into an inner layer (cytotrophoblast) and an outer layer (syncytiotrophoblast) (Figs 3.4 and 3.5), and then the blastocyst can attach to the endometrium and gain nourishment from it.

Proliferation continues to occur in the inner cell mass and two further cysts are derived from it. The cyst lying peripherally and adjacent to the trophoblast becomes the amniotic cavity, while that lying centrally becomes the yolk sac. Separating these two structures is a cellular layer containing ectoderm and mesoderm, derived from the amnion and endoderm of the yolk sac. From these primitive cells the fetus and umbilical cord will develop, and they are present by the 7th day.

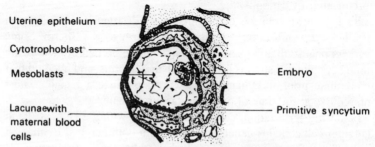

Fig. 3.5 An early human embryo which is differentiating into syncytial cytotrophoblastic and mesoblastic tissue. Lacunae are forming in the syncytium and maternal red cells can be identified in the tissue which will form the placenta.

Simultaneously, the trophoblast has developed villous tufts on its outer surface, which give it a fluffy appearance. Each villus is penetrated by a central core of mesenchyme — the trophoblast becomes the chorion and the villi are now chorionic villi. This occurs by the 14th day. By the 21st day blood vessels have formed in the mesenchyme of the villi, body stalk (cord) and embryo. The villi eventually disappear from the surface of the blastocyst, with the exception of that area adjacent to the endometrium; this will form the placenta.

The blastocyst is usually embedded in the endometrium by the 6th and 7th day following fertilization (Fig. 3.6), and commences to secrete minute quantities of human chorionic gonadotrophin (HCG), which is both luteinizing and luteotrophic. This maintains the corpus luteum, producing oestrogen and progesterone; the endometrium becomes decidua and amenorrhoea begins.

3.6 SYMPTOMS AND SIGNS DETECTED DURING PREGNANCY

Rise in basal temperature

Progesterone, released from the follicle after ovulation, is thermogenic. A persistent elevation of basal temperature for longer than 14 days is presumptive evidence of pregnancy.

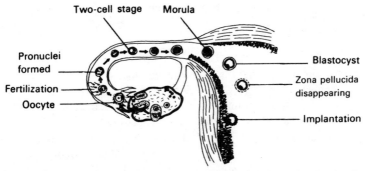

Fig. 3.6 Passage of the fertilized egg through tube to implantation in decidua (six days).

Pregnancy test

When performed on early-morning samples of urine, the tests can indicate the presence of HCG as early as 8 days after fertilization. However, false negative results may occur, and the customary time to perform the test is at 6 weeks of amenorrhoea. False positive results can occur due to cross-reaction with luteinizing hormone (LH) and a more specific test is by means of radioimmunoassay of the beta subunit of the HCG molecule in the serum.

Amenorrhoea

This occurs secondary to the luteotrophic and luteinizing effects of HCG. However, bleeding can occur from the decidua vera in early pregnancy, as the gestation sac does not completely fill the uterus until 12 weeks of amenorrhoea.

Nausea

Although nausea during pregnancy is traditionally called 'morning sickness', it may occur at any time during the day or night — and may, in fact, occur throughout both. It usually disappears before 12 weeks of amenorrhoea, but may persist longer, even throughout pregnancy. Occasionally it can recur in late pregnancy. The nausea experienced by some pregnant women is presumably associated with the appearance of new hormones, or the increased levels of existing hormones, that occur during pregnancy. It can occur in the absence of a fetus, as for example in the presence of a hydatidiform mole or an anembryonic pregnancy. Occasionally, severe vomiting may occur, and hospitalization and rehydration are then indicated.

Breast changes

Increases in size, vascularity and heaviness may all be early symptoms of pregnancy. The breasts, especially the nipples, may become sensitive or even painful to touch or pressure. These changes are presumed to be due to the effects of oestrogen, progesterone and possibly human placental lactogen (HPL). The areola enlarges and becomes darker, as does the nipple. Montgomery's tubercles become prominent. Colostrum usually appears spontaneously by the 28th week, but may be expressed as early as the 16th week of amenorrhoea.

Bladder symptoms

Frequency, both diurnal and nocturnal, usually commences in about the 6th week and subsides in the middle trimester. These symptoms are due to bladder hyperaemia and irritation of the bladder by the enlarging uterus.

Frequency commonly recurs late in pregnancy and is due to bladder compression by the uterus and the presenting part of the fetus.

Urinary stress incontinence is a common symptom during pregnancy, which almost always subsides during the puerperium.

Uterine changes

The cervix softens and may become bluish, secondary to oestrogen-induced increased vascularity. The normal cervical and vaginal discharge increases in amount. The uterus enlarges steadily, but its shape may be irregular in early pregnancy due to implantation in one particular site in the uterus.

Palpable uterine enlargement is best compared with everyday objects:

- Small lemon size: 6–8 weeks.
- Orange size: 8–10 weeks
- Grapefruit size: 12–14 weeks

Hegar's sign is difficult to elicit and uncomfortable for the patient; it should not be used.

At about 12 weeks the uterus is usually palpable above the symphysis pubis in a woman of average build whose uterus is anteverted or anteflexed. Thereafter the uterus enlarges rapidly and reaches the umbilicus at about 22–24 weeks of amenorrhoea.

Vaginal and vulval changes

Due to increased vascularity, the vaginal epithelium becomes darker and vaginal secretion increases.

Abdominal discomfort

This may take a variety of forms. In early pregnancy the woman may experience the feelings she normally has with menstruation but, of course, there is no bleeding.

A feeling of distension and tightness of clothing is common, even in the absence of obvious abdominal enlargement.

Brief sharp pains are often experienced in one of the iliac fossae, and may continue during pregnancy. The reason for these pains is not clearly understood, but they are usually explained as being due to 'pressure', 'uterine enlargement', and other such general causes.

Fetal movement (quickening)   16 - 24 WKS

In a primigravid patient, movement is first felt as a 'fluttering' or 'wind' in about the 20th to the 22nd week. After that time, definite movements are noticed. In the multigravida who is familiar with the sensation, movements are commonly noticed from about the 18th week onwards. The patient should note the date of onset of fetal movement, as this may help to confirm the duration of pregnancy.

The commonest form of antenatal fetal monitoring is by charting the fetal movements perceived by the mother.   "KICK CHART"

Audible fetal heart sounds

These may be detected as early as 24 weeks with a monaural stethoscope — of course, with a Doppler they can be detected at 14 weeks or even earlier.

Palpable fetal parts   22 - 24 wks

Depending on the thickness of the patient's anterior abdominal wall and the position of the placenta, fetal parts may be palpable abdominally from the 22–24th week onwards.

Changes in the skin and subcutaneous tissues

Brownish pigmentation of the nipples and areola occur early in pregnancy. Later the linea nigra develops in the midline between the umbilicus and pubic hair. Patchy brown discoloration of the facial skin — known as chloasma — may also develop in some women. Assoc Pill.

Fat deposition occurs, especially over the buttocks, thighs and upper arms. Sebaceous secretion may increase and skin lesions, especially acne-form types, may curiously be either exacerbated or diminished. Cutaneous haemangiomas may develop; presumably these are secondary to high oestrogen levels.

Striae gravidarum may develop on the skin of the abdomen, buttocks, thighs and breasts. Their formation is frequently preceded and accompanied by pruritus. Striae are due to changes in the deeper layers of the skin and initially are red or purple in colour. However, they fade with time to a silver colour, and are then relatively inconspicuous.

Other symptoms

Giddiness and faintness, and at times even fainting, may occur during pregnancy, especially in crowded, stuffy rooms.

Epistaxis and bleeding from the gums may occur in late pregnancy. The gums may hypertrophy to a small extent.

Headaches (usually 'tension' headaches) are not uncommon in the first half of pregnancy. Although they do not respond to commonly used analgesics, diazepam (Valium) is effective.

Muscular cramps are reasonably common after the 24th week, and may respond to calcium lactate (300 mg t.i.d.) or diazepam. They are due to the failure of the peripheral circulation to clear metabolic waste products.

Backache, especially sacro-iliac pain, is common in late pregnancy, particularly in multigravidas. This is attributed to altered posture and the softening of the pelvic ligaments that occurs in late pregnancy. A maternity girdle may be helpful.

Constipation is a common occurrence during pregnancy due to the effect of progesterone on the smooth muscle of the colon. A diet containing fruit, bran and cereals may be helpful.

Varicose veins and haemorrhoids may also occur, especially where there is a family history of these complaints. They are due to the effect of progesterone on the muscularis coat of veins, and the increased venous pressure in the lower part of the body as the uterus enlarges and compresses the inferior vena cave. Supportive stockings are most helpful in relieving any discomfort, and their prophylactic use should be recommended to women with a positive family history.

Psychological changes

A variety of psychological changes also occurs. In the early stages of pregnancy a feeling of dejection may occur, especially if the discomforts of pregnancy are great — a 'cheated' feeling is not uncommon.

As pregnancy progresses, a number of women feel extremely well and active.

In late pregnancy, when it is more difficult to move quickly or to bend and stoop, the woman feels cumbersome. As her abdomen enlarges and her weight increases, she may feel unattractive. The patient finds it difficult to become comfortable, especially at night, so that sleeping is disrupted. These problems often provoke a feeling of 'I wish it were all over'. The expression of such feelings must never be seen by obstetricians as an opportunity to offer elective induction.

Sexuality may also alter during pregnancy: for some women libido increases, whilst for others it may decrease. Provided there is no vaginal bleeding or other contra-indication like a cevical suture, intercourse need not be restricted. After this time, antepartum haemorrhage and premature labour may possibly be related to intercourse.

During a pregnancy a woman will undergo a tremendous number of physical, physiological and psychological changes. She may be able to cope with all of them or very few. The obstetrician must always be willing to answer any questions the couple may have and, when necessary, to offer help and reassurance. Patient education is very important, for both the patient and the doctor, because a lot of time is saved by answering questions fully and by explaining what is likely to occur.

3.7 THE FIRST ANTENATAL VISIT

The routine for taking the history is described in Chapter 1. Remember that this is the best time to establish rapport with the patient. On the first visit the diagnosis of pregnancy is usually established; and the patient's memory is then also most clear as to recent events, especially her last menstrual period. This is the time to recognize current or previous illness, or other factors that could influence the course of the pregnancy and labour.

The majority of risk factors related to a pregnancy can be established at this first visit. These factors include:

1. Age: younger than 16 or older than 35.
2. Parity: grand multiparity (fifth or subsequent pregnancy).
3. Poor economic circumstances.
4. Drug taking: smoking, salicylates, methadone, amphetamines, heroin and alcohol.
5. Poor obstetric history: infertility, recurrent abortion, premature labour, stillbirths and neonatal deaths.
6. Previous postpartum or antepartum haemorrhage.
7. Previous Caesarean section or difficult delivery.

8. Chronic maternal disease: hypertension, renal disease, cardiac disease, anaemia, diabetes mellitus and other endocrine disorders.
9. Short stature: problems with cephalopelvic disproportion are more likely to arise when the patient's height is 152 cm (5 ft) or less.
10. Rhesus iso-immunization.

A general physical and pelvic examination are performed at the first visit. The uterine size is assessed and correlated with the stated period of amenorrhoea. The presence of other pelvic tumours is sought, as these may produce problems during pregnancy or obstruction during labour. Their detection and removal (if they are ovarian tumours) can forestall many complications. Pelvimetry is not performed at this stage. The cervix is inspected and a cervical smear taken.

Advice should be given at this stage about obvious avoidable factors.

1. Obesity. The overweight woman should be given a low-kilojoule (calorie) diet when seen early in pregnancy, as obesity is a risk factor of pregnancy.
2. Smoking. Women who smoke more than ten cigarettes per day are more likely to produce babies of lower birth weight than women who do not smoke at all. They are also more likely to come into labour prematurely, and statistically are more likely to have a stillborn baby or neonatal death.
3. Medications. The pregnant woman should be told that all drugs cross the placenta, so medications should only be taken after ensuring their lack of harmful effect on the fetus. She should be warned about taking excessive amounts of analgesic or tranquillizing drugs.
4. One glass of alcohol each day is permissible and is probably best taken as wine with meals. However, many women become intolerant to alcohol whilst pregnant.

3.8 SUBSEQUENT VISITS

The woman should be seen every four weeks until 28 weeks, then fortnightly until 36 weeks and thereafter weekly until confinement.

The visits between 28 and 32 weeks are especially important because at this stage multiple pregnancy is most likely to be diagnosed, and pre-eclampsia can be detected.

During antenatal visits:

1. All question should be satisfactory answered.
2. General enquiries should be made about health, fetal movement, vaginal discharge, bleeding or pain.
3. Weight, blood pressure and fundal height should be recorded. After 28 weeks the lie, presentation and position of the fetus are checked, as are the fetal heart sounds.
4. Generalized oedema is looked for.
5. Urinalysis is performed.

If after 38 weeks the head is not engaged in a primigravid and doubt exists regarding the capacity of the pelvis, or if a breech presentation persists after 36 weeks, X-ray pelvimetry should be ordered.

3.9 GENERAL ADVICE

The woman should be encouraged to pursue her normal activities, but to avoid obviously hazardous activities such as water-skiing, horse-riding or body surfing. Sexual intercourse is permissible up to the onset of labour if there are no contra-indications such as antepartum haemorrhage and/or premature labour. Achieving orgasm during pregnancy is not harmful, and this can be done in late pregnancy by oral sex or masturbation if so desired.

Advice should also be given about diet, iron and vitamin supplements and what facilities are available for childbirth education and breast care.

Iron supplement should be given to all pregnant women from the beginning of the second trimester until they cease breast feeding.

Diet

Extra nutrition is required during pregnancy, as the mother's basal metabolic rate rises and the needs of the fetus and mother increase.

The usual nutritional requirement in pregnancy is about 10 500 kilojoules (2500 calories) daily, with a distribution of approximately 100 g protein, 100 g fat and 300 g carbohydrate. More specific diets can be found in booklets which are easily accessible.

Calcium supplements are necessary. If the woman dislikes dairy products, calcium tablets can be taken. Fluoride should be taken during the second half of pregnancy.

Supplemental iron and folic acid should be given, as the requirements for these substances increase during pregnancy. The administration of supplements can avoid the development of anaemia.

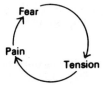

Fig. 3.7 Illustrating how fear, pain and tension produce a vicious circle of activity

Childbirth education

In more recent times, the concept put forward by Grantley Dick-Read (Fig. 3.7) has gained wide acceptance. Programmes aimed at educating parents about pregnancy and labour, coupled with the teaching of relaxation techniques, have done much to allay the anxiety of pregnant women. Apart from the more conventional programmes offered by hospitals, alternative methods of education and relaxation by methods such as psychoprophylaxis have much to offer.

3.10 ESTIMATION OF THE DATE OF CONFINEMENT

Over the last 150 years the method mostly used to determine the estimated date of confinement (EDC) is Naegele's method, which allows for an average pregnancy of 280 days from the commencement of the last menstrual period (LMP).

More recent work has shown that the average duration of pregnancy is 283 days from LMP so a quick calculation can be made of the expected date of confinement, by adding 10 days and 9 months to the first day of the LMP. This assumes, however, that every woman has a regular cycle and ovulates at approximately the 14th day of her cycle. Allowance must be made for cycle length, e.g.

28-day cycle	LMP 10-5-87	EDC 20-2-88
22-day cycle	LMP 10-5-87	EDC 14-2-88
42-day cycle	LMP 10-5-87	EDC 6-2-88

One must also be cautious when the LMP is a withdrawal bleed associated with an oral contraceptive as ovulation is not infrequently delayed in such an instance. Bleeding at the time of implantation or an early threatened abortion is also a source of confusion, and so the duration of amenorrhoea must always be compared to the uterine size.

3.11 INVESTIGATIONS PERFORMED DURING PREGNANCY

At the initial visit the following tests are made:

1. Blood tests
   (a) Haemoglobin: an initial screening to detect anaemia. If it is found, further investigations should ensue to determine the nature of the anaemia. Anaemic women are more likely to produce babies of low birth weight and they tolerate antepartum and postpartum haemorrhages poorly.
   (b) Blood grouping: ABO and Rhesus (Rh) grouping.
   (c) Antibody screen: all patients (both Rh+ve and Rh−ve) should be screened. Antibodies that can cause haemolytic disease may occur in Rh + ve women (e.g. Kell). In addition, antibodies such as anti-Lewis may be detected, which may produce difficulties with the cross-matching of blood.
   (d) Rubella antibody titre: a titre of 1 in 20 or greater is evidence of previous rubella infection. The test also provides a baseline for future comparison in the unprotected if infection is suspected.
   (e) VDRL: a screening test for syphilis. Untreated syphilis can cause congenital infection of the fetus which, if recognized antenatally, is readily treated. If a positive VDRL is found, further investigations should be performed to ensure that it is not a false positive.
   (f) Hepatitis B is screened for since antigen-positive women are a risk not only to those involved in their care, but also their newborn.
2. Urine tests
   (a) Routine urinalysis: traditionally an early-morning specimen of urine is tested to exclude orthostatic proteinuria. If protein is found, a midstream specimen of urine should be tested to exclude contamination by vaginal secretions.
   (b) Bacilluria screening test: 6% of pregnant women have asymptomatic bacilluria. If untreated, one-third of these women will develop acute pyelonephritis during pregnancy. This can be prevented by detection and treatment. Some workers claim a higher incidence of low birth weight babies and pre-term labours amongst women with untreated asymptomatic bacilluria.
3. Cervical smear. This will ensure that any overt cervical lesion is noted.

At 28 and 36 weeks a haemoglobin estimation, and Rhesus screen should be performed.

Tests of fetal well-being

Even in a normal pregnancy, obstetricians may wish to perform investigations to ensure that all is well.

Often, the uterus appears to be either too large or too small for the period of amenorrhoea. The simplest investigation to perform is an ultrasonic examination, which can measure fetal size, confirm or deny the presence of a multiple pregnancy, and give information about the placental site and amniotic fluid volume.

A plain radiograph of the abdomen may be used if a multiple pregnancy is suspected.

It is also helpful after 30 weeks of amenorrhoea to measure the girth of the mother at the level of the umbilicus. Failure of the girth measurement to increase after 34 weeks has a strong association with low birth weight babies, as does failure of the mother to gain weight. Static or falling maternal weight after 34 weeks also may indicate fetal growth retardation.

[handwritten annotations: Fetal assessment USS — hr rate — umbilical cord flow — pools of liquor — Size of fetus — estimated weight — subcutaneous tissue — look for structural abnormality*]*

Cardiotocography

During late pregnancy, the fetal heart rate (FHR) can be monitored by using an ultrasonic transducer applied to the mother's abdominal wall, and uterine contractions can be recorded by an external transducer.

Variations in the FHR may be noted in response to Braxton Hicks contractions if the ability of the fetal cardiovascular system to compensate is diminished, such as in prolonged pregnancy, hypertension or antepartum haemorrhage.

The information obtained from measurements of FHR can be used, in conjunction with clinical findings and other measurements of fetal well-being, to determine the optimal time for delivery in certain situations where the fetus may be at risk.

3.12 PLACENTAL FUNCTION

The placenta appears to have several functions:

1. Respiratory exchange.
2. Nutrition.
3. Hormone production.

4. In certain situations, it acts as a barrier to abnormal environmental agents.

The first two functions require transport of substances to and fro across the placenta, and to achieve this four types of transport mechanisms have been described: simple diffusion (e.g. of oxygen); facilitated diffusion (e.g. of glucose); active transport (e.g. of amino acids); and special processes, such as pinocytosis (e.g. leakage of large molecules up to cellular size) and iron transport.

The concept that the placenta acts as a barrier to protect the fetus from damaging agents has been shown to be largely incorrect. Apart from the rubella virus, vaccinia, Cytomegalovirus (CMV) and Cendehill virus have all been shown to cross the placenta. In addition, *Toxoplasma gondii*, *Mycobacterium tuberculosis*, *Treponema pallidum* and malarial parasites may also reach the fetus. In the case of *Treponema*, however, there is protection up to the 16th week, before which time no case of congenital syphilis has been reported.

All drugs, except heparin, some muscle relaxants and a small proportion of insulin cross the placenta. Drugs such as thalidomide have been proven to produce fetal malformations, whilst several other drugs have been linked by strong circumstantial evidence. Although it is possible that the placenta may prevent potential teratogens from reaching the fetus, it is probably wiser to exclude fetal protection as a placental function.

Haemodynamics of placental blood flow (Fig. 3.8)

There is a gradually increasing flow of blood through the utero-placental unit until, by the 32nd week, the amount of blood passing through the placenta each minute reaches 500–700 ml. Any reduction in this placental blood flow (exercise, spasm of arteries or fibrin deposition) may interfere with the nutritional transfer mechanisms of the placenta. Thus, infants born to mothers who suffer from a reduced placental blood flow will have reduced levels of glucose and glycogen, amino acids and protein, and fatty acids. These infants are often described as being dysmature and have reduced chances of survival.

Hormonal functions of the placenta

Two types of hormones are associated with the placenta:
1. Protein hormones
   (a) Human chorionic gonadotrophin (HCG).

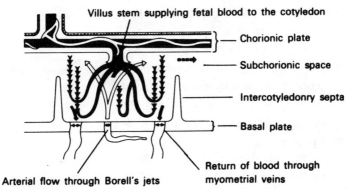

Fig. 3.8 Haemodynamics of the placenta. Approximately 500–700 ml of maternal blood enter the placental 'lake' each minute, spurting like an intermittent fountain to reach the chorionic plate before diffusing back past fetal villi and finally out through maternal sinuses in the decidua.

(b) Human placental lactogen (HPL).

(c) Other, less well-understood hormones such as human chorionic thyrotrophin and pregnancy-specific β-globulin.

These hormones are never found in the absence of trophoblastic tissue and they are transferred directly to the maternal circulation; very small amounts are found in fetal blood. They consist of two basic units, alpha and beta, the latter giving the hormone its specificity.

2. Steroid hormones

(a) Progesterone.

(b) Oestrogens.

Although progesterone is produced by the placenta, the oestrogens are not. In pregnancy the major oestrogen is oestriol. The placenta does not possess all the enzymes necessary to synthesize oestriol, but suitable enzymes in the fetal liver and adrenals enable this synthesis to occur. Because of the contributions from both the fetus and placenta, the concept of the feto-placental unit was put forward in relation to oestriol biosynthesis, and has since been expanded.

HUMAN CHORIONIC GONADOTROPHIN

HCG is a glycoprotein, and its exact site of formation within the placenta is still uncertain.

Similar HCG concentrations are found in the placenta, maternal blood and urine from the 11th day after ovulation, and urinary

excretion reaches a peak level between 11 and 12 weeks of amenorrhoea, and then declines.

The main actions of HCG are:

1. Maintenance of the corpus luteum (luteotrophic action), until the
   placenta produces sufficient progesterone.
2. Differentiation of Leydig cells in the fetal testis.

Higher than normal levels of HCG are found when more trophoblast is present (e.g. in multiple pregnancy or hydatidiform mole).

The main clinical use of HCG is in the diagnosis of pregnancy and
trophoblastic tumours, and in monitoring the response of the latter to
treatment. HCG determinations in the management of threatened
abortion is of little use, as levels will persist whilst there is retained
placental tissue.

Because of the immunological similarity of HCG to gonadotrophic
hormones, a false positive pregnancy test can occur at the time of ovulation and in relation to the menopause.

HUMAN PLACENTAL LACTOGEN

HPL is a polypeptide, and is immunologically and chemically similar to
human growth hormone (HGH). It is produced by the syncytiotrophoblast and levels increase steadily to term. After labour, the HPL level
falls rapidly.

The major functions of HPL include:

1. Diversion of glucose from the mother to the fetus.
2. Mobilization of fat stores in the mother.
3. Nitrogen retention.
4. Effects on the breast and a role in the initiation of lactation.
5. Antagonistic action to maternal insulin.

There is little clinical application for HPL assays, except in pregnancies complicated by hypertension. After 30 weeks of gestation, an
HPL level of less than 4 µg/ml is associated with a perinatal mortality
rate of about 50%.

PROGESTERONE

Plasma concentrations of progesterone rise rapidly after conception.
Although progesterone is initially produced by the corpus luteum, the

placenta soon becomes the sole source. Progesterone is usually assayed in maternal serum.

The effects of progesterone include:

1. Reduction of uterine activity.
2. Reduction of smooth muscle tone generally (e.g. of the stomach, colon and ureter).
3. Thermogenic. The basal temperature is raised after ovulation and thereafter.
4. Stimulation of growth of breast alveoli.
5. There is some evidence to show that a fall in progesterone precedes the spontaneous onset of labour.

There is no practical value currently in estimating progesterone levels during pregnancy.

OESTROGENS

The three major oestrogens found during pregnancy are oestriol, oestradiol and oestrone — and of these, oestriol is the most important quantitatively. Precursors from the fetal adrenals undergo changes in the fetal liver and in the placenta, and ultimately are excreted in the mother's urine as oestriol.

Urinary oestriol excretion has been exhaustively studied, and plasma oestriols have recently been found to have a similar significance. Oestriol levels rise steadily after the 10th week to term.

The actions of oestrogens during pregnancy are considered to be:

1. Stimulation of protein synthesis at a cellular level.
2. Myometrial hypertrophy, to accommodate the enlarging conceptus.
3. Fluid retention, especially by increasing the hygroscopic properties of collagen and other connective tissues.
4. Alteration of serum protein levels.
5. Stimulation of growth of the breast duct system.
6. Increase in uterine blood vessel diameter.

Clinical applications

Urinary oestriol levels may be used to monitor the state of the fetus in late pregnancy. However, there is a large fluctuation in the amount of oestriol produced each day under normal circumstances. Decisions regarding the management of a pregnancy should not be made on the basis of a single low result; repeated estimations should be made, so

that a trend is established. The causes of low urinary oestriol levels
are:

1. Hypertension in pregnancy.
2. Pre-eclampsia.
3. Abruptio placentae (accidental haemorrhage).
4. Renal infection.
5. Diabetes.
6. Maternal hypoglycaemia.
7. Placental insufficiency due to other causes.
8. Fetal anencephaly, and other congenital defects of fetal adrenals
   and liver.

In the US, ultrasound and fetal monitoring techniques have largely
replaced the use of biochemical monitoring.

Deviations from normal pregnancy

Colin Fisher
Revised by *Michael Bennett*

4.1 GENERAL INSTRUCTIONAL OBJECTIVE

The students should recognize deviations from normal pregnancy and understand their effects on mother and fetus so that they can initiate management.

4.2 SPECIFIC BEHAVIOURAL OBJECTIVES

1. Identify abnormalities of uterine size and shape, or lie and presentation of the fetus, by clinical examination of the abdomen of a pregnant patient, and discuss their significance.
2. Identify by history and examination the causes of vaginal bleeding in early pregnancy and discuss their significance.
3. Examine and counsel a patient with vaginal bleeding in early pregnancy.
4. Identify by history and clinical examination the differences between placenta praevia, accidental haemorrhage and bleeding due to other causes.
5. Discuss the principles of the immediate management of the patient with antepartum haemorrhage.
6. Identify hypertension, proteinuria, oedema and abnormal weight gain in a pregnant patient and discuss their significance.
7. Discuss the investigation of suspected fetal growth retardation.
8. Describe the application, risks and information to be derived from the use of amniocentesis, radiology, ultrasound and radioisotopes in pregnancy.

9. Discuss the significance and management of urinary tract infection in pregnancy.
10. Discuss the significance of heart disease in pregnancy.
11. Discuss the significance of glycosuria and diabetes in pregnancy.
12. Diagnose clinically, and with the aid of laboratory studies, the presence of anaemia in pregnancy and indicate appropriate therapy.
13. Discuss the management of rhesus iso-immunization in pregnancy and stress the prophylaxis.
14. Discuss the symptoms, signs, significance and management of convulsions and their prodromata in pregnancy and the puerperium.
15. Describe the causes of threatened premature labour in a patient and discuss her management.
16. Counsel and provide emotional support where necessary to a patient with an abnormal pregnancy.
17. Identify medical and psychiatric conditions in pregnant patients that necessitate specialist care.

4.3 REASONS FOR STUDYING DEVIATIONS FROM NORMAL PREGNANCY

Two factors should be borne in mind:

1. Deviations from normal may occur due to disease processes present in the mother prior to conception. Knowledge of these conditions will enable the practitioner to seek advice early and form a plan of management. As with normal pregnancies, the aim should be the prevention of complications.
2. The majority of problems that occur, however, are *not* associated with pre-existing conditions. Once again, their incidence can be reduced by thoughtful observation of and advice to the pregnant patient.

Most complications that occur during pregnancy can either be eliminated or at least minimized by careful antenatal care. Where complications do arise, they should be recognized *because* they are deviations from normal. If this concept (i.e. deviation from normal) is followed, complications will be detected earlier and so risks to the mother and fetus can be minimized.

Remember, obstetrics is an exercise in preventive medicine.

4.4 BLEEDING IN LATE PREGNANCY

Bleeding from the genital tract after the 20th week of pregnancy is referred to as antepartum haemorrhage (APH). The significance of this condition lies in its importance as a cause of maternal mortality and morbidity, and in its contribution to perinatal mortality.

Classification of APH

1. Accidental haemorrhage (Fig. 4.1). The word 'accidental' refers to bleeding occurring by chance (or accident) and not due to trauma, and refers to bleeding related to a placenta that is normally situated (i.e. in the upper segment of the uterus). Accidental haemorrhage (abruptio placentae) is the condition present when bleeding occurs from the decidua, behind the placenta. If the bleeding tracks down behind the membranes and appears through the cervix it may be described as 'revealed', but if it remains retroplacental it is described as 'concealed'.

   APH may also occur from the edge of the placenta (marginal haemorrhage), and in this instance the bleeding is always 'revealed'.
2. Placenta praevia (Fig. 4.2) refers to a placenta that is lying partially or wholly within the lower uterine segment and, according to the extent to which it intrudes into the lower segment, the degree of placenta praevia is classified as: lateral, marginal or central.

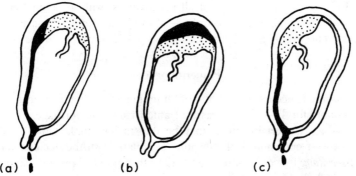

(a)   (b)   (c)

Fig. 4.1 (a) Partial detachment following retroplacental haemorrhage followed by external blood loss; (b) Complete detachment following retroplacental hae-morrhage near the centre of the placental attachment site — no external blood loss; (c) Marginal blood with little detachment of the placenta, but early bleeding seen externally.

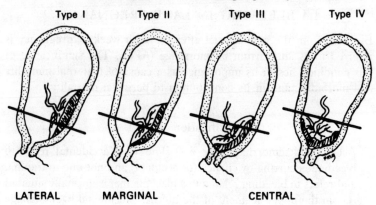

Fig. 4.2 Anatomical classification of placenta praevia. Type I. A minor portion of the placenta lies below the lower uterine segment. Type II. Most of the placenta lies below the lower uterine segment, but the placenta does not cover the internal os. Type III. The placenta covers the internal os when the os is closed but not when dilated. Type IV. The placenta completely covers the internal os even when dilated.

3. 'Of uncertain origin' is the third major category of APH. This group covers marginal haemorrhage, vasa praevia and those cases that cannot be confidently diagnosed as either abruptio placentae or placenta praevia.

Incidence

APH occurs in about 3% of all pregnancies, with an almost equal occurrence of all three categories — abruptio, placenta praevia and the uncertain group.

Placenta praevia

Incidence: It occurs in 1–1.5% of all pregnancies after 28 weeks, and accounts for 15–20% of cases of antepartum haemorrhage.
Aetiology: Uncertain, but it may be due to low implantation of the blastocyst or fusion of the decidua capsularis with the decidua vera.
Association: It occurs more often in uteri that have had previous surgery particularly Caesarean sections.

CLINICAL SYMPTOMS AND SIGNS
Painless, recurrent, bright red bleeding.

Usually this occurs after 28 weeks, but may occur earlier. Any antepartum bleeding should be viewed with suspicion. The bleeding may be of small or large volume, and the patient's condition will reflect the amount of blood lost.

Uterine contractions result in the shearing off of the placenta from the myometrium and decidua.

In about one-third of cases, placenta praevia is associated with an unstable lie, an abnormal presentation or a high presenting part.

DIAGNOSIS

1. History (painless, recurrent bright red bleeding).
2. Soft uterus without areas of tenderness.
3. Usually no associated hypertension.
4. Unengaged presenting part.

Do not perform a vaginal examination

Confirmation of the diagnosis can be made in almost all cases by the use of an ultrasonic examination. Isotope and X-ray placentography are no longer used.

MANAGEMENT

1. Admission to a hospital that is equipped to deal with such an emergency.
2. Bed rest.
3. Blood should be cross-matched and kept available.
4. Perform ultrasound examination to confirm diagnosis.

The main aim is to prolong the pregnancy until the fetus is mature (37–38 weeks).

Repeated minor bleeding as well as more severe bleeding, may produce anaemia, thus transfusion may be indicated.

Where a major degree of placenta praevia is diagnosed and the diagnosis confirmed, delivery should be by Caesarean section without vaginal examination.

Examination under anaesthesia before Caesarean section should be reserved for lateral-type placenta praevias or where the diagnosis is in doubt, and is rarely performed today.

Postpartum haemorrhage is more common with placenta praevia because of the poor ability of the lower segment to retract.

Accidental haemorrhage (abruptio placentae)

Associated factors occur in a small number of cases:

1. Hypertension and proteinuria.
2. Trauma.

Bleeding occurs from the decidua basalis separating the placenta from its attachment. As the volume of blood increases, placental separation occurs. After delivery, a clot may be found adhering to the maternal surface of the placenta. In severe forms of abruptions, the uterine muscle is suffused with blood and presents a very dark congested appearance (Couvelaire uterus).

CLINICAL FEATURES

These vary depending on the site and extent of bleeding and, as described previously, bleeding may be: revealed, concealed, or mixed.

Three grades of accidental haemorrhage are described: mild, moderate, or severe.

MILD

Only a small area of placental separation occurs and blood loss is usually less than 200 ml. There may be some abdominal discomfort or pain. Occasionally the uterus may be tender.

Management

1. Admission to hospital.
2. Bed rest.
3. Cross-match blood.
4. Localize placenta.
5. Inspect cervix.

If bleeding settles and does not recur, the patient may be discharged after 4–5 days. Intercourse should be avoided. The pregnancy should be followed thereafter using ultrasound examination, fetal growth patterns and fetal cardiac monitoring.

MODERATE

A greater area of the placenta separates (up to one-third) and the bleeding is more severe (200–600 ml). Pain is always present and the uterus will be locally tender. The patient does not usually have symptoms and signs of hypovolaemia, but will have a tachycardia and be understandably anxious. Fetal heart sounds are present and the uterus is frequently irritable.

Management

As for mild abruptio. Premature labour can often follow a bleed of this magnitude. The patient should not be discharged from hospital. Placental localization is indicated with ultrasound growth patterns, fetal growth pattern and fetal cardiac monitoring is essential.

Labour should be induced no later than term, or earlier if the fetus appears to be endangered.

SEVERE

More than half the placenta separates. Abdominal pain is more severe and the uterus is tender and rigid. Fetal heart sounds are muffled or often absent. Fetal movements may have ceased.

The patient is shocked, and is often in a worse condition than expected from the observed blood loss.

Management

Remember the two major complications: coagulation disorders and renal failure.

1. Withdraw blood for cross-matching and estimation of clotting time.
2. Insert CVP catheter.
3. Administer morphine (10 mg intravenously).
4. Give blood and fluids according to CVP reading.
5. Insert indwelling catheter into bladder.
6. If fetal heart sounds are present, assess the cervix — if favourable, perform an amniotomy; if unfavourable, perform a Caesarean section *after* restoring central venous pressure and ensuring that clotting time is normal.

Beware of postpartum haemorrhage, as the uterine muscle cannot retract efficiently.

If the correct steps in management are taken, the maternal mortality will be minimal. Fetal mortality may be as high as 75%, mainly due to immaturity and hypoxia.

Uncertain APH

This includes bleeding from a marginal placental sinus, circumvallate placenta where the trophoblast extends beyond the major placental mass, and vasa praevia.

Vasa praevia is associated with a velamentous insertion of the cord, so that fetal blood is lost.

The bleeding may be due to local causes, such as ectopic columnar epithelium, cervical polyps and carcinoma of the cervix. However, bleeding should not be attributed to these conditions unless they are actually found to be bleeding on inspection.

4.5 RENAL DISEASES ASSOCIATED WITH PREGNANCY

Renal infection

Of the various forms of renal disease occurring in pregnancy, renal infecton is by far the commonest. It is mostly thought of as an acute pyelonephritis, but may in fact be a subclinical renal infection which, because it is asymptomatic, is not often diagnosed unless special screening tests are performed. The significance of renal infection in pregnancy lies not so much with the pyrexia, nausea, vomiting and dehydration of acute infection, nor with the chronic lethargy and bone marrow depression of subclinical renal infection, but with the effect the renal infection has on the outcome of the pregnancy.

Renal infection is associated with an increased risk of abruptio placentae (5–10 times higher), premature labour (3–4 times higher) and increased perinatal loss (5–10 times higher). Elimination of kidney infection will assist in reducing the morbidity and mortality of pregnant mothers.

Because only 1–2% of women present with acute renal infection in pregnancy, a search must be made for those others who have subclinical pyelonephritis. It is probably best identified by performing a screening test for organisms in urine (asymptomatic bacteriuria). About one-third of those women with a positive screening test for organisms in urine have subclinical pyelonephritis. The actual incidence of renal infection is significant — about 2–3%.

Renal infection causes premature labour, antepartum haemorrhage and intrauterine death. There is controversy over the significance of the various other types of urinary tract infection, and the causes of the complications.

Types of urinary infection

There are three major groups of urinary infection seen in pregnancy:

1. Asymptomatic bacteriuria (incidence 3–5%). This condition is the presence of significant numbers (more than 100 000) of organisms in urine without any associated symptoms. Although about 3–5% of pregnant women have asymptomatic bacteriuria, this condition is not a disease of pregnancy — the same incidence of the disease is found among non-pregnant women who may have associated conditions, such as chronic interstitial fibrosis in the kidney, stones, obstruction, reflux and diverticulae, to explain the persistent presence of organisms.

2. Acute cystitis (incidence 2–3%). In pregnancy, the changes in the anatomy, physiology and biochemistry of the urinary tract and urine predispose to retention of urine and to the rapid growth of organisms. If these organisms multiply at a rate greater than the bladder wall has the capacity to reject them, then acute inflammation occurs, particularly of the trigone and urethra, and leads to the symptoms of frequency and dysuria. The major reason for the increase in number of organisms is the increased nutrients (glucose, amino acids) found in the urine of pregnant women.

   The physiological stasis and dilatation of the urinary tract, the anatomical changes in the position of the trigone and the ureters, and hyperaemia and softening of the pelvic fascia predispose to infection. Trauma and introduction of bacteria to the bladder are more frequent, so that eventually the natural defences (complete emptying of the bladder, vesical antibacterial activity) are overcome.

   The organisms producing cystitis may have been present in the bladder as asymptomatic bacteriuria or may have been introduced during such activity as intercourse, a gynaecological examination or catheterization.

3. Pyelonephritis (incidence 1–2%). Once organisms enter the bladder, they will ascend to the kidney if there is reflux of urine. Reflux may be associated with congenital abnormality of the uretero-vesical junction, with anatomical changes as in pregnancy, or with infection in the bladder causing oedema and fibrosis of the ureteric opening. Once reflux occurs in pregnancy, the

hydroureters and urinary stasis then increase the risk of the infection in the calyceal region of the kidney.

CLINICAL AND LABORATORY EVIDENCE OF URINARY INFECTION

all women - urynalysis at eac antenatal visit for PROT/SUGAR/RC

Patients with asymptomatic bacteriuria have no symptoms related to the urinary tract. Urine examination will disclose a bacteriuria of more than 100 000 organisms.

Cystitis will produce frequency and dysuria, associated with a positive urine culture and an increase in urinary white cell count, epithelial cells, occasionally red cells and mucous secretions. Acute pyelonephritis may present with fever, nausea, vomiting, loin pain and tenderness. In pregnancy it may become difficult to differentiate from hyperemesis gravidarum, acute renal infections, hepatitis or appendicitis. Laboratory investigations will demonstrate a positive urinary culture.

EFFECT OF URINARY INFECTION ON PREGNANCY

It has been shown that untreated acute pyelonephritis is associated with a 25% fetal loss due to intrauterine death, premature labour, accidental haemorrhage and neonatal death. However, this mortality has fallen dramatically over the past 40 years due to the use of appropriate chemotherapy and hydration soon after a patient presents with symptoms — but there is still a 3–4 times greater fetal morbidity and mortality when a mother develops pyelonephritis in pregnancy. If subclinical pyelonephritis is present, the risks appear to be greater because the disease is not usually detected early.

DETECTION OF SUBCLINICAL RENAL INFECTION

Asymptomatic bacteriuria and cystitis account for about 80% of all cases of urinary infection in pregnancy and when present should be appropriately treated with antibiotics.

DIAGNOSIS OF RENAL INFECTION IN PREGNANCY

Women with symptoms will usually present early, and a mid-stream specimen of urine should be taken for microscopy and culture of organisms, before beginning chemotherapy.

However, whilst cystitis and pyelonephritis account for about one-third of urinary infections in pregnancy, the incidence of asymptomatic bacteriuria is far greater. Whilst only one-third of these cases of urinary infection are potentially dangerous to the mother and infant, it is important that they be detected early and adequately managed.

Early detection can be accomplished by carrying out a bacteriuric screening test (BST) at the first antenatal visit. It appears that most of the significantly positive bacteriuric women can be detected at this stage, and appropriate therapeutic measures can then be taken.

DO NOT USE TETRACYCLINES or ANTI FOLATES eg TRIMETHOPRIM SULPHONY

TREATMENT

1. Cystitis. This should be treated by using a chemotherapeutic agent that is specifically concentrated in urine and renders the urine sterile. The most commonly used agents are nitrofurantoin (Furadantin), nalidixic acid (Negram) and methenamine mandelate (Mandelamine). All are given for 10–14 days, and after cessation of treatment the urine is recultured for organisms.

2. Pyelonephritis. When renal infection is present, the chemotherapeutic agents of choice are indicated by *in vitro* testing. If nausea, vomiting and dehydration require admission to hospital, then the appropriate antibiotics may be administered by the parenteral route. However, care must be taken that renal function is adequate and that the dosage and extent of therapy is not so great as to cause harm to the fetus or the mother.

3. Asymptomatic bacteriuria. This should be initially managed as for cystitis.

LENGTH OF TREATMENT COURSE

If the initial 1–2 week course of chemotherapy clears the urine of organisms, and there is no further evidence of infection, then the antibiotics should be ceased.

However, if further urine cultures show a recurrence of infection, persistence of casts and red cells, or an elevated leucocyte excretion rate (LER), then continuation of chemotherapy is indicated. It may be necessary to maintain antibiotics throughout the whole of the antenatal period. If this is indicated, then the various chemotherapeutic agents should be alternated and the urine checked regularly for organisms and leucocytes.

SPECIAL INVESTIGATIONS

Blood urea and serum creatinine estimations should be performed regularly on all pregnant patients who have pyelonephritis. A persistent raised urinary white cell count, casts or red cells is an indication to carry out an intravenous pyelogram. This investigation may be performed using only three radiographs taken at the optimum time, to determine if there is an underlying pathological lesion that may require special management.

FOLLOWING DELIVERY

All patients who have developed urinary infection in pregnancy should be followed up 8–12 weeks after delivery. At this time a full urine culture and examination should be performed. Any persistent abnormality merits further investigation. Approximately 20% of women with persistent renal infection in pregnancy will be found to have some evidence of an abnormality by pyelography and a large number of these women will have a surgically correctable lesion.

CONCLUSION

Approximately 7–9% of pregnant women will be found to have urinary infection in pregnancy due to pyelonephritis, cystitis or asymptomatic bacteriuria.

Treatment can eliminate the infection and reduce the risk to the fetus. Thus investigation and management of all pregnant women should include an adequate screening test to detect organisms in the urine.

Acute glomerulonephritis in pregnancy

This is relatively rare compared to renal infection, but should be suspected when hypertension, oedema, proteinuria and haematuria occur about 10–12 days following an acute streptococcal sore throat. It is more common in early pregnancy, but may be confused with severe pre-eclampsia. However, microscopy to show red cells, granular casts and increased white cell count, together with a high antistreptolysin titre, should confirm the diagnosis. Acute glomerulonephritis is often associated with spontaneous abortion and premature labour, as well as an increased incidence of fetal loss. The maternal mortality is about

2–3% and if the renal problem appears to be severe, it is advisable to terminate the pregnancy.

Chronic glomerulonephritis

This in pregnancy usually presents with hypertension, occasionally cardiovascular problems and renal insufficiency. Although pregnancy does not appear to make the disease process worse, it has a poor prognosis for the fetus. There is a high risk of intrauterine death, growth-retarded infants, prematurity and severe hypertensive problems. It is wise to induce labour early in such cases.

Nephrosis in pregnancy

This is due to such diseases as diabetes, amyloidosis and lupus erythematosus. It is very rare, and the general effect on mother and fetus is to increase mortality. Unless the disease is well controlled and managed, it is often advisable to terminate the pregnancy early.

Surgical problems

Such problems as large calculi, polycystic kidney or congenital abnormalities should not be treated in pregnancy unless they actually obstruct or interfere with the normal delivery process or are causing acute problems (renal calculi in a ureter).

Acute renal failure

This is seen when less than 500 ml of urine are passed in 24 hours. It may follow obstetric, medical or traumatic conditions. It is common in association with gram-negative infection (endotoxic shock), blood loss, trauma and drugs. The maternal and fetal prognosis is often poor, but is improved when the mother is transferred early to a renal unit to receive highly specialized therapy. Care must be taken in the anuric or oliguric phase that fluid requirements are carefully monitored and maintained, that diuretics are not used and that electrolyte balance is maintained. The prognosis for cases treated by inexperienced medical practitioners is very poor. The ideal management is in specially equipped renal units.

4.6 ANAEMIA IN PREGNANCY

Anaemia in pregnancy is significant because of increased risks to both mother and fetus:

1. Maternal
   (a) Inability to withstand haemorrhage.
   (b) Susceptibility to infection.
   (c) Developing heart failure if the anaemia is severe.
2. Fetal
   (a) Hypoxia — less oxygen is carried to the placenta by maternal blood.
   (b) Premature labour is more common.

Anaemia is present when the circulating haemoglobin mass is reduced. An arbitrary figure of 10.5 g% is often used as an indication that investigation for anaemia should be undertaken.

Changes seen during pregnancy

Both the plasma volume and red cell mass increase during pregnancy, but the rise in plasma volume (45%) greatly exceeds that of the red cell mass (15%). The resulting haemodilution allows for easier blood flow. If follows that the red cell count and packed cell volume fall during pregnancy and the haemoglobin will appear to be low.

Red cell size and haemoglobin content are unaffected and so the MCV and MCHC remain constant. Serum iron levels rise because the amount of iron-binding protein, like all plasma proteins, increases.

During pregnancy there is an increase in the amount of iron metabolized and its distribution is as follows:

- Excess red cell formation: 320 mg
- Increased uterine myoglobin: 50 mg
- Transferred to fetus: 200 mg
- Transferred to placenta: 100 mg

Types of anaemia

1. Iron deficiency. The patient may enter pregnancy with iron deficiency due to:
   (a) Inadequate intake.
   (b) Poor absorption.
   (c) Excessive losses from too frequent pregnancies, menorrhagia.

This initial deficiency may be aggravated by the extra demands for iron imposed by the pregnancy. Iron-deficiency anaemia is the most common type seen in Australia.

2. Thalassaemia minor. This is the second most common anaemia seen in pregnancy — 6% of Greek-born and 4% of Italian-born patients carry this trait. There is a genetically determined abnormality in β chain production, resulting in fewer red cells whose life span is reduced.

3. Folic acid deficiency. This is no longer common. Folic acid is necessary for amino acid metabolism, and increased amounts are needed for dividing cells. It usually manifests itself late in pregnancy.

4. Renal disease. This is a rare cause of anaemia, but when no obvious cause is found for a normochromic, normocytic anaemia, it may well be present.

Symptoms and signs

As in the non-pregnant state, the symptoms are non-specific and include lassitude, dyspnoea, palpitations, giddiness, fainting and oedema. These symptoms may have a gradual onset (iron deficiency) or a rapid onset (folic acid deficiency). Iron deficiency or β-thalassaemia can produce symptoms at any time during the pregnancy, but it is rare for folic acid deficiency to cause symptoms before 26 weeks — symptoms are usually first seen after 30 weeks.

Pallor is common, and oedema, raised jugular vein pressure and bounding pulse are normally seen in pregnancy. Nail and hair changes are rare. Occasionally, especially with folic acid deficiency, symptoms and signs of cardiac failure can occur.

Management

Prophylaxis: iron and folic acid supplements are routinely given during pregnancy. Fefol-2 given daily provides 270 mg of ferrous sulphate and 300 µg of folic acid.

Increased amounts of folic acid should be given in multiple pregnancy and to women taking phenytoin (Phentoin or Dilantin).

Investigations

1. Haemoglobin estimation. This should be done routinely at the first antenatal visit, at 28 weeks and 34 weeks. If this value is below acceptable limits, further investigations are performed.

2. Blood film. Abnormal red cell size, shape and haemoglobin content can be readily observed.
3. Packed cell volume. This is an unreliable test during pregnancy, but its determination is necessary in order to calculate red cell indices:
   (a) Mean corpuscular volume (packed cell volume (PCV)/red cell count). This is diminished in iron deficiency.
   (b) Mean corpuscular haemoglobin (haemoglobin concentration/ red cell count). This is diminished in iron deficiency.
   (c) Mean corpuscular haemoglobin concentration (haemoglobin concentration/packed cell volume). This is decreased in iron deficiency, and is probably the most significant test for iron-deficiency anaemia in pregnancy.
4. Serum iron and iron-binding capacity. The serum iron levels fall and the iron-binding capacity rises.
5. Serum folate and red cell folate. Levels fall with folic acid anaemia.
6. Haemoglobin electrophoresis. This will detect elevated levels of HbA_2 and HbF in thalassaemia minor.
7. Bone marrow examination. This is indicated in unresponsive cases or where blood studies are non-specific or suggest leukaemia.

Treatment

1. Iron deficiency. Either oral iron or total dose infusion with iron dextran (Imferon).
2. Packed cells. These may be given prior to or in labour if haemoglobin levels are below 8 g% and a rapid rise is needed. Provided the cells are infused slowly with added frusemide, no complications should occur.
3. Folic acid anaemia. Folic acid (5–15 mg daily by mouth) will produce a fairly rapid rise in haemoglobin levels.
4. Thalassaemia minor. Usually these patients are not iron deficient, but iron therapy may be indicated in certain cases. Ensure that folic acid is being taken (5 mg/day). Blood should only be given for acute blood loss.

In addition to specific measures, the importance of a well-balanced diet should be stressed to the mother. This measure, together with routine iron and folic acid supplements, has served to diminish the incidence of anaemia in pregnancy.

4.7 HEART DISEASE IN PREGNANCY

Deaths due to heart disease are the fourth most common cause of maternal mortality, and are the most common cause of death not due solely to obstetrical factors. Additionally, the perinatal mortality is at least doubled and in the most severe forms can be as high as 33%.

Incidence

Approximately 0.9% of pregnancies occur in patients with heart disease or who have previously had cardiac surgery.

Previously, rheumatic heart disease was by far the most common form seen, but its incidence has declined to a level similar to that of congenital heart disease.

Other types of heart disease encountered are cardiomyopathy, ischaemic and hypertensive heart disease.

Assessment

The severity of heart disease is commonly assessed by grading of symptoms:

1. No breathlessness on exertion.
2. Breathlessness with moderate exertion.
3. Breathlessness with slight exertion.
4. Breathlessness at rest.

In addition, the following points should be determined from history and examination:

1. Outcome of any previous pregnancy.
2. Previous episodes of heart failure.
3. The precise nature of the cardiac lesion.
4. Presence of arrhythmias.

In almost all cases, the co-operation of a cardiologist is desirable in both initial assessment and subsequent management.

Effect of pregnancy on heart disease

Cardiac output rises by up to 40% during pregnancy, the greater part of this rise occurring in the first 20 weeks. There is an increased blood flow to all areas of the body except the liver. Cardiac output remains at this elevated level until the commencement of labour, and increases even further during the first and second stages of labour. The increase in cardiac output increases the amount of cardiac work, and also the risk of women developing left ventricular heart failure.

Antenatal care is largely devoted to avoiding complications that may lead to heart failure, and to improving the grade of disability.

Obesity, hypertension, anaemia and multiple pregnancy may be deleterious factors, as can the development of a cardiac arrhythmia, especially atrial fibrillation. If any signs of heart decompensation develop, immediate admission to hospital and conventional management are indicated.

Patients on prophylactic anticoagulants following cardiac surgery should continue with this treatment. Warfarin sodium (Coumadin) however, may be teratogenic — so phenindione (Dindevan) is to be preferred. Both these agents, however, cause haemorrhagic disease of the newborn. Heparin should be substituted in the last 6 weeks of pregnancy, as it does not cross the placenta.

Labour should not be induced, nor Caesarean section undertaken, unless there is an obstetrical indication. If heart failure develops, it should be controlled before there is any obstetric interference.

Management during labour

Endocarditis: women with structural heart disease are exposed to infection during labour. Antibiotic cover should be given during labour and for at least 4 days afterwards.

The patient's head and shoulders should be kept propped up and it is best to avoid delivery in the conventional lithotomy position.

For patients with minor degrees of heart disease, lumbar epidural block is helpful as it will greatly diminish the additional increase in cardiac output during labour. With the more severe types of heart disease where patients are likely to develop left ventricular heart failure, more caution is advisable.

If acute pulmonary oedema develops, it is treated by conventional methods; the patient is propped up, 80–120 mg of frusemide (Lasix) are given intravenously, and digitalization may also be necessary.

Delivery

With minor degrees of heart disease, there is no reason why a normal vaginal delivery cannot be achieved, however, a prolonged second stage should be avoided.

With more severe forms of heart disease, forceps delivery is indicated to minimize maternal effort.

Caesarean section is only performed for obstetrical reasons.

Oxytocic agents

Normally these drugs are given prophylactically to prevent postpartum haemorrhage. Following the third stage of labour, there is an injection of up to 500 ml of blood into the circulation from the uterus. In certain instances the use of oxytocic agents is contra-indicated (i.g. in women with incipient left ventricular heart failure).

Ergometrine should be withheld, for in addition to its oxytocic properties, it also increases peripheral resistance and therefore the work of the heart.

However, if postpartum haemorrhage occurs, use intravenous ergometrine (0.125–0.25 mg), as it is often simpler to treat pulmonary oedema than postpartum haemorrhage.

Following delivery, the patient must be closely watched during the first 24 hours for the development of heart failure. However, after this time the blood volume commences to fall and as the return towards pre-pregnancy levels continues, the likelihood of heart failure diminishes.

Breast feeding is only contra-indicated in women with severe forms of heart failure.

4.8 PRETERM LABOUR

Preterm labour is labour commencing before the 38th week of amenorrhoea. The onset of preterm labour may be either spontaneous or induced — spontaneous preterm labour occurs in approximately 7% of all pregnancies.

Causes

1. Idiopathic — by far the largest group.
2. Secondary to premature rupture of membranes.
3. Overdistension of the uterus — multiple pregnancy, polyhydramnios.
4. Placental abruption.
5. Severe hypertension, and other situations where the fetus is at risk.
6. Cervical incompetence — where the sphincteric action of the cervix is lost due to previous trauma.

7. Uterine malformations.
8. Acute febrile illnesses in the mother.
9. Intrauterine fetal death.

Management

In some instances labour should be allowed to proceed normally without any interference. These include: severe antepartum haemorrhage, severe maternal hypertension, and intrauterine fetal death. Excluding these situations, an attempt should be made to arrest the progress of labour so that therapy can be instituted in an attempt to mature the fetal lungs.

If the period of amenorrhoea exceeds 24 weeks and the uterine size is either commensurate with, or larger than, dates:

1. Ascertain that the fetal heart beat is present.
2. Distinguish between true and false labour. If labour is false, there will not be any 'show' nor will the cervix be effaced or dilated.
3. Determine whether or not there are uterine contractions, either by palpation or an external pressure transducer attached to a fetal monitor.
4. If the membranes are ruptured, take a high vaginal swab for culture.

If painful contractions are occurring at a rate of one every 10 minutes and the cervix is dilated:

1. Commence an intravenous infusion of salbutamol (25 mg/l) and titrate the dose according to the maternal and fetal responses.
2. Providing the pregnancy has not exceeded 34 weeks, and that the mother is not hypertensive, corticosteroids are given. For instance, 1 g of betamethasone (Celestone Chronodose) is given intramuscularly, and then once more 24 hours later to assist in maturing the fetal lungs.
3. If the membranes are ruptured, the mother may be given antibiotics. For instance, 1 g of Cephalexin (Keflex) is given intravenously, and then 6 hourly whilst the infusion is running. Continue a similar oral dosage after the infusion is removed for a further 4 days.

Such a regime will inhibit labour in approximately 80% of cases where cervical dilatation does not exceed 4 cm before the commencement of treatment. The success rate is less when dilatation is greater than 4 cm or when the membranes are ruptured.

False labour occurs when uterine contractions are distressing to the mother in the absence of cervical effacement or dilatation.

In most instances explanation of what is occurring will be sufficient. to allay symptoms and if not, sedation with 10 mg Valium orally is effective.

4.9 COUNSELLING IN RELATION TO AN ABNORMAL PREGNANCY

When a pregnancy deviates from its normal course, a great responsibility falls on the obsterician to explain to the patient and her husband the exact situation, with regard to both the mother and baby.

Where premature induction of labour is planned on behalf of either mother or the fetus, care should be taken to explain:

1. Why induction is necessary.
2. What may happen if the pregnancy is prolonged.
3. How induction will be undertaken.
4. What will happen if it is unsuccessful.
5. What will happen to the baby following delivery.

Whilst a lot of people will take advice uncritically and unhesitatingly, with a response such as 'do whatever you think best', some people will question methods of management, and a frank and simple explanation will be expected.

Fetal malformation

Occasionally a fetal malformation may be diagnosed in late pregnancy. Usually there are gross malformations incompatible with life, such as anencephaly.

The parents should be told and offered the alternative forms of management. In such a situation this will consist of either induction of labour, or awaiting its spontaneous onset.

A great number of women find the second alternative intolerable and wish to have labour induced. Usually induction is successful, but the parents must be told what may happen if induction is unsuccessful.

When the baby is delivered, the parents should be asked if they wish to see the baby or if they would like it christened. Most parents will see the baby if given the choice, thereby ascertaining for themselves what the abnormality is. On no account should parents be dissuaded from looking at their baby in such a situation.

Intrauterine fetal death

The basic principles of counselling should be followed. The baby should be given to the parents to see or touch if they wish. In all instances, the cause of death should be explained to the parents. The risk of recurrence should also be ascertained and told to the parents. In most instances a post mortem is indicated.

Establishing an exact diagnosis

In all instances of stillbirth or neonatal death, an exact diagnosis should be made if possible, especially if there is any fetal malformation.

It is only by establishing a precise diagnosis that you can answer such questions as: Will it occur again? If so, what are the chances of recurrence? Can the condition be diagnosed antenatally? Such information is not only important to the parents, but also to their siblings who may be contemplating having children, and to future generations of their family.

4.10 CONVULSIONS IN PREGNANCY AND THE PUERPERIUM

Generalized convulsions may occur at any time during pregnancy and the puerperium, and may be caused by specific disorders of pregnancy (by far the most common) or by disorders unassociated with pregnancy.

Specific disorders of pregnancy

1. Hypertensive encephalopathy, associated with hypertension of pregnancy. Usually seen in late pregnancy, associated with fluid retention and proteinuria. It may, however, occur during labour or postnatally, especially in the first 24 hours following delivery.
2. Generalized convulsions can occur for the first time during pregnancy, and may be apparently precipitated by pregnancy in the absence of severe hypertension. This is much less common than hypertensive encephalopathy.

Convulsions specifically associated with pregnancy are known as eclamptic convulsions. The frequency of these convulsions is equally distributed between antepartum, intrapartum and postpartum periods.

Disorders unassociated with pregnancy

1. Idiopathic epilepsy. Phenytoin metabolism is altered considerably during pregnancy, and increasing amounts are needed as pregnancy progresses to maintain therapeutic levels in the plasma. Consequently subtherapeutic levels are more commonly found and the tendency for convulsions increases.
2. Hypoxic encephalopathy. Fainting is a common symptom of pregnancy and unless the person who faints is laid down, an hypoxic convulsion may ensue.
3. Water intoxication and hyponatraemia. This is more commonly seen with high-concentration oxytocin infusions, such as with the induction of a mid-trimester abortion, or induction of labour following intrauterine fetal death. Such conclusions are wholly preventable.
4. Associated with hypoglycaemia. This is mostly seen in cases of diabetes mellitus, where the insulin dosage is increased according to blood glucose levels. It can occur in early pregnancy when nausea prevents an adequate intake of nourishment.
5. Rupture of a cerebral artery aneurysm. This is usually seen post-natally, and does not always produce a convulsion.
6. Barbiturate and alcohol withdrawal.
7. Cerebral tumour. Problems in this instance are again usually seen postnatally, associated with haemorrhage into the tumour.

Symptoms and signs

1. Sudden loss of consciousness.
2. Crying out.
3. Falling, if the patient is upright.
4. Tonic movements of the tongue and limbs.
5. Clonic movements of the tongue and limbs.
6. Occasional sphincteric incontinence.

When there has been cerebral damage, localizing signs can be demonstrated in addition to coma or altered levels of consciousness. When there is no damage, the most common sign (apart from alteration of the levels of consciousness) is bilateral upgoing plantar reflexes.

Treatment
(see also the section on pre-eclampsia, section 4.19.)

1. Maintain the airway.
2. Ensure adequate oxygenation.
3. If status epilepticus is present, given intravenous diazepam (Valium).

   The most common cause is hypertensive encephalopathy, thus the following treatment is given:

4. The level of hypertension is reduced, for example by drugs such as diazoxide (Hyperstat-IV, 300 mg intravenously). Magnesium sulphate as an intravenous infusion reduces both the blood pressure and the level of cerebral irritability.
5. If the convulsion has occurred antepartum or intrapartum, the baby is delivered in order to minimize the risk to both mother and baby.
6. When clinical examination confirms an intracranial lesion, dexamethasone such as dexamethasone sodium phosphate (Decadron) (8 mg intravenously) should be given to reduce intracranial pressure.

   When an intracranial lesion is suspected or where a convulsion has occurred *de novo* during pregnancy, further investigations should be undertaken to exclude life-threatening lesions.

4.11 CHRONIC ILLNESS

The obstetrician should identify medical and psychiatric conditions in pregnant patients that necessitate specialist care. As a good general principle, patients with a chronic illness (either physical or psychological) should seek advice before embarking on a pregnancy.

Advice should be given relating to:

1. The likely effect of pregnancy on the mother in both the short and long term.
2. The effect of the mother's condition on the fetus, and the likelihood of any disabling disorder occurring.
3. The effects on the fetus of any medication needed by the mother.

Any decisions regarding the patient's management should only be made after discussion with the woman and her medical attendant. Frequently more specialized knowledge is required and a consultation should be sought.

Women with chronic illness who embark upon a pregnancy as a rule should be managed in a large centre, and close co-operation between the obstetrician and other physicians is essential.

4.12 RHESUS ISO-IMMUNIZATION AND HAEMOLYTIC DISEASE

The Rhesus (Rh) factor was first described by Landsteiner and Wiener in 1940. Fisher (1944) discovered that individual antigens made up the Rh factor.

There are three pairs of Rh antigens inherited by six separate genes (C, c, D, d, E, e), three from each parent. It is the presence or absence of D antigen that alone determines if a person is Rh-positive or Rh-negative.

Of Europeans, 83% are Rh-positive, 50% are heterozygous (Dd), and 33% are homozygous (DD) for the D antigen. Rh-negative persons are uncommon in Asians and Polynesians.

Rh iso-immunization accounts for 98% of haemolytic disease of the newborn and of these 95% are due to D antigen.

Immunization may occur:

1. When a Rh-negative woman is pregnant with a Rh-positive fetus.
2. Following an incompatible blood transfusion.
3. Following intramuscular injection of blood. *Why would you do this?*
4. *With needle sharing by IV drug abusers.*

Feto–maternal haemorrhage is most likely to occur during labour when the placenta separates. It may also occur following therapeutic abortion, spontaneous abortion, placental abruption or Caesarean section, chorionic villus sampling, amniocentesis, or spontaneously. *External cephalic version.*

Maternal antibody formation depends on the size of the feto–maternal haemorrhage, the stage of pregnancy at which it occurs, the individual sensitivity of the mother and on the ABO blood grouping. If there is ABO incompatibility between the mother and fetus, the fetal cells are rapidly destroyed by the mother's anti-A and/or anti-B antibodies.

It is rare for a first pregnancy to sensitize a woman. Previously, one in ten Rh-negative women were sensitized by two such pregnancies. In recent years, the incidence of Rh iso-immunization has declined markedly due to the introduction of anti-D globulin (see Prophylaxis, page 94).

When sensitization occurs, two major types of antibody appear in the maternal blood:

1. Immunoglobulin M (IgM) — does not cross the placenta.
2. Immunoglobulin G (IgG) — does cross the placenta. Detected by indirect Coombs' test.

Effects on the fetus

When IgG crosses the placenta, it attaches to the fetal red cells and enables them to be broken down. Anaemia results, and the fetus compensates by increasing haemopoiesis. This results in fetal hepatosplenomegaly. Red cell breakdown occurs mainly in the spleen, and accentuates splenomegaly.

There is increased bilirubin production — some bilirubin crosses the placenta and is metabolized by the mother, and some enters the amniotic fluid to give increased bilirubin levels in the fluid. These increased levels are detected by light-absorption studies, which helps assessment in the management of haemolytic disease.

If anaemia is mild, the fetus can compensate. However, imbalance may occur and increasingly severe anaemia develops. In the most severe forms, anaemia leads to hypoxia, with ultimate fetal death due to heart failure (hydrops fetalis).

Management

PROPHYLAXIS

At the first antenatal visit, blood group and antibody screen must be ordered in all instances. Where the patient is Rh-negative, antibodies should be looked for again at 28 weeks and if absent, she should receive 250 or 300 micrograms of Anti-D globulin.

If no antibodies are found in Rh-negative women during pregnancy, then two samples of cord blood should be collected following delivery. Fig. 4.3 shows the sequence of determinations to be followed.

If the cord blood tests indicate haemolytic disease due to Rh isoimmunization, the baby should be assessed for the severity of its effects by haemoglobin and plasma bilirubin estimations, and then managed accordingly.

Anti-D globulin should also be given to Rh-negative women who abort spontaneously, have a therapeutic abortion or tubal pregnancy, or undergo amniocentesis (except for haemolytic disease due to Rh).

Anti-D globulin is about 98% effective in preventing Rh isoimmunization. However, its exact mechanism of action is uncertain.

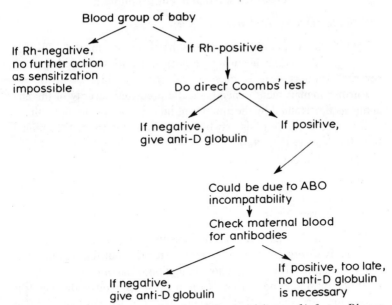

Fig. 4.3 Sequence of steps to be taken following delivery of infant to Rhesus negative mother.

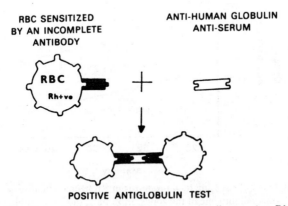

POSITIVE ANTIGLOBULIN TEST

Fig. 4.4 The direct Coombs' test. The fetal red cells carrying Rh-positive antigens are coated with maternal incomplete antibodies. Addition of anti-human globulin antiserum leads to an agglutination of these cells, giving a positive result. This indicates both the presence of maternal iso-immunization and potential fetal haemolysis.

SENSITIZED PREGNANCY

If antibodies are found during the antenatal course, this indicates that haemolytic disease is likely but it does not indicate the degree of severity. Amniocentesis is indicated to determine this.

Further management depends on the predicted severity of the anaemia as determined by the amount of bilirubin in the amniotic fluid.

Repeated amniocentesis may be necessary to determine the optimal time for delivery (Fig. 4.5).

The mainstays of treatment are:

1. Premature induction of labour.
2. Exchange transfusion.
3. Phototherapy.

Occasionally, fetal intrauterine transfusion is indicated when the anaemia is severe enough to warrant treatment, but the pregnancy is not sufficiently advanced to allow induction of labour.

Other antibodies apart from Rh may cause haemolytic disease. It is important to remember that these may occur in Rh-positive *as well as* Rh-negative women. The antibodies include:

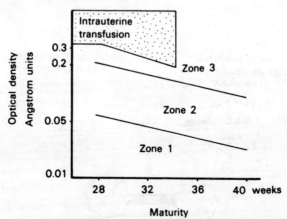

Fig. 4.5 Chart for assessing fetal prognosis in Rh haemolytic disease. Amniocentesis results fall into one of the zones. In Zone 1, the baby is mildly affected and can safely be allowed to go to 38 weeks. In Zone 2, multiple amniocentesis may be required to determine in which direction the trend is developing. Early induction may be required. In Zone 3, after 34 weeks immediate delivery should be undertaken, whilst prior to 34 weeks, intrauterine transfusion will be necessary.

1. Kell (usually due to an incompatible blood transfusion).
2. Duffy.
3. MNS antibodies.

Remember, *all* pregnant women should be screened for antibodies, likely to cause haemolytic disease at their first antenatal visit.

4.13 GLYCOSURIA AND DIABETES MELLITUS

Glycosuria

During pregnancy the renal blood flow increases by 50% and the glomerular filtration rate by 45% above non-pregnant values. As a result, more glucose is presented to the renal tubules for reabsorption and often the T_m for glucose is exceeded and glycosuria occurs.

When 1% of glucose is found on two successive visits, a glucose tolerance test should be performed. Glucose tolerance tests should also be performed on potential diabetics when they are pregnant, such as women:

1. Who have an identical twin who is diabetic.
2. Whose parents are diabetic.
3. Who have one diabetic parent, and the other parent has diabetic siblings or parents.
4. Who have borne a live or stillborn child whose birth weight exceeded 4.5 kg.
5. Who have borne a stillborn child with islet cell hyperplasia not associated with Rh incompatibility.
6. Who weigh over 80 kg at conception.

There is a better likelihood of finding an abnormal response to a glucose tolerance test if the test is performed in the second half of pregnancy or if the women who are tested are over 30 years of age.

When the diagnosis of diabetes mellitus is made initially during a pregnancy, the patient is classified as a gestational diabetic.

Effects of pregnancy on glucose metabolism

1. Glycosuria — previously described in the physiology of tubular reabsorption of glucose.
2. Human placental lactogen exerts an anti-insulin and lipolytic effect, which increases plasma glucose levels and makes more glucose available to the fetus.

3. Steroid hormones (oestrogens and progesterone) also have a mild anti-insulin effect.
4. Some insulin is probably destroyed by the placenta.

The net effect is a rise in maternal glucose levels throughout pregnancy, and in some women this is excessive and produces gestational diabetes.

Incidence of diabetes mellitus in pregnancy

Of the total population, 3% suffer from either juvenile or mature-onset diabetes mellitus. One-sixth of these people are women of child-bearing age, so that about one pregnancy in 400 is complicated by diabetes.

Effects of diabetes on pregnancy and vice versa

1. The infertility rate is slightly increased.
2. Hypoglycaemia is more common, due to nausea of pregnancy.
3. Ketoacidosis is more likely due to vomiting of early pregnancy.
4. Urinary tract infection is more common — 18% of pregnant women have asymptomatic bacteriuria (three times the usual rate).
5. Moniliasis is more common, and is often severe.
6. Pre-eclampsia is more common.
7. Polyhydramnios is more common.
8. Insulin requirements increase steadily during pregnancy, and it is easy to lose control of the diabetes.
9. Perinatal morbidity and mortality is increased.
   (a) There is a 6% incidence of major congenital malformations (three times the average rate).
   (b) Sudden intrauterine death may occur in late pregnancy.
   (c) Birth trauma may occur due to larger than average babies, predisposing to dystocia.

Management of insulin-dependent diabetes mellitus

1. A team approach ensures continuity of treatment by experienced people. The team includes obstetricians, physicians, paediatricians, dietitians, social workers, and pathology and nursing staff.
2. An early assessment of obstetrical and medical condition is necessary. In addition to usual investigations, renal function must be assessed.
3. Plasma glucose levels are used to regulate insulin dosage, rather

than urinary glucose. The aim is to keep plasma glucose levels below 5 mmol/1. Fortnightly visits are indicated.

4. Fetal maturity should be checked by ultrasound at 20 weeks.
5. Twice daily biphasic insulin should be given from 16 weeks.
6. Admission may be required during this time for stabilization of diabetes or investigation of obstetric complications.
7. Admission at 32 weeks is indicated, for bed rest to increase placental flow.
   (a) Thrice weekly, 2-hour postprandial plasma glucose levels are determined.
   (b) Regular fetal movement charting is performed.
   (c) Serial ultrasound examinations are taken.
   (d) Daily weighing and girth measurements are made.
   (e) External cardiotocography is performed.
   (f) Vaginal delivery at 37–38 weeks is preferable.
   (g) The lecithin/sphingomyelin (L/S) ratio may be needed.

Delivery

1. If cervix favourable: amniotomy and oxytocin drip.
2. If cervix unfavourable: Caesarean section.

Postnatal

1. Maternal insulin requirements drop suddenly.
2. Postnatal insulin requirements are much lower.
3. Lactation can be successfully established.

Baby

The baby is more prone to hypoglycaemia, so is fed at 1-hour intervals and regular plasma glucose levels are determined. Diabetic babies are also more prone to hyaline membrane disease, so should be monitored daily for this complaint.

With this routine, the perinatal loss can be reduced to 5–10%. With less strict regimes, the incidence of diabetic and obstetrical complications increases.

Gestational diabetes

Where the diagnosis of diabetes is made during pregnancy, initially control should be attempted through diet.

1. If diet is successful. Make fortnightly estimations of plasma glucose. Do not allow pregnancy to progress past term.
2. If diet not successful. Insulin (not oral hypoglycaemics) is needed. The routine for insulin-dependent diabetics should be followed.

4.14 AMNIOCENTESIS IN PREGNANCY

Amniocentesis is the withdrawal of fluid from the amniotic cavity. This involves passing a needle through the anterior walls of the mother's abdomen and uterus, always under ultrasound control.

Amniocentesis may be performed:

1. Early in pregnancy for:
   (a) Therapeutic abortion.
   (b) Antenatal genetic diagnosis.
2. Late in pregnancy for:
   (a) Determining fetal lung maturity (L/S ratio).
   (b) Management of Rh iso-immunization.

The ideal time for amniocentesis in early pregnancy is 15 weeks.

Antenatal diagnosis

It is possible to diagnose a variety of conditions, either directly from the amniotic fluid or as a result of cells cultured from the fluid. Such conditions include:

1. Chromosomal abnormalities. These occur either:
   (a) When the mother has previously had a baby with a chromosomal abnormality.
   (b) When the mother or the father is a mosaic carrier.
   Or may arise:
   (c) As the mother's age advances towards 40 years.
2. Neural tube defects. Anencephaly, iniencephaly, encephalocoele, myelomeningocoele and spina bifida can be diagnosed when the fetal lesion is not skin covered. Approximately 90% of cases of spina bifida, can be detected by estimating the levels of alpha-fetoprotein (AFP) in amniotic fluid. AFP levels may also be raised when there is a large exomphalos or cystic hygroma, so it is not entirely specific for neural tube disorders. Hydrocephaly cannot be diagnosed by this procedure.
3. Biochemical disorders. A variety of such disorders are inherited as

autosomal recessive genes. These may also be diagnosed. For example, adrenogenital syndrome, mucopolysaccharide disorders, some amino-acidurias.

4. X-linked disorders. Sexing of the fetus can be achieved by amniotic cell culture. Male children are aborted in the presence of X-linked disorders, such as haemophilia, and muscular dystrophy.

5. Haemoglobinopathies. These can be diagnosed by fetal blood sampling at the time of amniocentesis.

Lecithin/sphingomyelin ratio determination

The most common cause of respiratory distress syndrome in the newborn is hyaline membrane disease. Whether or not a baby develops this condition depends on the amount of surfactant in the lung alveoli. The appearance of surfactant in fetal lungs in sufficient amount to prevent hyaline membrane disease coincides with a sudden increase in the amount of lecithin in amniotic fluid.

Lecithin is a phospholipid, and its concentration and its relation to that of another phospholipid, sphingomyelin, is expressed as a ratio (L/S ratio).

As a rule, the increase in lecithin occurs at 35–36 weeks (Fig. 4.6),

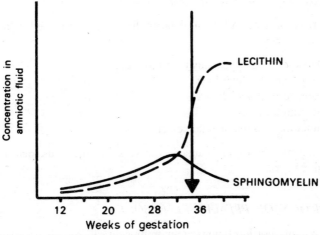

Fig. 4.6 Amniotic fluid levels of lecithin and sphingomyelin indicate fetal lung maturity. After 36 weeks of gestation, there is usually a dramatic rise in lecithin levels compared to sphingomyelin, indicating that the fetal lung is mature and will probably easily sustain respiration after delivery.

but may occur earlier or later than this, depending on fetal maturation of adrenal tissue.

Factors known to accelerate surfactant production in certain cases include:

1. Repeated small antepartum haemorrhage.
2. Maternal heroin addiction.
3. Prolonged premature rupture of the membranes.
4. Stress situations to the fetus.

Factors that may delay lung maturation include:

1. Maternal diabetes mellitus.
2. Severe Rh iso-immunization.

Rhesus iso-immunization assessment

The severity of fetal haemolytic anaemia can be assessed by estimation of the amount of bilirubin in the amniotic fluid (see Rhesus iso-immunization page 93).

Complications of amniocentesis

FETAL DAMAGE OR DEATH

A variety of types of fetal damage have been reported following amniocentesis:

1. Damage of one eye, causing blindness ⎫
2. Gangrene of a fetal limb   ⎪
3. Damage to brachial plexus   ⎬ all very rare.
4. Pneumothorax   ⎪
5. Puncture of a major fetal vessel   ⎭

Death may be due to damage to a vessel in the fetus, placenta or umbilical cord.

ABORTION OR PREMATURE LABOUR

The risk of abortion following an amniocentesis in early pregnancy is ±1% — only slightly higher than the normal incidence of midtrimester abortion (0.7%).

Premature labour follows amniocentesis in late pregnancy in about

5% of cases, and is more likely to occur the closer the pregnancy is to term.

INFECTION

Amniocentesis is an invasive procedure and an aseptic technique is necessary to prevent the development of amnionitis.

MATERNAL MORBIDITY

This is a rare occurrence, but complications due to maternal bleeding and formation of haematoma in the uterus have been recorded.

4.15 RADIOLOGY IN PREGNANCY

Because of the potential hazards of radiation and the emergence of diagnostic ultrasound, the role of radiology in obstetrics has diminished considerably. Attention to the possible teratogenic effects of radiology was first raised in the 1920s in relation to fetal microcephaly.

The effect of radiation to future generations because of irradiation of fetal gonads has not yet been evaluated. However, radiological examination is indicated in late pregnancy in certain situations.

Radiology related to pregnancy

1. Pelvimetry. Where cephalopelvic disproportion is suspected or there is a breech presentation during the last 3 weeks of pregnancy. The most useful view is a lateral radiograph of the pelvis with the mother standing erect. This will provide information about the following:
   (a) Angle of inclination of the pelvic brim.
   (b) Shape of the sacrum.
   (c) Antero-posterior diameters of the pelvis.
   In some instances (e.g. previous fractured pelvis), a Thom's view of the pelvic brim is indicated.
2. Fetal maturity. Radiology will show any ossification centres. Distal femoral epiphysis appears at about 36 weeks, proximal tibial at about 40 weeks. If both epiphyses are seen, the fetus is most likely to be at or near term. However, the appearance of ossification centres is frequently delayed in growth retardation, the very situation where the information is most frequently required.

3. Where the uterus is larger than dates. Multiple pregnancy may be diagnosed, as well as skeletal malformations that may be associated with polyhydramnios. Ultrasound has largely replaced X-rays for this indication.

Radiology incidental to pregnancy

When the pregnant woman develops an illness in which radiology would normally be used radiology is indicated in special circumstances. These situations include:

1. Severe chest pain.
2. Pneumonia.
3. IVP for haematuria or suspected ureteric colic (single exposure only).
4. Suspected perforated viscus.
5. Suspected fractures.

4.16 ULTRASOUND IN PREGNANCY

Ultrasound is sound of a frequency greater than 2 mHz. It is a safe procedure for both mother and fetus. Two types of ultrasound are used during pregnancy:

1. Continuous ultrasound. Use is made of the Doppler effect to pick up fetal heart movement. This is used in the portable fetal heart detectors, as well as by the external transducers found on fetal monitors.
2. Pulsed utrasound. Impulses are released at several millisecond intervals and are reflected by the body tissues at differing speeds, depending on the density of the tissue. The reflected sound can be converted to dots of light and a picture is subsequently built up on a storage tube oscilloscope. Transverse and longitudinal tomograms are then used to build up a three-dimensional picture of the uterus and its contents.

Uses in early pregnancy

1. Diagnosis and prognosis of threatened abortion and diagnosis of missed abortion.
2. Diagnosis of hydatidiform mole.
3. Examination of the uterus that is apparently larger or smaller than dates.

4. Differential diagnosis of pelvic tumours.
5. Prior to amniocentesis.
6. Estimation of fetal age — between 14 and 24 weeks, fetal size and fetal age (duration of pregnancy) correlate with a great degree of accuracy ($\pm$ 7 days). After this time the correlation between fetal size and age becomes less accurate using a single examination. However, serial examinations are helpful.

Uses in late pregnancy

1. Estimation of fetal age (see item 6 above).
2. Serial measurements of fetal size. These will give valuable information about the rate of fetal growth. If three readings are made at intervals of 10–14 days, the correlation with fetal size is accurate to 250 g in over 80% of cases.
3. Diagnosis of multiple pregnancy.
4. Investigation of polyhydramnios. Ultrasound can be very helpful in detecting both skeletal and non-skeletal conditions associated with polyhydramnios.
5. Diagnosis of fetal abnormalities.
6. Determination of abnormalities of fetal presentation, lie and position.
7. Placental localization. Ultrasound can accurately diagnose placental position in about 98% of cases. Any difficulties encountered are usually associated with posterior wall placentas. Because ultrasound is harmless and the method is accurate, it has superseded other methods of placental localization.

4.17 RADIOISOTOPES IN PREGNANCY

The principal use of radioisotopes was placentography. The technique is now redundant. Radioisotope scanning is only used in pregnancy to confirm a diagnosis of pulmonary embolism.

4.18 INVESTIGATION OF SUSPECTED FETAL GROWTH RETARDATION

Fetal growth retardation is suspected when the size of the uterus is less than expected in relation to the period of amenorrhoea during the last trimester. To make this assumption, however, the date of the last menstrual period should be accurately known and corrections should have been made for:

1. Variations in menstrual cycle length.
2. Taking of oral contraceptives prior to conception.
3. Maternal height. Where a mother is taller than average, the fundus of the uterus will not reach the usual landmarks at the anticipated time. The uterus frequently appears smaller than dates would suggest. With a small woman, the uterine size may appear to be larger than dates.

Causes of fetal growth retardation

Fetal growth velocity can be expressed as a simple equation:

Velocity of fetal growth = Intrinsic growth potential ×
Growth support

Intrinsic growth potential is genetically determined. Thus two small parents will produce a small baby, whilst two large parents will produce a large baby. The growth potential can be altered in certain situations:

1. Chromosomal abnormalities. The total body cell number may be reduced.
2. Damage to the embryo during organogenesis. For example, the effect of rubella or drugs diminish the number of cells by damage or cell death.

Growth support is a measure of the amounts of nutrients and oxygen supplied to the fetus by the mother and placenta, and the amounts of waste products and carbon dioxide removed. Factors that interfere with these processes will diminish growth support. In the case of multiple pregnancy, the nutrients and oxygen supplied may be sufficient to maintain a single fetus in optimal conditions, but they may not be enough for more than one fetus.

Management

Initially this includes an adequate history to discover the likelihood of fetal abnormality by determining such factors as drug exposure and transplacental infection. In addition, the woman's own birth weight and her situation in her own family is important, as there is good correlation between fetal and maternal birth weights.

Menstrual cycle length and exposure to oral contraceptives should be noted, and these factors taken into account when correlating uterine size with the duration of amenorrhoea at the first antenatal visit.

If there is a discrepancy noted, an utrasonic examination before the uterine fundus reaches the umbilicus will help to acertain fetal maturity accurately.

In instances other than these, growth retardation may be suspected from physical findings in the third trimester.

When the uterus is smaller to palpation than expected:

1. Check available information with regard to such factors as duration of amenorrhoea and cycle length.
2. Assess maternal weight gain. Growth retardation is often associated with a low weight increase of the mother during pregnancy.
3. Check growth of the fundus by measuring the pubis to fundus distance serially.
4. Measure the mother's girth at the umbilicus and relate this to her weight, by using one of the available charts.
5. If these parameters are abnormal, repeat the assessments at subsequent visits.
6. Commence serial ultrasound measurements of the fetus.

Ultrasound growth patterns

These will show one of three types:

1. Normal. This is usually found in larger women, and especially those in whom palpation is difficult due to obesity.
2. Where growth has originally been satisfactory, but then proceeds slower than normal. These charts correlate with:
   (a) Genetically small, but normal children.
   (b) Fetuses whose growth potential has been altered by: chromosomal or genetic problems, exposure to transplacental infection, exposure to drugs including alcohol and nicotine, or malnutrition.
3. Where growth has proceeded normally until late pregnancy and has then slowed. This indicates failure of growth support, such as in:
   (a) Hypertension.
   (b) Repeated antepartum haemorrhage.
   (c) Chronic maternal disease (excluding diabetes mellitus).

Where growth retardation is proven the mother should rest in bed to improve uterine blood flow. The optimal time of delivery is determined by:

1. Clinical information.
2. Ultrasonic growth patterns.

3. Daily fetal movement charting.
4. Antenatal cardiotocography can be helpful in order to prolong a pregnancy where the fetus is retarded but immature.
5. An L/S ratio will help in trying to determine the optimal time to deliver the baby without the risk of hyaline membrane disease.

4.19 PRE-ECLAMPSIA AND ECLAMPSIA

Pre-eclampsia and eclampsia are diseases dependent on the presence of trophoblastic tissue. Their incidence is higher in conditions where the volume of trophoblast is greater than normal, such as diabetes mellitus, multiple pregnancy, Rh iso-immunization, and large hydatidiform moles.

Pre-eclampsia results in more admissions to hospital in the antenatal period than any other condition. In its more severe forms, it is a cause of both fetal and maternal morbidity and mortality.

Diagnosis

The diagnosis is made when any two of the following three signs are observed:

1. Hypertension.
2. Generalized oedema. less imp^t
3. Proteinuria.

The first two signs almost invariably precede proteinuria. Additionally, generalized oedema may be accompanied by a sudden increase in maternal weight.

Elevation of the blood pressure above 140/90, with the patient in the left lateral position, or a rise in the diastolic pressure of 15 mmHg above pre-pregnancy or early pregnancy levels, should be regarded as significant.

The detection of proteinuria on routine testing should be followed by boiling a mid-stream specimen of urine. A common cause of small amounts of proteinuria is the contamination of urine by vaginal secretions, or a urinary tract infection.

Generalized oedema, which produces puffiness of the face and hands, is more significant than dependent oedema. However, dependent oedema will occur when oedema is generalized.

The presence of proteinuria during pregnancy has long been associated with a poor outcome for both the mother and the fetus. Women are encouraged to bring an early-morning sample of urine for testing in order to avoid false positive results due to orthostatic proteinuria. About fifty years ago, the detection of proteinuria was an indication to take the mother's blood pressure. This practice continued until it was observed that with the exception of renal disease, hypertension occurring during pregnancy precedes proteinuria.

Incidence

In Australia about 6% of pregnancies are complicated by pre-eclampsia, but its occurence is twice as common in primigravid women.

Aetiology

The aetiology is unknown, but obviously is related to the presence of functioning trophoblast, and presumably placental hormones are responsible.

? Male factor — can occur in parous pt who never had it before if partner changed.

Pathology

The following conditions are known to be found in patients with pre-eclampsia:

1. Diminished plasma volume.
2. Increased extracellular fluid.
3. Vasospasm. *esp arterioles of kidney + uterus.*
4. Disseminated intravascular coagulation in very severe cases.
5. Ischaemic changes in various organs, when the disease is severe.

Diminished plasma volume is probably associated with the increase in extravascular fluid. This results in increased vasopressin and aldosterone secretion, in an effort to maintain intravascular volume — and vasospasm occurs. *? Altered response to Angiotensin all sea*

The resultant diminished renal blood flow causes increased renin secretion and glomerular damage, thus causing proteinuria. Diminished uterine blood flow will affect placental perfusion and fetal growth. Reduction in cerebral and hepatic perfusion can produce ischaemic change in these organs.

Disseminated intravascular coagulation will further diminish the calibre of small vessels, thus increasing blood pressure and further diminishing organ perfusion.

When left untreated, the following complications can arise:

1. Fitting (Seizures) (eclampsia): related to cerebral hypoxia and oedema.
2. Cerebral haemorrhage: hypertension.
3. Left ventricular heart failure: hypertension and ischaemia.
4. Renal failure: ischaemia.
5. Liver failure: ischaemia.
6. Death: from any of the above causes, or due to failure of coagulation.

Fetal loss increases as the disease becomes more severe, and can be as high as 50% if the mother fits. The causes of perinatal death are hypoxia, placental separation and immaturity following premature delivery.

Classification

Pre-eclampsia can be classified according to blood pressure measurements:

- Mild: diastolic BP less than 100 mmHg
- Moderate: diastolic BP less than 110 mmHg
- Severe: diastolic BP more than 110 mmHg or more than 100 mmHg with proteinuria.

Management

Prophylaxis: A past history of pre-eclamptic toxaemia (PET), hypertension or renal disease, or a family history of the same conditions, may predispose to eclampsia.

Regular checks should be made of weight, blood pressure and urine during pregnancy, and greater vigilance is required for those mothers at risk, as determined from the history.

Early admission to hospital is indicated when there are abnormal findings.

Mild and moderate pre-eclamptic toxaemia

1. Bed rest. This will result in increased uterine and renal blood flow. A diuresis will almost always be achieved with bed rest.

2. Regular 4-hourly blood pressure recordings and urinalysis, together with daily weighing, are required.
3. Occasionally, sedation will benefit the patient. For example, phenobarbital (60 mg), Valium (diazepham) (5 mg 6-hourly) or Dormicum or Mogadon (nitrazepam) at night. Some have discouraged the use of diazepam-like products during pregnancy.

There is no indication for diuretics unless nerve compression syndromes (e.g. carpal tunnel) are present.

In mild cases, the blood pressure and oedema subside readily and after 3–4 days the patient may be discharged from hospital after a period of mobilization. Usually further management is on an outpatient basis. If readmission is required, the patient should remain in hospital.

In moderate cases, rest in hospital should continue if the blood pressure does not fall below 90 mmHg. Hypotensive agents are rarely, if ever, indicated unless the blood pressure remains above 100 mmHg. Besides the routine observations, the pregnancy should be monitored by fetal movement charts, cardiotocography and serial ultrasound. Induction of labour may be necessary between 37 and 40 weeks.

Severe pre-eclamptic toxaemia

Severe PET (or pregnancy-induced hypertension) is an obstetric emergency requiring intensive care both before and after delivery. Most patients recover quickly, usually after transient episodes of extreme hypertension or oliguria. If further complications arise, e.g. eclampsia, renal failure or intravascular coagulation, recovery may be delayed. Although PET is relatively common, most obstetricians will only see an occasional severe case.

Blood pressure recording

Before commencing management, it is important to standardize the recording of blood pressure. Due to hydrostatic pressure differences blood pressure should aways be taken with the arm at the level of the heart. Thus patients in hospital should have their blood pressure taken as follows — the patient should lie on her back. If more than 26 weeks gestation, she should roll her lower abdomen and hips 45° to her left to prevent compression of the vena cava and aorta. The cuff is placed on the left arm with a pillow under the elbow. A pillow may also be placed under the abdomen.

Management of severe PET (BP higher than 110 mmHg diastolic, 1/3 proteinuria) where delivery is indicated

1. Admit to Labour Ward.
2. Allocate *one* nurse to look after the patient.
3. Inform a physician and a paediatrician.
4. Deliver by the most expeditious means.
5. Fetal observation:
   Continuous CTG in labour.
6. Maternal observations:
   (a) Strict fluid balance chart.
   (b) Blood pressure — every 15 minutes.
   (c) Special nurse.
   (d) Urinalysis — 4-hourly.
   (e) Urine output — hourly measure with indwelling catheter.
   (f) CVP — measure hourly. To be inserted by anaesthetist and check with chest radiology.
   (g) Pathology — Full blood count and platelets.
   　　　　　　　　　Clotting time.
   　　　　　　　　　Fibrinogen, fibrin degradation products.
   　　　　　　　　　Urea, creatinine, electrolytes and uric acid.
   　　　　　　　　　Cross-match blood.
   Albumin, total protein, liver function tests may be performed later.
7. (a) Maternal treatment:
   Strict bed rest in a single, quiet, dark room.
   (b) Anticonvulsant therapy:
   Diazepam (Valium) infusion via IVAC infusion pump.
   Commence at 5 mg/h after initial statim dose. In the US, magnesium sulphate 4 g IV is much preferred.
   (c) Hypotensive therapy:
   If patient is conscious, continue previous hypotensive agents.
   If unconscious, or blood pressure high, use:
   hydrallazine (Apresoline), 20 mg parenteral *or* labetolol (Trandate), or magnesium sulphate IVI
   (i) Epidural block is sometimes used if patient is labouring.
   (ii) Urine output maintain at more than 25 ml/h. If output less than 25 ml/h and CVP less than 12 mm use concentrated albumin.
   　　If output less than 25 ml/h and CVP more than 16 mm use frusemide (Lasix) 40 mg IV.

8. Remain in Labour Ward until blood pressure and urine output satisfactory — most patients become worse immediately postpartum, then eventually improve.

Patients in hospital requiring hypotensive therapy

1. Inform physicians and paediatricians.
2. Fetal observations:
   (a) Fetal movement chart and monitoring.
   (b) Serial CTGs.
   (c) Serial ultrasound.
   (d) Oestriols, HPLs.
   (e) L/S ratio if necessary.
3. Maternal observations:
   (a) Fluid balance chart.
   (b) Weigh daily.
   (c) Blood pressure every 4 hours.
   (d) Pathology — as for severe PET, including uric acid and liver function tests.
   (e) 24-hour urine protein.
4. Maternal treatment:
   (a) Bed rest.
   (b) Hypotensive agents. Continue previous treatment. If blood pressure rises: hydralazine (Apresoline) or, labetolol (Trandate).
   (c) Sedation — preferably nil. Otherwise diazepam (Valium) or phenobarbitone.
5. Deliver if there is:
   (a) Rising blood pressure.
   (b) Rising proteinura.
   (c) Fetal maturity.
   (d) Fetal compromise.
6. Continue treatment at least 48 hours postpartum.

Delivery

If the cervix is favourable, amniotomy should be performed and an oxytocin infusion commenced. If the cervix is unfavourable, Caesarean section should be performed.

Following delivery of the baby the maternal condition should be monitored until blood pressure returns to normal. This is frequently rapid, but may take several days. Remember that fitting (seizures) may recur at any time, but especially within the first 24 hours. In the long term, the mother should be observed for evidence of hypertension or renal disease.

Outcome

Eclampsia is still a cause of maternal mortality, usually associated with cerebral haemorrhage.

Fetal mortality is in excess of 50% when the mother has fitted either due to hypoxia *per se* or secondary to placental separation.

4.20 INTRAUTERINE FETAL DEATH

Fetal death may occur at any time during pregnancy due to a variety of causes, including:

1. Maternal hypertension (especially pre-eclamptic toxaemia).
2. Placental separation.
3. Transplacental infection.
4. Cord entanglement (rarely).
5. Rh iso-immunization.
6. Maternal diseases, such as diabetes mellitus and chronic renal disease.

In a great number of instances, no obvious cause can be found.

Symptoms and signs

There may be a preceding history of one of the causes of fetal death. A loss of fetal movement is noted, which sometimes may be heralded by a period of unusual fetal activity. Fetal heart sounds are absent. After several days the uterus commences to shrink due to resorption of amniotic fluid.

Robert's Sign

Confirmation

1. Radiology. Radiology is performed within 24–36 hours, gas may be seen in the fetal heart, great vessels and even the umbilical cord. Overlapping of the fetal cranial bones (Spalding's sign) takes about 3–10 days to develop, and is usually preceded by obvious separation of the cranial sutures.

2. Ultrasound. No heart movement will be detected either with a Doppler sensor or M-mode echography.

Outcome

Labour usually commences within a few days or a week of the episode that kills the fetus. However, if labour has not commenced within 3 weeks of fetal death then disseminated intravascular thrombosis may occur in the mother.

The mechanism for such coagulation is thought to be thromboplastin entering the maternal circulation from the degenerating placenta, causing widespread fibrin deposition. This is a chronic event that usually takes about 4 weeks to develop. As intravascular fibrin deposition occurs, there is a compensatory response from the plasma to convert plasminogen to plasmin. This in turn causes a further breakdown of fibrin and fibrinogen. The result of intravascular thrombosis and fibrinogen utilization is to produce hypofibrinogenaemia. Normal fibrinogen levels of 0.45 g/l fall slowly to under 0.1 g/l.

Management

If spontaneous labour does not ensue, it is natural for the parents to ask that labour be induced. Induction should not be embarked upon unless coagulation studies are normal.

The usual method of induction is by high-dose oxytocin infusion. The membranes are usually not ruptured due to the high risk of intrauterine infection. EXTRA AMNIOTIC PGE₂ if Cx not favourable 200 ml/2hr

After delivery, if there is no obvious cause, the mother should be investigated to exclude syphilis, iso-immunization or diabetes mellitus.

4.21 COAGULATION DEFECTS IN OBSTETRICS

These defects may be either chronic or acute.

1. Chronic, due to:
   (a) Fetal death *in utero*.
   (b) Missed abortion.
2. Acute, due to:
   (a) Severe placental abruption.
   (b) Severe pre-eclampsia and eclampsia.
   (c) Septic shock.
3. Amniotic fluid embolism.

The principle of management is the same, although the method is different. *Never* undertake a surgical procedure until the bleeding defect is corrected.

Investigations

1. Platelet count.
2. Fibrinogen and fibrin degradation product estimation.
3. Coagulation time.
4. Prothrombin index.

Chronic coagulation disorders

The patient should be given heparin. This will inhibit fibrin deposition and allow fibrinogen and platelet levels, as well as other coagulation factors, to return to normal over a period of 48 hours.

Acute coagulation disorders

Transfusion with ultrafresh whole blood under central venous pressure control. This will provide not only haemoglobin, but also all other coagulation factors including platelets (which are not present in stored blood).

Stored plasma protein substrate (SPPS) can be given whilst waiting for fresh blood.

If there is a fibrinolytic effect from plasmin production, then epsilon-aminocaproic acid (EACA) may be given to inhibit this reaction.

Normal labour and delivery

Barry G. Wren
Revised by *Leo R. Leader*

5.1 GENERAL INSTRUCTIONAL OBJECTIVE

The students should understand perinatal anatomy, physiology and psychology that occurs in both mother and baby so that he/she appreciates the principles of management of labour and knows how to supervise a spontaneous delivery.

5.2 SPECIFIC BEHAVIOURAL OBJECTIVES

1. Describe the anatomy of the female pelvis and the fetus relevant to labour and delivery.
2. Describe the uterine physiology and the mechanisms of labour.
3. Conduct a normal third stage of labour, examine the placenta, cord and membranes and describe the findings.
4. Discuss normal placental separation and the drugs affecting uterine muscle activity.
5. Provide emotional support to a woman in normal labour.
6. Recognize the onset of labour and the normal progress of labour by history, abdominal and vaginal examination and record the findings.
7. Assist with the conduct of a normal delivery.
8. Discuss the nutritional and fluid requirements of the mother during labour and be aware of how to assess them clinically.
9. Assess and discuss the condition of the fetus during labour.
10. Demonstrate a knowledge of pain relief with drugs and other measures during labour, and discuss the possible effects on the fetus and mother.
11. Describe the management of an assisted breech delivery.
12. Discuss the indications for and the technique of episiotomy, and the principles of repair of episiotomy or lacerations.

5.3 REASONS FOR UNDERSTANDING NORMAL LABOUR AND DELIVERY, AND RESUSCITATION OF THE NEWBORN

The basis of obstetrics is to care for a woman during her pregnancy, to assist with the delivery of an infant who is born in an optimal condition, and to prevent any complications occurring to either mother or baby during this process. To achieve this skill in practice requires an understanding of the physiological processes and the mechanisms of labour, as well as the techniques of management of labour, delivery, resuscitation of the newborn and the management of the puerperium. This chapter will be involved in providing the basic information necessary for students to understand these processes.

5.4 ANATOMY OF THE FEMALE PELVIS

The obstetric anatomy of the female pelvis is divided into the bony structure of the pelvis and the soft tissues that line the pelvis, including the uterus, cervix, vagina, pelvic fascia, ligaments, muscles and perineum.

The obstetric pelvic bones are divided into three obstetrically significant sections:

1. The inlet or brim is bounded in front by the symphysis pubis, at the sides by the pubic crest, pectineal eminence, ilio-pectineal line, sacro-iliac joint and the ala of the sacrum, and posteriorly by the sacrum itself.
2. The midcavity is the true pelvis, and is that area lying between the pelvic brim or inlet and the pelvic outlet. It is bounded in front by the lower border of the back of the symphysis pubis, by the ischial spines laterally, and by the lower border of the last sacral vertebra posteriorly.
3. The outlet is bounded by the lower border of the symphysis pubis, the ischial tuberosities and the coccyx.

Diameters of the obstetric pelvis

1. The true conjugate diameter of the brim extends from the centre of the back of the symphysis pubis to the sacral promontory. In a normal gynaecoid pelvis, this normally measures about 11.5 cm.
2. The oblique diameters of the pelvic brim extend from the sacro-

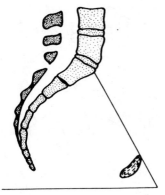

Fig. 5.1 Illustrating that in the erect position the plane of the pelvic brim makes an angle of 55° with the horizontal.

iliac joint to the diagonally opposite pectineal eminence. Normally, in a gynaecoid pelvis, this distance is about 12.5 cm.

3. The transverse diameter of the pelvic brim extends across the pelvis at its widest point. It normally measures about 13.5 cm.

In a gynaecoid pelvis, the average diameters in the midcavity generally measure about 12 cm, whereas at the obstetric outlet the diameters are the reverse of the brim — with the antero-posterior diameter being 13.5 cm and the transverse or bi-ischial diameter being about 11.5 cm.

The plane of the brim is an imaginary plane at the obstetric inlet which, in the erect female with a gynaecoid pelvis, makes an inclination of 55° to the horizontal (Fig. 5.1).

The axis of the pelvis is a line drawn through the midcavity of the pelvis from the brim to the outlet. Normally it curves forward through 90° in the midpelvis (Fig. 5.2).

Pelvic brim shapes

Caldwell and Moloy in 1934 performed anatomical studies on female pelves and were able to describe four major categories of pelvic shapes. Although there are many variations on these basic brim shapes, most women will have a pelvis that is described by one of these major subdivisions. The shape and size of the obstetric inlet dictates the mechanisms of labour and influences the progress in labour. It is important to understand these variations in pelvic shapes (Fig. 5.3).

The commonest type (45%) of pelvic brim shape among females is

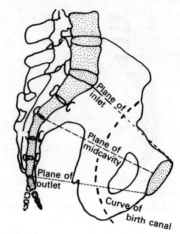

Fig. 5.2 Showing the three planes of the pelvis — brim, midcavity and outlet
— and illustrating that the coccyx will bend backwards to accommodate a large
fetal head.

the gynaecoid pelvis, where there is a basically rounded brim. This
brim shape is usually accompanied by a well-rounded sacral curve, an
adequate pelvic cavity, a well-rounded subpubic arch and an adequate
obstetric outlet.

The anthropoid pelvis is also common (35%) and is characterized
by a long antero-posterior diameter, a normal transverse diameter and
a deep pelvic cavity. The obstetric diameters are generally large and
the subpubic angle is well-rounded.

The android pelvis occurs in about 15% of women and is associated
with a generally triangular brim shape, with the transverse diameter
close to the posterior portion of the obstetric inlet. There is usually a
flattened sacrum, convergent pelvic walls and a narrow subpubic arch.

The platypelloid pelvis is relatively uncommon and is characterized
by a shortened antero-posterior diameter and wide transverse diameter of the brim, with a shallow pelvic cavity having divergent walls and a
wide subpubic arch. Obstetric problems usually are encountered at
the brim only.

Soft tissues of birth canal

The pelvic floor comprises those muscles, ligaments and fascia that fill
in the pelvic outlet and support the intrapelvic viscera. During the process of labour, these soft tissues stretch and dilate to allow the fetus to

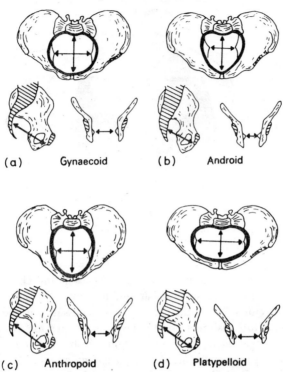

(a)   Gynaecoid   (b)   Android

(c)   Anthropoid   (d)   Platypelloid

Fig. 5.3 Common types of pelvic brim shapes. (a) Well-rounded brim. Rounded sacral curve, parallel pelvic side walls; (b) Triangular-shaped brim. Flattened sacrum, narrow sacro-sciatic notch. Convergent pelvic side walls; (c) Large pelvic brim with long antero-posterior diameter. Wide but deep sacrum. Parallel side walls; (d) Flattened pelvic brim with small antero-posterior diameter. Short but good pelvic curve. Parallel side walls.

pass through the bony pelvis (Fig. 5.4). The uterus and cervix form a muscular sac in which the muscle bundles are arranged to produce an efficient expulsive unit, which forces the fetus through the pelvis, stretching the soft tissue in the pelvic floor during the process.

The main anatomical soft structures of the pelvis are:

1. The levator ani muscles and their investing fascia, which slope forwards, downwards and inwards. By this inclination, they exert an important influence on the movement and rotation of the fetal head as it passes down the pelvis (Fig. 5.5). The levator ani muscle arises from a broad expanse over the sides of the pelvis, extending from the ala of the sacrum, the ileo-pectineal line and around to the front

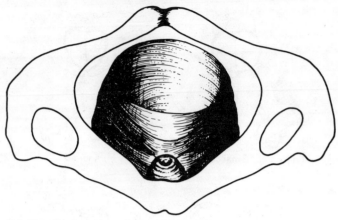

Fig. 5.4 Showing how the soft tissues of the pelvis become elastic and form a birth canal through which the fetus passes during birth.

of the pelvis behind the symphysis pubis. The muscle fibres pass down to insert into the fascia around the anus. The anterior fibres pass on either side of the vagina, some decussating in the perineal region before inserting into the fascia of the perianal region.

2. The endopelvic fascial condensation which form the transverse cervical ligaments, the utero-sacral ligaments and the pubo-cervical ligaments. With the surrounding fascia, these support the uterus, cervix and upper third of the vagina (Fig. 5.6).

3. Below the levator ani are the bulbo-cavernosus and ischio-cavernosus muscles, as well as the transverse perinei muscles,

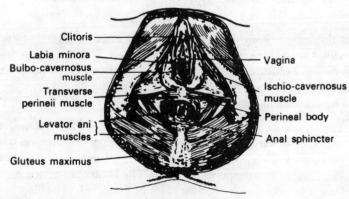

Fig. 5.5 Soft structures of the pelvic floor.

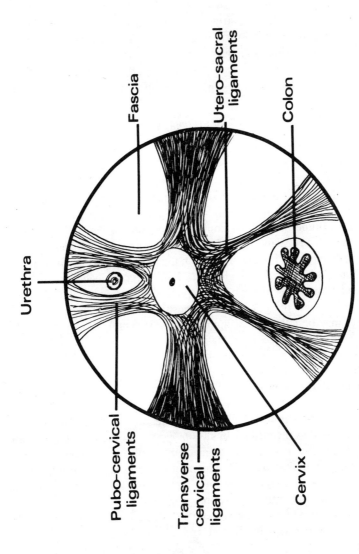

Urethra

Pubo-cervical
ligaments

Transverse
cervical
ligaments

Cervix

Fascia

Utero-sacral
ligaments

Colon

Fig. 5.6 Ligamentous supports of the cervix and uterus.

which together with the fascia investing these muscles make up the remainder of the support for the vagina and introitus (see Fig. 5.5).

Normally, all those soft structures composing the support for the pelvic floor are softened, stretched and dilated during labour. However, during difficult deliveries (such as prolonged labour, disproportion and forceps delivery) tears, overstretching or cuts may occur to produce anatomical weakness or deficiency. If these are not properly managed, a permanent deficiency may occur, predisposing to prolapse.

5.5 THE FETUS

Normally the fetus presents by the head (95%), so the anatomical arrangement of the fetal skull is important in understanding the process and mechanisms of labour.

The fetal head is generally oval in shape and will pass through the pelvis relatively easily when in an ideal attitude and position.

The attitude of the fetal skull is usually one of flexion, so that the suboccipito-bregmatic diameter (9.5 cm) will enter the pelvic brim. This is the presenting diameter when the head rotates into an occipito-anterior position so that the fetal head may pass through the pelvis and extend from under the symphysis pubis. If the head is deflexed and presents in an occipito-posterior position then the presenting diameter may be either suboccipito-frontal (10.5 cm) or occipito-frontal (11.5 cm). In a face presentation, the diameter is the submento-bregmatic (9.5 cm) whereas in a brow presentation it is mento-vertical (13.5 cm) (Fig. 5.7).

The skull is composed of the bones forming the base, the face and the vault. Those bones at the base and in the face are firm and incompressible, whereas the skull bones of the vault are soft cartilaginous plates joined at their edges by fibrous tissue. These fibrous joints are called sutures. This arrangement of the vault bones allows for considerable moulding or overlapping of these bony plates during labour. The sutures easily identified on a fetal skull are the sagittal, frontal, coronal and the lambdoid sutures (Fig. 5.8).

The anterior fontanelle is diamond shaped and is formed by the junction of the sagittal, frontal and coronal sutures. The posterior fontanelle is much smaller and triangular shaped and the junction of the sagittal and lambdoid sutures.

The vertex is a point that lies midway between the anterior and the posterior fontanelle: It is usually the leading point of the well-flexed head as it passes down the pelvis.

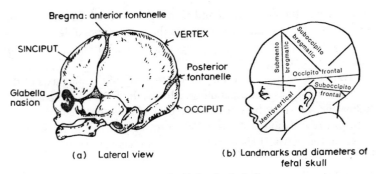

Fig. 5.7 Landmarks and diameters of the fetal skull.

The occiput (the posterior vault bone) extends from the lambdoid sutures to the foramen magnum. Because of its size and the occipital ridge, it is easily identified and is used as a point of reference (denominator) when identifying the position of a fetus in relationship to the maternal pelvis.

Definitions of importance regarding the fetus in its relationship to the mother prior to and during labour

Fetal attitude is the term applied to fetal parts in their relationship to each other. Normally a fetus is universally flexed with the head flexed

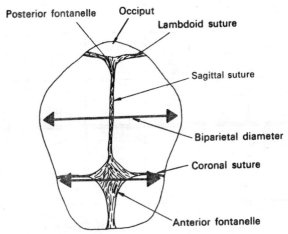

Fig. 5.8 Sutures and fontanelles of the fetal skull.

on the trunk, the back flexed and all the limbs flexed. In this position of universal flexion, the fetus presents the smallest possible diameters to the pelvic brim (suboccipito-bregmatic and biparietal diameters of skull — 9.5 cm).

Fetal lie is the term given to the relationship of the long axis of the fetus to the long axis of the mother. Mostly, the fetus takes up a longitudinal lie, but may have a transverse or oblique lie.

Fetal presentation is the term given to the part of the fetus that is lowest in the pelvis. This is usually the head (cephalic) but may be the breech, shoulder, abdomen, etc., depending on the lie of the fetus.

Fetal position is defined as the relationship of the denominator of the presenting part of the fetus to the maternal pelvis. When the head is presenting, there are two possible denominators (occiput and mentum). Because the mentum or chin is only used as the denominator in relation to the fully extended head (face presentation), most reference will be to the occiput. Normally at the onset of labour, the fetus presents with the head in the occipito-lateral position (OL, 65%), right or left occipito-anterior (OA, 23%), right or left occipito-posterior (OP, 10%) and direct occipito-anterior (OA) or occipito-posterior position (OP) (2%).

Engagement of the fetal head is said to occur when the widest transverse diameter of the head (biparietal diameter 9.5 cm) has passed through the pelvic brim. On vaginal examination the head will be at the level of the ischial spines. Descent of the fetal head is usually assessed abdominally. The head is divided into fifths below the pelvic inlet (Fig. 5.9). Descent of the presenting part is probably the result

5/5	4/5	3/5	2/5	1/5	0/5
'FLOATING' ABOVE THE BRIM	'FIXING'	NOT ENGAGED	JUST ENGAGED	ENGAGED	DEEPLY ENGAGED

Head level 'in fifths' palpable above the brim.

Fig. 5.9 Showing the assessment of descent of the fetal head into the pelvis, measured in fifths.

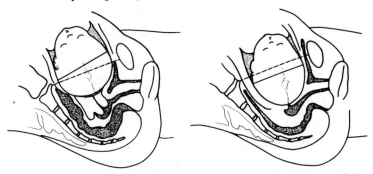

Fig. 5.10 Demonstrating how a head may enter the pelvic brim by asynclitism, with first one parietal bone presenting and then, following pressure and moulding, the other parietal bone sliding through the pelvic brim.

of increased uterus activity as well as formation of the lower uterine segment. This develops from the anatomical isthmus of the uterus. The fetal head engages earlier in primigravid patients but may not engage in multiparous patients until they are in labour. Asynclitism occurs when the sagittal suture of the fetal skull does not lie midway between the sacral promontory and the symphysis pubis once the parietal bones will present instead of the vertex. The head usually engages by lateral flexion. This phenomenon occurs in association with occipito-lateral positions, cephalopelvic disproportion and with a platypelloid pelvis (Fig. 5.10).

5.6 PHYSIOLOGICAL PROCESS IN LABOUR (THE POWERS)

Physiology of labour

1. Effective labour contractions are initiated by a complex process beginning in the fetus. It appears that maturation of fetal adrenal tissue produces cortisone, which acts on the placenta to produce a change in the oestrogen/progesterone ratio, and which also appears to initiate the production of increased amounts of prostaglandins. The prostaglandins produce not only increased amplitude in the uterine contractions, but also an increase in the rate of contractions. Eventually, as well as softening the cervix with partial effacement, contractions force the presenting part onto the lower uterine segment and as this is thinned out and stretched, a reflex (Ferguson's

reflex) initiates the production of oxytocin from the posterior pituitary. Stretching of the cervix in turn also leads to prostaglandin
production. These hormones enhance uterine contractions by increasing the rate, tone and amplitude of contractions, and so labour
becomes established.

2. Painful contractions. The pain of labour contractions is almost entirely cervical in origin and is associated with the resistance of the
cervix to the dilating forces. As labour progresses pain is felt as
soon as the intrauterine pressure rises above 25 mmHg (Fig. 5.11).

In well-established labour, a uterine contraction lasts for about
50–60 seconds and occurs every 2–4 minutes. During contractions the intrauterine pressure varies from 50 to 70 mmHg in the
late first stage, thus the pain lasts for the entire duration of the contraction whereas in early labour the pain may be only mild and
occurs near the peak of the uterine contraction.

As labour progresses, the spiral muscles of the fundus of the
uterus become more dominant, pulling up and thinning the cervix
and lower segment. Normally, in a primipara, the cervix is shortened before beginning dilatation, whereas in a multigravida the
cervix begins to dilate as the lower segment and cervix are pulled
up.

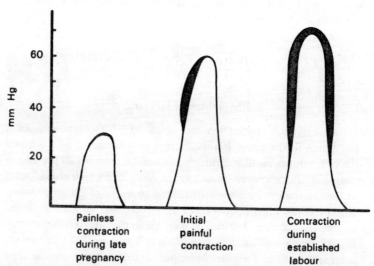

DURATION OF 'PAIN' SHOWN BY THICKENED LINE

Fig. 5.11 Showing pain in relation to amplitude of contraction.

As the cervix dilates in early labour, the mucous plug blocking the endocervical canal is dislodged. This, together with some bleeding that occurs as the chorionic membrane 'shears' off the lower segment, forms a bloodstained 'show'.

The uterus and cervix are an active unit of muscular power providing the force by which the fetus (passenger) is pushed through the pelvis (passage).

Secondary powers in labour

When the presenting part reaches the pelvic floor (usually after full dilatation), the distension of the vagina and pressure on the rectum produces a sensation that results in the expulsive 'bearing down' exertion. During this process the diaphragm is fixed, and the thoracic and abdominal muscles are contracted to assist in expelling the fetus. The pressure on the fetal skull during this stage may reach 100–120 mmHg.

5.7 MECHANISM OF LABOUR

The mechanism of labour is the mechanical changes that take place throughout the process of labour and delivery. These are physiological processes and occur spontaneously without any operator assistance. The following steps normally occur for a fetus with a cephalic presentation:

1. Flexion. Most fetuses present in the occipito-lateral position at the onset of labour. Uterine contractions exert pressure on the upper pole of the fetus to produce flexion of the head on the neck and so reduce the presenting diameter (Fig. 5.12).
2. Descent. The next stage in the mechanism is descent into the pelvic brim. When the head is well flexed, the presenting diameters (biparietal 9.5 cm, suboccipito-bregmatic 9.5 cm) pass easily through the brim and descent is rapid. Delay may occur when extension of the head persists (occipito-posterior position), the head is abnormally large, the pelvis is of an abnormal shape (android brim) or the pelvis is small in size.
3. Internal rotation. The underlining principle in rotation is that whichever part of the fetus hits the pelvic floor first, will rotate anteriorly. If the fetal head is well flexed the occiput hits the pelvic floor first and then rotates anteriorly. This is called 'internal

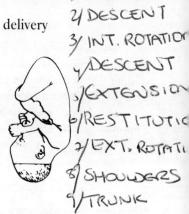

1/ FLEXION
2/ DESCENT
3/ INT. ROTATION
4/ DESCENT
5/ EXTENSION
6/ RESTITUTION
7/ EXT. ROTATION
8/ SHOULDERS
9/ TRUNK

Fig. 5.12 Flexion: resistance at the pelvic brim and the asymmetry of the fetal head encourages flexion of the neck. d_1 and d_2 — distances to foramen magnum. R = resistance of pelvic brim. $R \times d_1$ is greater than $R \times d_2$, thus resulting in flexion.

rotation' and varies from 45 to 90° depending upon whether the head was in an occipito-lateral or occipito-anterior position. If the head rotates through 45° then the shoulders at this stage remain unchanged in their position. Should the head rotate through 90° the shoulders will rotate to 45° (Figs 5.13 and 5.14).

4. Descent. Further descent of the presenting part now occurs.
5. Extension. The head, as it passes out of the birth canal, extends with the symphysis pubis as a fulcrum. This process is called crowning and leads to delivery of the fetal head (Fig. 5.15).
6. Restitution. As the head is no longer being flexed inside the birth canal, it now rotates through 45° to return to the position that it

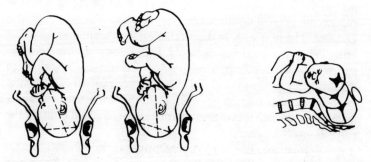

Fig. 5.13 Showing that descent occurs as the head flexes. It usually enters the pelvic brim in the occipito-lateral position and then undergoes internal rotation deep in the pelvic cavity.

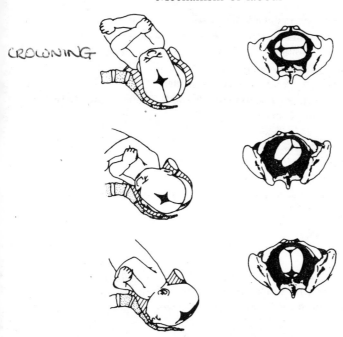

CROWNING

Fig. 5.14 Demonstrating how internal rotation occurs deep in the pelvic cavity, so that the occiput normally comes to lie in an anterior position.

held prior to internal rotation. At this stage the head is once again at right angles to the shoulders.

7. External Rotation. There is now further descent until the leading shoulder reaches the pelvic floor where it rotates anteriorly. This leads to further rotation of the head to 45°. This is called external

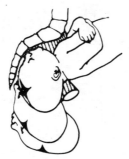

Fig. 5.15 Demonstrating how the head extends as it descends and is born from under the symphysis pubis.

rotation as it occurs outside the pelvis and is visible to the observer. The sagittal suture is now in the transverse position.

8. Birth of the shoulders. The anterior shoulder comes into view under the symphysis pubis where it remains whilst the posterior shoulder is born by anterior lateral flexion.

9. Birth of the trunk. The remainder of the trunk is also born by posterior lateral flexion.

Moulding

As labour progresses the shape of the fetal head alters to better fit the maternal pelvis. This leads to overlapping skull bone and assists in producing a smaller head diameter.

Caput succedaneum

If the fetal scalp is compressed against the cervix or the pelvic soft tissue, it interferes with venous return. This in turn leads to oedema of the small portion of the scalp which is known as caput succedaneum.

Third stage of labour

This is the shortest and the most hazardous stage of labour for the mother. It commences with the delivery of the infant and is completed

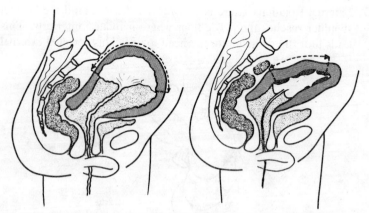

Fig. 5.16 Showing how the placental site of attachment is drastically reduced following the end of the second stage, thus aiding separation of the placenta from the uterus.

with the delivery of the placenta. It is concerned with separation and expulsion of the placenta and control of haemorrhage from the placental site (Fig. 5.16).

Separation of the placenta is accomplished by marked uterine contractions. This leads to a reduction of the internal surface area of the uterus by over 50%. The placenta, however, which has been firmly adherent by the trophoblastic invasion of the decidua has a fixed mass. It is unable to reduce its surface area and so begins to separate from the uterus. The site for separation occurs in the decidua with many small cleavage sites. Blood collects in the small cleavage sites forming small pools behind the placenta. In some instances this retroplacental bleeding will also help to shear the placenta from the uterine wall. Some of this bleeding traps behind the chorionic membranes and appears in the vagina as a 'show'.

Placental expulsion

Uterine contractions expel the placenta into the vagina 5–20 minutes after delivery of the infant. This is usually indicated by a gush of blood from the vagina and lengthening of the cord as the placenta descends into the upper vagina. The now empty and firmly contracted uterus rises up on the full vagina to form a 'large ball' at the level of the umbilicus. Removal of the placenta can then be completed either by bearing down of the mother or by applying traction to the umbilical cord and lifting the uterus off the placenta (Brandt–Andrews technique).

Control of haemorrhage

This is effected by contraction and retraction of the myometrium after the placenta has been expelled. Although contraction of the muscle compresses the vessels and it stops bleeding at the time of placental separation, the permanent arrest of haemorrhage is due to retraction which causes a permanent shifting and shortening of the muscle fasciculi. This compresses the vessels which pass between the muscle bundles and effectively stops bleeding.

5.8 NORMAL LABOUR

Throughout pregnancy, the uterus contracts in a rhythmic fashion but these are impalpable and undetected by the mother. After the 32nd week of pregnancy, these contractions become more dominant and are known as Braxton Hicks' contractions. They are usually not painful and do not lead to any permanent shortening of muscle fibres (retraction) and therefore there is no cervical dilatation. These contractions usually lead to formation of the lower uterine segment and need to be distinguished from labour contractions which are usually painful.

Labour is said to begin when the uterine contractions are strong enough to cause pain (more than 25 mmHg) and lead to the shortening of the muscle and cervical dilatation.

Admission

Women are advised to present to the hospital for admission when the uterine contractions are painful and occurring regularly at intervals of less than 10 minutes, when the 'waters break', or if there is any fresh bleeding. In 10% of patients rupture of the membrane precede the onset of labour.

Each woman admitted to the labour ward will:

1. Have a relevant obstetric history taken.
2. Be examined to determine the state of pregnancy and labour.
3. Be given a suppository or enema only if the bowel is full.

History

The history on admission will include previous pregnancies, the relevant information regarding the present pregnancy, when the labour commenced and whether the membranes are ruptured or not.

Examination

Examination will include palpation of the fetus for size, lie, presentation, position and engagement. The strength, duration and interval of contractions are also determined. The maternal blood pressure is recorded and urine is tested for sugar, protein and ketones. The fetal heart rate is also recorded before, during and after contractions.

Management of labour

Although the entire labour should be regarded as a continuum, for convenience it is divided into the following stages.

First stage of labour

The first stage of labour commences when uterine contractions are sufficiently efficient to lead to cervical dilatation and ends when the cervix is fully dilated. Established labour is considered to have occurred when uterine contractions are painful and last more than one-third of a ten-minute period of time. Contractions should be regular, last more than 45 seconds in duration and occur every 2–3 minutes with good relaxation in between. The patient usually experiences pain once the intrauterine pressure rises more than 25 mmHg. Once the pressure reaches 40 mmHg, the uterus is now no longer indentible. This is the maximum pressure that can be palpated or determined using external tocodynomometry. For labour to progress in the first stage, intrauterine pressures of 50–70 mmHg are required. In between contractions, the intrauterine pressure should not exceed 10 mmHg as this is the pressure above which chororio-decidual bloodflow ceases.

The first stage of labour is divided into two phases:

1. Latent phase. This commences at the onset of contractions and is completed when the cervix reaches 3 cm of dilatation. In a primigravid patient this takes approximately 8 hours, whilst in a multigravid patient it lasts an average of 5 hours.
2. Active phase. This commences when the patient reaches 3 cm of dilatation, and is completed when the patient is fully dilated. The average duration of labour in a primigravid patient is 12 hours, whilst in a multigravid patient it is 7 hours. Primigravid patients will progress approximately 1–2 cm per hour during the active phase, whilst multigravid patients progress 2–3 cm per hour during the active phase of labour.

During this stage the mother should be encouraged to keep herself occupied by reading or watching television and where the father is present, he should be involved in activities to provide support and encouragement. Once admitted to the labour ward, the patient's observations are charted on a partogram (Fig. 5.17). This is a graphical recording of all the patient's observations which include:

1. Fetal heart rate observations before, during and after each contraction and recorded every 15 minutes.
2. Strength, duration and frequency of uterine contractions recorded over a 10-minute period of time.
3. Observation of the presenting part with regard to its descent and engagement as well as its position.

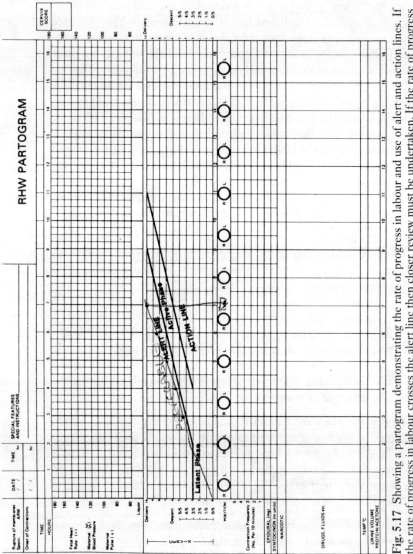

Fig. 5.17 Showing a partogram demonstrating the rate of progress in labour and use of alert and action lines. If the rate of progress in labour crosses the alert line then closer review must be undertaken. If the rate of progress is even slower and crosses the action line then some positive steps must be taken to expedite delivery.

4. Maternal pulse rate and blood pressure are recorded every hour, but temperature is taken every 4 hours.
5. Observations of maternal fluid intake must be recorded as well as the urinary output and its chemical analysis.
6. Any drugs given to the mother are recorded on the partogram.

A vaginal examination is done every 4 hours unless there is an indication to do it more frequently.

Use of the partogram (Fig. 5.17)

Once the patient's cervix reaches 3 cm of dilatation (the active phase), the minimum rate of dilatation should be 1 cm per hour and a line is drawn to mark this rate. This is known as the *alert line*. Studies have shown that active intervention is rarely required in patients whose rate of dilatation exceeds this. A parallel line is drawn 2 hours later than the alert line and this is called the *action line*. Once the rate of dilatation, as recorded on the partogram, crosses the alert line, a vaginal examination should be done after a further 2 hours. If at this stage, progress has been satisfactory no further intervention is required. If the labour has not progressed at the second examination, and the action line is crossed, then a critical review of the patient, her labour and her fetus are needed. It needs to be established by means of a vaginal examination as to whether there is obvious cephalo-pelvic disproportion, relative cephalo-pelvic disproportion due to a malposition or the rate of progress has been due to inadequate uterine activity.

1. The vaginal examination should determine the degree of cervical dilatation, descent and position of the presenting part whether there is caput or moulding and to ensure that the membranes have ruptured.
2. An intravenous syntocinon infusion may be required if uterine contractions are inadequate. Uterine contractions can be measured by means of external tocodynomometry or if this presents difficulty by direct intrauterine pressure recording.
3. The fetal heart rate should be monitored continuously using a cardiotocograph.
4. Intravenous drip of dextrose/saline to rehydrate and provide adequate nutrition for the mother.
5. Adequate analgesia should be provided, preferably by means of an epidural anaesthetic, but if this is not possible, parenteral analgesics will suffice.

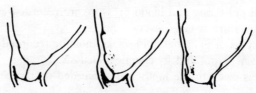

Fig. 5.18 Showing that as labour progresses the cervix becomes shorter and dilates slowly until about 5 cm, following which effacement and dilatation occur more rapidly.

6. Blood should be taken for cross-matching.
7. Should an abnormal fetal heart rate pattern be present, then a fetal scalp blood sample analysis may be necessary to determine fetal pH, pCO_2 and base deficit levels.

Cervical dilatation

Normally, the cervix dilates slowly up to about 5 cm, after which the progress is more rapid. When the cervix reaches full dilatation (10 cm) the cervix and lower segment of the uterus are usually thinned out and thus easily drawn out round the presenting part of the fetus. Once the cervix is fully dilated, the first stage is said to have been completed. During the late first stage of labour pain and discomfort increases as the head passes through the cervix into the vagina. This causes increased rectal pressure and a sensation of 'bearing down' or the desire to push (Figs 5.18, 5.19, 5.20).

Analgesia

During the first stage analgesics such as nitrous oxide may be administered by a face mask or the patient may require intramuscular analgesics such as pethidine (meperidine) or morphine to provide pain

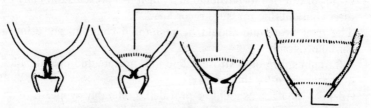

Fig. 5.19 Dilatation of the cervix in a primigravid is usually slower because the cervix must shorten before it begins to dilate.

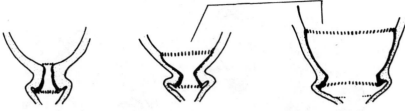

Fig. 5.20 Dilatation of the cervix in a multigravid is usually more rapid than in a primigravid because the cervix is usually shorter and slightly dilated before the onset of labour.

relief. If, however, the pain becomes more severe later in labour, an epidural anaesthetic may be the only way of providing adequate relief.

Local anaesthesia

Local anaesthesia, such as perineal infiltration or a pudendal block, provides adequate analgesia for delivery but does not provide relief for women in late first stage. The longer the labour lasts, particularly in late first stage, the more anxiety and tension are created in the mother. The pain, the low backache and the feeling of helplessness, may cause the mother to become hysterically anxious and distressed. If this distressful situation continues, the obstetrician may also be under severe pressure to bring about completion of the labour, perhaps performing otherwise unnecessary procedures. This situation can be avoided by the judicious use of epidural anaesthesia to provide adequate pain relief and the administration of Syntocinon by intravenous infusion to enhance uterine contractions.

It is most important to reassure the mother that all is under control even though the labour may be proceeding slowly. Knowledge, empathy, understanding and sympathy will probably do more to protect a mother from a poor obstetric outcome than the most sophisticated technical aids.

Second stage of labour

The second stage of labour lasts from full dilatation of the cervix to delivery of the infant. In primigravid women, this normally takes about 1 hour whilst in a multigravid patient the time is usually halved.

Once the cervix is fully dilated, the fetus will proceed through the pelvis with the aid of uterine contractions and maternal expulsive

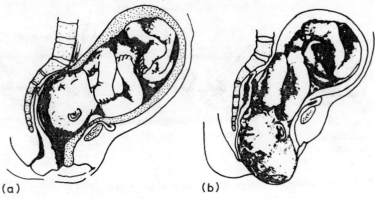

(a) (b)

Fig. 5.21 (a) Descent; (b) Extension.

efforts. The head flexes, descends, moulds and undergoes internal rotation so that the occiput comes to lie anteriorly under the symphysis pubis. From this position, expulsive efforts assist the fetal head undergoing extension and delivery from under the symphysis pubis (Fig. 5.21).

Normal uterine pressure during contractions and in association with internal (bearing down) may increase the uterine pressure to 100–120 mmHg and assist delivery of the infant.

As the head delivers, the perineal tissue will stretch and may tear. If this seems likely it is wise to perform an episiotomy under local anaesthesia.

Episiotomy

An episiotomy is a cut in the perineum that enlarges the vaginal introitus. It aids delivery by removing the peripheral resistance of the perineum. It is usually used for primigravid women whose perineum is less elastic and less dilated than that of a multigravid woman. It also may be indicated in a patient who has delay in the second stage of labour or where there is any complication associated with delivery.

The most common form of episiotomy is the medio-lateral type. This divides the vaginal and perineal epithelium, the transverse perinei muscle, the posterior fibres of the bulbo-cavernosus muscles and the decussating fibres of the levator ani muscle. It begins in the midline of the fourchette and extends along a line that would run just lateral to the external anal sphincter. The advantages of an episiotomy are:

1. It avoids tears and rupture of the anal sphincter or tears into the rectum.
2. It hastens delivery when the head is arrested on the pelvic floor.
3. It assists in preventing future prolapse by avoiding over-distension and tearing of vaginal tissue.
4. It avoids undue pressure on the fetal tissue, particularly in pre-term infants.
5. It makes vaginal manipulations (such as rotation and forceps delivery) easier to perform.

Indications for an episiotomy are:

1. To prevent perineal tears.
2. Avoid arrest of the presenting part at the perineum.
3. When delivering small premature infants.
4. When delivering large babies who are at risk of shoulder dystocia.
5. When performing obstetric manipulations such as rotations or forceps delivery.
6. When fetal distress necessitates a rapid delivery.

The repair of an episiotomy (Fig. 5.22) should be performed with care, as an inadequate repair may lead to haemorrhage, infection, haematomas, painful scars, tight vagina or severe dyspareunia. The incision is sutured in layers, using minimal amounts of tension with the thinnest possible suture material. *CAT GUT (CHROMIC)*
Initially the vaginal cut should be completely visualized and care

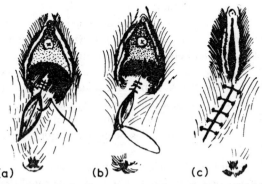

Fig. 5.22 Episiotomy repair. Demonstrating the technique of: (a) Sewing the vaginal epithelium from apex of cut to introitus of vagina. Then uniting transverse perinei muscle; (b) Uniting fascia of perineal body; (c) Suturing skin of episiotomy.

taken to close the first suture high in the vagina at the apex of the incision. A continuous fine chromic catgut suture or synthetic absorbable suture can be used to unite the vaginal epithelium as far as the introitus, making sure that the hymenal remnants are opposed at the introitus.

When the vagina is intact, the levator ani, transverse perinei and bulbo-cavernosus muscles are united in that order, together with their investing fascia by means of interrupted sutures.

Finally, the skin is resutured using a subcuticular absorbable suture or with interrupted sutures.

A rectal examination is always done afterwards to ensure that no sutures have inadvertently penetrated the rectal epithelium.

Delivery of the baby

The natural method for delivery is for the mother to squat on her haunches. This allows the maximum intra-abdominal pressure to be generated by the mother and also the alteration of the angle of inclination of the pelvis leads to an increased surface area being available to the advancing presenting part. However, it is usually more convenient for the obstetrician to assist or manipulate during delivery if the mother is in the dorsal or lateral position. In most developed countries as a result of adequate maternal nutrition the relationship between the fetal size and brim area is such that alteration of the angle of inclination is not critical for a normal delivery. The mother usually lies on her back, her legs and abdomen are draped with sterile towels and the obstetrician stands at the side.

In this position the obstetrician can use one hand to guide the vertex as it 'crowns' and is born from under the symphysis pubis, whilst the other hand feels deep between the anus and the coccyx for the fetal chin. Once the chin has been 'caught', the patient is asked to stop bearing down whilst the obstetrician assists delivery of the head by extension. To relieve pain at this stage, the woman may be given nitrous oxide to inhale unless an injection of local anaesthetic into the perineum or a pudendal block has been given prior to this stage (Fig. 5.23).

Once the head has been delivered by extension, the nasopharynx is sucked free of mucous and fluid. The neck is palpated to ensure that the cord is not wrapped around it — if it is, it is freed by slipping it over the head or shoulders. If, however, it is tight or encircles the neck two or more times it should be clamped and cut. By this stage restitution

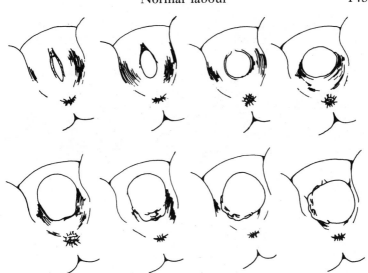

Fig. 5.23 Crowning, extension and delivery of the fetal head.

will have occurred and with further descent, external rotation will take place and the occiput rotates to present to the obstetrician. The obstetrician then places both hands on either side of the fetal skull, over the ears and parietal bones, ensuring that no pressure is placed on the infant's carotid arteries (Fig. 5.24). Firm pressure is then exerted in a posterior direction to aid the delivery of the shoulder. By pulling out and downwards the anterior shoulder should slide under the symphysis pubis. A finger can then be inserted into the axilla from behind and by lifting the head upwards as the baby is delivered, the posterior shoulder will also slide out. Once the shoulders are free, the baby is easily delivered. The baby is then placed on the mother's abdomen, the cord is clamped and cut. Mother is encouraged to touch and hold her baby. After a short while the baby is wrapped in a warm blanket and given to the mother to hold.

Routine following delivery of the baby

1. The baby is checked immediately for gross abnormalities and the name of the mother is painted on the baby's chest with an identification tag tied around the baby's ankle.
2. Cord blood is obtained for the infant's blood group, antibodies and haemoglobin.

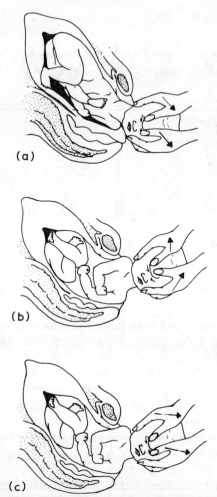

Fig. 5.24 (a) Demonstrating the technique of delivering the anterior shoulder. Stand on the side to which the occiput is pointing and with a hand pressing firmly over either parietal bone, pull the head out and down to deliver the anterior shoulder; (b) Demonstrating the technique to deliver the posterior shoulder. With the hands grasping the head on either side of the parietal bones, the head is lifted upwards until the posterior shoulder slides out of the vagina; (c) Once the shoulders have delivered, the body of the baby is delivered in a downward and outward motion.

3. The fundus of the uterus is checked to ascertain whether signs of placental separation have occurred.

Third stage of labour

The third stage of labour commences from the time of delivery of the infant and ends with the delivery of the placenta. It normally lasts 5–20 minutes. Separation of the placenta normally occurs when the uterus contracts and the muscle retracts following delivery of the fetus.

STEPS IN MANAGEMENT

1. When the anterior shoulder of the fetus is born from under the symphysis pubis, Syntocinon (5 units) is usually given by intramuscular injection. This results in uterine contractions after 3–4 minutes.
2. The vaginal introitus is observed so that the 'show' of blood and lengthening of the cord (which indicates separation and expulsion of the placenta into the upper vagina) can be noted.
3. The uterus is gently palpated so that when the placenta separates and is expelled from the upper vagina, the firmly contracted small uterus can be identified just above the level of the umbilicus.
4. When the placenta has been identified to have separated and passed from the uterus into the upper vagina, the cord is grasped firmly in one hand whilst the uterus is steadied by the other hand and lifted off the placenta. This technique of delivery is known as the Brandt–Andrews technique.
5. Following delivery of the placenta, the patient's blood pressure is checked and if not elevated, ergometrine (0.25–0.5 mg) is given by intramuscular injection.

Action of oxytocics

1. Oxytocin is absorbed rapidly from an intramuscular injection site and will produce a uterine contraction within 2–3 minutes. It is rapidly broken down by the enzyme oxytocinase. By intramuscular injection, ergometrine will only produce uterine contractions after 5–6 minutes and its action lasts a number of hours.
2. Oxytocin produces contractions of higher amplitude than ergometrine.

3. Oxytocin produces contractions with an intervening relaxation phase, thus simulating physiological contractions.
4. Ergometrine produces contractions of high tone and frequency, but of small amplitude. Because of the longer duration of action ergometrine provides more reliable contractions and aids in preventing postpartum haemorrhage.

These differing properties of oxytocin and ergometrine are used to advantage in the third stage of labour. By giving oxytocin on delivery of the anterior shoulder, physiological contractions occur that aid in separation and expulsion of the placenta. Following expulsion of the placenta, ergometrine then provides prolonged tetanic contraction that helps to prevent postpartum haemorrhage.

If the patient is at risk from postpartum haemorrhage (e.g. from multiple pregnancy, grandmultiparity, antepartum haemorrhage, etc.) then an intravenous infusion should be commenced during labour. The oxytocin or ergometrine can be given directly intravenously. If postpartum bleeding occurs due to uterine atony (e.g. from retained placenta, prolong labour, APH, etc.) then ergometrine (0.25–0.5 mg) can be given directly intravenously or an oxytocin infusion (40 units in 1 litre Hartman's solution) can be commenced.

5.9 BREECH DELIVERY

Breech presentation in labour occurs in 4–5% of all deliveries. It should be managed as for a woman with a cephalic presentation. However, because of the greater risks associated with complications of a breech delivery, it should take place in a well-equipped hospital with an experienced obstetrician in attendance.

Before labour is allowed to proceed, care should be taken to ensure that the maternal pelvis is adequate. Ideally the patient should be multiparous with a large, well-formed pelvis whose dimensions are known (by the use of a standing lateral and a Thom's radiograph). The fetus should have extended legs and the ideal weight for a breech delivery is between 2500 and 3500 g. If there are any doubts as to the adequacy of the pelvic dimension, then an elective Caesarean section should be performed between 38 and 40 weeks.

Care should be taken to maintain intact membranes, as premature rupture of the membranes is associated with a high incidence of cord prolapse.

Most breech presentations will progress to a normal vaginal delivery, so the management includes the following principles:

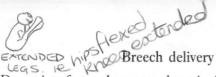

1. Do not interfere, unless some obstetric situation (such as fetal distress) indicates that this is necessary.
2. The fetus should be monitored continuously throughout labour using external cardiotography or if the membranes are ruptured a scalp electrode may be placed on the buttocks.
3. Keep the patient in bed throughout the labour.
4. Do not rupture the membranes in the early stage of labour.
5. Maintain an intravenous drip and only use Syntocinon if the contractions are inadequate.
6. Judicious use of adequate analgesia, in particular epidural anaesthesia prevents the mother from bearing down before the cervix is fully dilated leading to entrapment of the fetal head.
7. Perform a vaginal examination regularly throughout labour or when the membranes rupture so as to exclude cord prolapse or other complications.
8. Ascertain that the nursing staff, medical staff and anaesthetist are notified of the presence of a breech in labour so that they may be readily summoned if needed.
9. Use of local anaesthesia and an episiotomy is necessary to assist easy delivery of the trunk and after-coming head.

Delivery technique

During each contraction the patient is encouraged to bear down so that the buttocks distend the perineum (Fig. 5.25). At this stage, if the patient has not had an epidural anaesthetic then local anaesthesia into the perineum is injected prior to performing an episiotomy. Contractions are allowed to proceed with bearing down, until the buttocks are delivered to the trunk and the umbilicus is seen. At this stage, a loop of cord is pulled down and the legs are freed from inside the vagina. It is now important to deliver the baby within 5 minutes to decrease the risk of hypoxia. A towel is wrapped around the limbs of the fetus to support it, and the mother is encouraged to bear down. Unnecessary traction on the fetal trunk may lead to extension of the fetal arms and their entrapment above the pelvic brim. If this occurs, then it may require rotation of the lower trunk in the reverse direction to allow the delivery of the shoulders from under the symphysis pubis (Lovset manoeuvre) (Fig. 5.26).

Once the shoulders have delivered the baby is allowed to hang by using its own weight to allow the head to engage. The head is then delivered either by means of the Mauriceau–Smellie–Viet manoeuvre

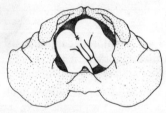

Fig. 5.25 Right sacro-anterior position in a breech with extended legs.

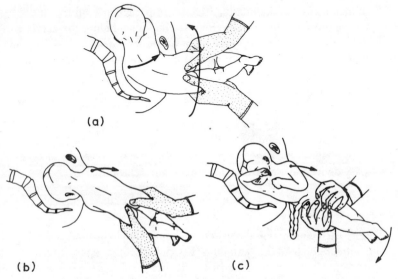

(a)

(b)   (c)

Fig. 5.26 The Lovset manoeuvre. (a) Hands grasp buttocks with thumbs over the sacrum. By pulling down and rotating the lower part of the body through 180°, the anterior shoulder slides from under the symphysis pubis.

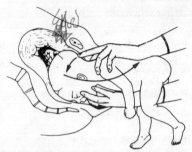

Fig. 5.27 The after-coming head of the breech delivered by the Mauriceau–Smellie–Viet manoeuvre.

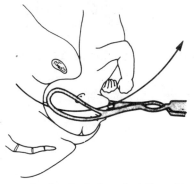

Fig. 5.28 The after-coming head of a breech delivered by forceps.

(Fig. 5.27) or by applying forceps to the after-coming head (Fig. 5.28). In the former a hand is passed into the vagina until the face and mouth are felt. A finger is placed in the fetal mouth to assist in maintaining flexion while the other hand exerts traction on the fetal shoulders. Major expulsive force in this manoeuvre should be from an assistant applying suprapubic pressure. More commonly, forceps are applied to control the delivery of the fetal head. An assistant holds the infant's legs in the air whilst the blades are applied. Slow and steady traction is applied to deliver the fetal head. It is important that the head should be delivered slowly as it is the sudden compression and expansion that leads to tentorial tears and intracerebral haemorrhage.

The newborn infant

Jagdish M. Gupta

6.1 GENERAL INSTRUCTIONAL OBJECTIVE

The students will develop competence in examining a normal newborn infant and recognize abnormalities which require investigation and treatment.

6.2 SPECIFIC BEHAVIOURAL OBJECTIVES

1. Take a perinatal history.
2. Examine and follow up normal newborn babies (including feeding).
3. Recognize minor abnormalities (in newborn infants) that require no treatment.
4. Examine and manage low birth weight babies.
5. Plan investigations and management of a jaundiced infant.
6. Plan investigations and treatment of an infant with infection.
7. Plan investigations and treatment of an infant with neurological problems.

6.3 EXAMINATION OF THE NEWBORN

It is the duty of the attendant at delivery to record the Apgar (Table 6.1) score at 1 and 5 minutes (and subsequently if the baby has problems with establishing regular respiration), and note the presence of major malformations (e.g. meningomyelocoele) which might cause difficulty to the baby in adapting to extrauterine life. All well babies must be examined (in the presence of the mother) as soon after birth as possible and again before discharge from hospital. The aim of the first examination is to reassure the mother that the baby is normal. The second examination aims to determine the progress of the infant and to detect any minor problems that may have surfaced or been overlooked at the first examination.

Table 6.1. Apgar scoring chart

Sign	0	1	2
Heart rate	Absent	Slow (below 100)	Over 100
Respiratory effort	Absent	Weak cry, hypoventilation	Good strong cry
Muscle Tone	Limp	Some flexion of extremities	Well flexed
Reflex response (i) Response to catheter in nostril (tested after oropharynx is clear)	No response	Grimace	Cough or sneeze
(ii) Tangential foot slap	No response	Grimace	Cry and withdrawal of foot
Colour	Blue, pale	Body pink, Extremities blue	Completely pink

History

Before examining the baby it is important to check the mother's notes to determine the history of pregnancy, labour and the state of the infant at birth. Nursing notes also give essential information regarding the birth weight of the infant, the changes in weight since birth, feeding pattern of the infant and observations such as colour, respiratory rate, heart rate, passage of meconium and urine. It is best to examine the baby in the mother's presence, as this will allow the examiner to demonstrate to her some of the normal findings in the newborn and also to answer any questions.

The examination of the baby is described systematically here, but this is usually not possible in the newborn. However, the same procedure should be used each time so as to avoid omissions, and a check list should be kept to ensure that no abnormalities are overlooked.

General observations

Much information is obtained by general observations which include posture, activity, peripheral perfusion, colour, type and rate of

Table 6.2: Assessment of gestational age

Characteristic	Gestational age in weeks			
	28–30	*32–34*	*36–38*	*40+*
Breast nodule development	Absent	Absent	3–5 mm	7 mm+
Sole creases	Absent	Single anterior creases	2–3 creases	Many creases
Ear lobe	No cartilage	No cartilage	Pliable, some cartilage present	Stiff
Male genitalia	Testis unpalpable: small, smooth scrotum	Testis in inguinal canal: small, smooth scrotum	Testis often descended: some scrotal rugae	Testis descended: scrotum fully rugose
Female genitalia	Prominent labia minora, labia majora flat	Prominent labia minora, labia majora flat	Labia majora almost cover labia minora, few rugae	Labia majora completely cover labia minora, marked rugae
Posture	Hypotonia	Some flexor tone at hips and knees	Some flexor tone at hips, knees and elbows	Marked flexor tone all joints
Scarf sign	Elbow past midline	Elbow past midline	Elbow reaches midline	Elbow does not reach midline
Toe to ear	Usual	Usual	Difficult	Impossible

respiration, shape and size of the skull, the presence of abdominal distension and features which indicate the maturity of the infant (Table 6.2).

Skull

Most full-term newborn infants examined in the first 24–48 hours will show some evidence of moulding of the skull. A caput succedaneum or a cephalhaematoma may be present in some cases. The occipito-frontal head circumference is measured routinely, but it may be difficult to interpret if severe moulding is present. The fontanelles are examined for size and tension and the sutures felt for overlapping, synostosis or separation.

Facies

Most newborn infants show some facial asymmetry. In facial nerve palsy there is evidence of flattening of the nasolabial folds in addition to facial asymmetry. If the appearance of the infant suggests dysmorphic features, a more detailed examination is indicated. This includes the palpebral slant, size of the orbits, the distance between the inner canthi (hypo- or hypertelorism), the position of the ears in relation to the outer canthi of the eyes (low-set ears), the appearance of the bridge of the nose, the size of the philtrum, mouth and chin. Unless measurements are carried out (e.g. distance between the inner canthi) and compared to normal standards it is very easy to draw wrong conclusions. If a specific condition is suspected (e.g. Down's syndrome), one should look for other stigmas of the condition.

The oral cavity is examined for the presence of abnormalities (especially posterior cleft palate) and infection (thrush). The hard palate usually has some small white nodules (Epstein's pearls) which consist of epithelial cells and should not be confused with monilia infection. The eyes are usually closed but will open if the baby is lifted above the examiner's head. There may be evidence of subconjunctival haemorrhage or infection (sticky eye). Unless the eyes are examined carefully (red reflex) it is very easy to miss abnormalities (e.g. congenital cataracts).

Chest

The chest circumference is within 0.5–1 cm of the head circumference. Abnormalities of the respiratory system would be suspected from the general observations. Normal respiration in the newborn is usually diaphragmatic. Percussion and auscultation of the chest in infants who are breathing normally are unlikely to reveal any abnormalities and are best omitted.

Cardiovascular system

The normal heart rate is 100–140 per minute and sinus arrhythmia is usually very marked. The sounds over the pulmonary area are louder than the aortic sounds. Systolic murmurs are not uncommon and vary from day to day and they do not necessarily indicate the presence of congenital heart disease. Conversely, the absence of murmurs does not exclude congenital heart disease. Femoral pulses should be examined to exclude coarctation of the aorta.

Abdomen

The abdomen usually appears distended, and a scaphoid abdomen may be the only sign of a diaphragmatic hernia. The abdomen should be palpated for the presence of masses, and in particular for enlargement of kidneys, liver or spleen. The liver is palpable 1–2 cm below the right costal margin in the midclavicular line. The umbilicus should be examined for infection and number of blood vessels. The hernial orifices should be checked and the genitalia and anal region examined.

Skeletal system

The spine should be examined carefully to exclude skin defects, small closed meningomyelocoele and sinuses. Most newborn infants have capillary naevi and some may have café-au-lait spots, the benign nature of which should be explained to the mother. Children of Asiatic, Mediterranean and Negroid descent may have a blue spot (Mongolian spot) over the back, which has no medical significance.

Skeletal anomalies such as polydactyly may be obvious. However, careful examination will be required to note the presence of sternomastoid tumour, fractured clavicle, paronychia, Sydney line or a Simian crease. Particular attention should be paid to the examination of the hips by the method described by Ortolani and by telescoping to exclude the presence of congenital dislocation of the hip. Other abnormalities to observe in the lower limbs include torsion of the femora or tibia and the presence of congenital talipes.

Nervous system

Well newborn infants will demonstrate the presence of primitive reflexes such as grasping, rooting, sucking, glabella tap, Gallant and Moro. Abnormalities of these reflexes do not necessarily indicate brain damage, but a more detailed neurological examination should be performed. The Moro reflex is probably the most useful guide to the infant's neurological status.

6.4 DEFINITIONS

● *Gestation* is regarded as being the time from the first day of the last menstrual period.
● The *low birth weight* baby has a birth weight of 2500 g or less irrespective of the gestation period.
● The *pre-term* baby has a gestation period less than 37 weeks (i.e. 36 weeks 6 days, or less).
● The *full-term* baby has a gestation period of 37 weeks to 41 weeks 6 days.
● The *post-mature* baby has a gestation period of 42 weeks or more.
● The *small-for-dates* baby has a birth weight below the 10th percentile for the gestation period.
● The *large-for-dates* baby has a birth weight above the 90th percentile for the gestation period.
● The *appropriate-for-gestation* baby has a birth weight between the 10th and 90th percentile for the gestation period.

Any of these combinations may be present in a particular infant. Unless the gestation period can be accurately determined, it is not possible to place an infant in a definite category. The gestational age of the infant may be determined from maternal history (last menstrual period), and checked by ultrasonic examination. After birth, gestational age can be estimated within an accuracy of 2 weeks by careful physical and neurological examination of the newborn. However, the neurological examination cannot be performed on a sick, depressed infant. The physical and neurological characteristics that are most useful in diagnosing gestational age are shown in Table 6.1.

6.5 PRE-TERM BABIES

Most pre-term (premature) infants also have a low birth weight (i.e. birth weight of 2500 g or less), but a premature infant may weigh more than 2500 g. A premature infant may also be small-for-dates if the birth weight is below the 10th percentile for the gestation period.

In the majority of cases, the cause of premature birth is not clear. Until the exact mechanism that causes the onset of labour is known it is unlikely that the cause of prematurity will be understood. However, it is well recognized that prematurity is associated with antepartum haemorrhage, multiple pregnancy, incompetent cervix, amnionitis, toxaemia of pregnancy, urinary tract infection of the mother and possibly malnutrition of the mother. Some of the features of prematurity are described in Table 6.1. Others include reddish skin due to lack of subcutaneous fat, presence of lanugo hair, oedema of the feet, large fontanelles with widely separated sutures, and poorly developed primitive reflexes.

Clinical problems

These are due to immaturity of organ function. The most serious of these is immaturity of the respiratory function, which results in difficulties in establishing regular respiration at birth, idiopathic respiratory distress syndrome (hyaline membrane disease), apnoeic attacks and periodic respiration. Respiratory problems may also result from aspiration of liquor amnii or meconium, retained lung fluid or infection.

Hepatic immaturity results in increased and prolonged jaundice, and immaturity of the nervous system predisposes the premature infant to kernicterus at a lower level of bilirubin than a full-term infant. Premature infants also have low protein levels, which further increases the hazard of bilirubin toxicity and also restricts the use of drugs that are bound to protein (such as sulphonamides and cloxacillin). As renal function is immature, drugs such as streptomycin, kanamycin or gentamicin must be used with caution.

Premature infants have very little subcutaneous tissue and brown fat which limits their ability to control their body temperature. They are also liable to increased risk of infection. Problems in feeding result due to poorly developed sucking and swallowing reflexes. Hypoglycaemia may result because of difficulties in feeding, and because of the presence of low energy stores in the form of fat and glycogen. Premature infants also have a greater tendency to develop cerebral birth trauma during delivery and intraventricular haemorrhage.

Management

As premature infants are more liable to infection, appropriate precautions should be taken by rigorous attention to the problem of cross-infection.

To help maintain body temperature, the pre-term infant should be nursed at a temperature much greater than that for the average nursery; even healthy babies may need to be nursed in an incubator. The smaller the baby, the higher the environmental temperature it will require to maintain normal body temperature. The temperature of the incubator is adjusted to the needs of the baby, and this is best achieved by the use of a thermostat attached to the abdomen of the infant. One pitfall in recording temperature of newborn premature infants is that their body temperature may be below 35°C. Unless a low-reading thermometer is used, it may not be apparent that the baby's body temperature is very low.

The management of other problems of premature infants is discussed later.

6.6 SMALL-FOR-DATES BABIES

Small-for-dates babies may result as a consequence of inadequate potential for growth (due to such factors as genetic, chromosomal, congenital abnormalities, congenital infections), in which case their head size is in proportion to the rest of the body. It has been suggested that these infants were small in size before the second trimester.

Other small-for-dates infants result from multiple pregnancy, maternal toxaemia, maternal hypertension, maternal heart disease, placental insufficiency, excessive maternal smoking, maternal malnutrition and high altitudes. These infants appear to have lost weight, have desquamated wrinkled skin and may show evidence of intrauterine hypoxia (meconium staining of the liquor, umbilical cord and skin). They usually have a skull circumference that is on a higher percentile than their body weight. It has been suggested that growth retardation may have occurred in the late second and third trimester of pregnancy. The principal problems of small-for-dates infants are hypoglycaemia (due to inadequate stores of fat and glycogen), hypocalcaemia, meconium aspiration, respiratory problems due to meconium aspiration, polycythaemia with or without increased viscosity of the blood (which may also cause respiratory problems) and a tendency to bleeding (particularly massive pulmonary haemorrhage).

6.7 LARGE-FOR-DATES INFANTS

Some large babies (usually born to large parents) are constitutionally large. Such infants do not have any problems other than complications of delivery. The commonest pathological cause for a large-for-dates infant is maternal diabetes mellitus, which may be gestational or permanent. The large size of the infant is thought to be due to increased production of insulin by the fetus in response to intermittent hyperglycaemia in the mother. Other known causes of large-for-dates infants include cyanotic congenital heart disease in the infant, haemolytic disease of the newborn and Beckwith's syndrome.

6.8 INFANT OF THE DIABETIC MOTHER

Diabetes mellitus in the mother is associated with subfertility, increased fetal and neonatal wastage, and increased incidence of congenital malformations (particularly of the central nervous system) in the infant. Characteristically the infant is large (due to increase in fat and generalized organomegaly), appears overfed, is plethoric and has a Cushingoid appearance. Though large in size, these infants may be born prematurely and have all the problems related to prematurity. There is also an apparent increase in the incidence of idiopathic respiratory distress syndrome (hyaline membrane disease) in these infants. Other problems include hypoglycaemia (due to increased circulating insulin and polycythemia. The latter is due to decrease in extracellular fluid and may lead to venous thrombosis.

6.9 INFECTIONS IN THE NEWBORN

Infections in the newborn may be acquired transplacentally from the mother. The baby may be born with the TORCH (Toxoplasma, Other, Rubella, Cytomegolovirus, Herpes simplex) syndrome: hepatosplenomegaly, jaundice, nervous system abnormalities, chorioretinitis and rashes. The diagnosis may be suspected from the maternal history, and routine examination of cord blood for immunoglobulin M (IgM). Viral studies and examination of cord blood for specific IgM will further help to elucidate the diagnosis.

Congenital syphilis can be acquired in the second and the third trimesters. Bacterial infections including septicaemia, pneumonia, pyelonephritis, meningitis and tuberculosis may also be acquired *in utero*, though they usually occur during parturition or postnatally.

Factors that predispose the newborn to infection include prolonged labour, prolonged rupture of membranes and manipulative and re-suscitative procedures on the infant. Other conditions that may pre-dispose to infection are immaturity, respiratory distress and invasive procedures such as intermittent positive-pressure ventilation, arterial and venous lines.

Newborn babies are susceptible to infection by most micro-organisms, but the local and systemic response to infection is poor: most infections become generalized and have non-specific symptoms. Clinical features that should arouse suspicion of infection include changes in behaviour (e.g. irritability, lethargy, poor feeding, and vomiting), or simply that the baby does not 'look well'. Other symp-toms include failure in temperature control (hypothermia or hyper-thermia), prolonged or unexpected jaundice (particularly in urinary tract infections and septicaemia), disturbances in respiration, ab-dominal distension due to ileus, and the presence of purpura and pustules on the skin. In the presence of specific signs, investigations are directed towards the appropriate organ system. However, in most cases it is necessary to do a 'septic work up' which includes swabs for culture of the ear and umbilical cord, full blood count (including differential and band count), blood, urine and cerebrospinal fluid cultures. Infants with infection develop secondary problems, and in severe cases it is necessary to measure blood glucose, serum bilirubin, acid–base balance and electrolytes.

The management of the newborn with suspected infection includes anticipating problems in 'at risk' situations, carrying out appropriate investigations and instituting treatment on clinical grounds (rather than relying on prophylaxis or bacteriological investigation). Antimi-crobial therapy is indicated if the infection is thought to be bacterial. The choice of antibiotics will depend on the sensitivity of the orga-nisms in a particular nursery, until bacteriological results are available. The usual practice is to use a combination of two drugs, such as a penicillin and an aminoglycoside. Supportive measures include nur-sing in a neutral thermal environment, adequate fluid and nutrition, and the management of the complications that occur in severe cases, such as anaemia, shock, hypoglycaemia and disseminated intravascular coagulation.

6.10 JAUNDICE IN THE NEWBORN

About one-half the infants in a postnatal nursery will show visible jaundice. It is therefore not surprising that its occurrence may be taken for granted by the medical attendants. However, it may be the only symptom that occurs in many serious illnesses in the newborn. The jaundice may be due to enzyme deficiencies in the liver, haemolysis, infection, metabolic disturbances and obstruction to the bile passage. High levels of indirect reacting bilirubin can cause brain damage, which may be so mild as to cause only disturbance of cognitive function or so serious as to cause kernicterus and deafness. Although 340 mmol/l is quoted as the level at which bilirubin toxicity may occur, factors such as the maturity of the infant, hypoxia, acidosis, rate of rise of bilirubin, and the presence of substances that compete with bilirubin for albumin-binding sites must also be taken into consideration when planning treatment for an infant with raised indirect bilirubin.

Physiological jaundice

This condition occurs in newborn infants and requires no treatment. It is mainly due to relative deficiency of the enzyme glucuronyl transferase, though red cell destruction and the enterohepatic circulation may be partially responsible. The infant is usually well, and the jaundice does not appear before the age of 24 hours and begins to wane by the 7th day in the full-term and by the 10th day in the pre-term infant. Usually it is maximum on the 3rd or 4th day in full-term infants and on the 5th or 6th day in pre-term infants. The serum level of unconjugated (indirect) bilirubin remains below 250 μmol/l, and the conjugated (direct) bilirubin level does not exceed 16–25 μmol/l.

Haemolytic jaundice

This may be due to blood group incompatibility (Rh, ABO and other rare blood groups), abnormalities of the shape of the red blood cells (e.g. hereditary spherocytosis) red blood cell enzyme deficiency (e.g. glucose-6-phosphate-dehydrogenase deficiency), or abnormal haemoglobins (e.g. Bart's). The haemolysis may also be secondary to the administration of drugs. It may occur in extravascular sites secondary to bleeding in the tissues, as in ecchymosis and caphalhaematoma.

Bacterial and viral infections

These may cause jaundice in the neonatal period, and the infection may be congenital or acquired. Bacterial infections (particularly septicaemia due to gram-negative organisms) should be considered in all cases of neonatal jaundice. In jaundice due to infection there is usually a rise in both direct and indirect bilirubin.

Metabolic conditions

Those that tend to cause hyperbilirubinaemia include hypoxia, hypoglycaemia, hypothyroidism, galactosaemia, alpha-1-antitrypsin deficiency, cystic fibrosis and many disturbances of amino acid metabolism. The mechanism of jaundice in these conditions is complex, and the type of bilirubin will depend on the underlying disease process. Other symptoms will sometimes aid in the diagnosis.

Bile-duct atresia

This type of jaundice is rarely recognized in the first week of life, and is difficult to distinguish from neonatal hepatitis. In both these conditions there are signs of obstructive jaundice (raised direct bilirubin, clay-coloured stools, bile in urine). Bile-duct atresia and neonatal hepatitis must be distinguished from other conditions causing a raised direct bilirubin (e.g. galactosaemia and cystic fibrosis).

Enzyme deficiencies

Certain congenital liver cell enzyme deficiencies cause neonatal hyperbilirubinaemia, but these conditions are rare. Crigler–Najjar syndrome is an example of unconjugated hyperbilirubinaemia due to glucuronyl transferase deficiency, and Dubin–Johnson syndrome is an example of direct hyperbilirubinaemia due to a defect of hepatic excretory function.

Bilirubin competitors

Many substances compete with bilirubin for conjugation by the liver and will tend to cause hyperbilirubinaemia in the neonatal period. Examples of some commonly used drugs in the perinatal period that compete are salicylates, water-soluble analogues of vitamin K, diazepam by injection which contains benzoate, certain sulphonamides and steroids.

Other drugs that have been implicated in the causation of neonatal jaundice include phenothiazines and oxytocin given to the mother.

The exact mechanism of breast milk jaundice is not clear though pregnanetriol and unsaturated fatty acids (which are bilirubin competitors) in the milk have been implicated in its causation. More recently, it has been shown that bilirubin reductase in breast milk breaks down conjugated bilirubin in the gut which increases bilirubin load via the enterohepatic circulation.

Management of hyperbilirubinaemia

There are many causes of hyperbilirubinaemia, so the investigations and treatment will depend on individual cases. Investigations aim to exclude haemolysis (blood group of infant and mother, direct Coombs' test, peripheral blood smear and enzymes), infection (urine and blood cultures) and metabolic conditions (reducing substances in urine).

Exchange transfusion is the most reliable and quick method for reducing bilirubin concentration, whatever the cause of hyperbilirubinaemia. However, phototherapy has greatly reduced the need for exchange transfusion in neonatal nurseries. The exact mechanism by which phototherapy reduces bilirubin is not clear, but so far two types of reaction have been demonstrated: photo-oxidation in which the bilirubin molecule is broken down into monopyrroles and dipyrroles and photo-isomerization in which the molecule remains intact and can be excreted without hepatic glucuronization in the bile. *In vitro* studies suggest that photo-isomerization is the more important reaction. Though phototherapy has been known to cause retinal damage, growth retardation and the early onset of puberty in experimental animals, no such problems have been reported in infants. It appears that these effects are mediated through the retina and it has been recommended that the eyes of newborn babies be shielded during phototherapy.

It has been observed that phenobarbitone given to the mother or the newborn infant activates the enzyme glucuronyl transferase over a period of approximately 48–96 hours. It is not a useful drug for reducing bilirubin levels, but in selected cases it may be given prophylactically to the mother prior to delivery.

6.11 HYPOGLYCAEMIA IN THE NEWBORN

Newborn infants have low blood sugar levels compared to those of an adult. However, a blood sugar level of less than 30 mg/100 ml (1.6 mmol/l) in the full-term infant, and of less than 20 mg/100 ml

(1.1 mmol/l) in the low birth weight infant is defined as neonatal hypoglycaemia. The condition may be asymptomatic. Reported signs are vague and may occur in infants who do not have hypoglycaemia. Signs are mainly respiratory (cyanosis, irregular respirations, apnoea) or neurological (tremors, jitteriness, convulsions, apathy, limpness, refusal to feed, eye-rolling and a high-pitched or weak cry). Neonatal hypoglycaemia is associated with low birth weight or small-for-dates infants, infants of diabetic mothers, infants with haemolytic disease of the newborn, hypoxia, respiratory distress syndrome, cerebral haemorrhage and difficult delivery. The diagnosis is usually made by routine monitoring of blood sugar levels by Dextrostix examination at frequent intervals in the babies at risk.

Management

Infants at risk should be fed early and their blood glucose monitored closely by 3-hourly Dextrostix examination before feeds. If the Dextrostix suggests a glucose level below 1.5 mmol/l, true blood glucose levels should be determined by the glucose oxidase method. In the event of absence of facilities for measuring true blood glucose, a blood specimen for glucose should be collected and the infant should be treated as for hypoglycaemia.

Infants with hypoglycaemia should be given 0.5 g of glucose per kg of body weight (2 ml/kg of 25% or 5 ml/kg of 10% glucose) intravenously immediately followed by a 10% intravenous glucose drip. Oral feeding is introduced as soon as possible, but the intravenous infusion should be continued until such time as feeding is established fully. If hypoglycaemia persists or recurs in spite of the above measures, plasma insulin levels should be measured before administering more glucose. In resistant cases hydrocortisone, glucagon and growth hormone may be indicated.

6.12 RESPIRATORY PROBLEMS OF THE NEWBORN

Respiratory failure causes more than 50% of the deaths of normally formed live-born infants during the first 48 hours of life. The respiratory failure may be central or peripheral. Central respiratory failure is characterized by apnoea and slow, irregular, gasping respiratory movements. It is associated with narcosis, perinatal anoxia, cerebral birth trauma and central nervous system anomalies. Peripheral respiratory failure is characterized by a rapid and increasing respiratory rate, chest recession and expiratory grunt. It is commonly seen with idiopathic respiratory distress syndrome (hyaline membrane disease), 'wet lungs', aspiration syndromes, pneumonia and congenital abnormalities such as lung cysts or diaphragmatic hernia. Other conditions that cause peripheral respiratory difficulty include pneumothorax under tension and congestive cardiac failure. Many inborn errors of metabolism present with deep and rapid breathing because of metabolic acidosis and are easily confused with peripheral respiratory failure.

Treatment of respiratory failure in the newborn is aimed at the underlying cause (e.g. antibiotics for pneumonia, and surgical treatment for diaphragmatic hernia), and is also symptomatic (oxygen, correction of acid–base balance, respiratory support in the form of positive airway pressure or intermittent mandatory ventilation). Other ancillary aids include provision of adequate fluid and nourishment, and nursing in a neutral thermal environment.

6.13 NEONATAL CONVULSIONS

Convulsions in the neonatal period most frequently are subtle (when they are easily overlooked) or obvious (multifocal clonic movements, focal clonic movements and tonic or myoclonic movements). Generalized convulsions are rare. Subtle manifestations include eye movements (horizontal deviation, jerking, blinking or fluttering), drooling, sucking, unusual limb movements ('rowing' or 'swimming') and apnoea. Jitteriness (rhythmic limb movements) which is fairly common in the newborn may be confused with convulsions. However, unlike convulsions, jitteriness is rhythmic, stimulus sensitive and is not accompanied by abnormalities of eye movements. Furthermore, jitteriness can be stopped by flexion of the affected limb.

Common causes of neonatal convulsions

CEREBRAL BIRTH TRAUMA

Hypoxic ischaemic encephalopathy, including oedema, haemorrhage and perinatal anoxia.

METABOLIC CONDITIONS

Hypoglycaemia (usually in the first 48 hours in low birth weight infants and within the first 24 hours in infants of diabetic or pre-diabetic mothers), hypocalcaemia (1st or 2nd day usually in association with maternal complications of pregnancy and delivery or 5th day in bottle fed babies), disturbances of amino acid metabolism (usually 24–48 hours after commencement of feeding) and miscellaneous conditions such as hypomagnesaemia, electrolyte imbalance, hyperbilirubinaemia and pyridoxine dependency.

DRUG WITHDRAWAL

Heroin, methadone, barbiturates (usually present within 48–72 hours of birth, though may present a week later).

INFECTIONS

Central nervous system (e.g. meningitis) or systemic.

INTRACRANIAL MALFORMATIONS

INTRAVENTRICULAR HAEMORRHAGE

In premature infants.

7

Abnormal labour

Barry G. Wren
Revised by *Leo R. Leader*

7.1 GENERAL INSTRUCTIONAL OBJECTIVE

The students should recognize deviations from normal labour and understand their effect on mother and fetus so that in an emergency they can initiate management.

7.2 SPECIFIC BEHAVIOURAL OBJECTIVES

1. Identify failure of progress in labour.
2. Identify the symptoms and signs that are suggestive of disproportion.
3. Describe the clinical features of a patient with obstructed labour.
4. Identify signs that may indicate fetal distress, and discuss their causes and the implications to the fetus.
5. Distinguish between normal and abnormal uterine action.
6. Identify the effects of prolonged labour on mother and fetus.
7. Assist in the management of a patient with a prolonged labour, and discuss the problems that are identifiable.
8. Discuss the signs of fetal distress and the use of continuous fetal heart rate monitoring.
9. Discuss the initial management of a transverse lie, cord prolapse and unsuspected second twin.
10. List the common indications for and the complications of Caesarean section.
11. List the criteria necessary for the safe application of forceps.
12. Discuss the causes of postpartum haemorrhage.
13. Examine a patient with a postpartum haemorrhage, diagnose the cause and initiate the appropriate emergency management.
14. List the causes of shock during labour and early puerperium, and indicate the emergency management of these patients.

15. Discuss the causes of intrapartum haemorrhage.
16. Discuss the causes and management of women who have a pre-term labour.

7.3 REASONS FOR STUDYING ABNORMAL LABOUR

Almost every labour progresses to delivery with some minor deviations from normal which do not produce any marked problems to the mother or fetus or which require minimal interference to correct. However, some labours become so abnormal that continuation may produce death or increased morbidity to the mother or fetus. It is important that the competent student will have the ability to recognize these deviations and to assess their significance and then to initiate the appropriate steps in management. Every student should spend as much time as possible in the labour ward, recognizing abnormalities in women during first and second stages of labour. The student should recognize these minor deviations and be prepared to discuss their observations with the obstetrician in charge. In this manner, major deviations become easier to define and management instituted at a more appropriate time.

7.4 DELAY IN LABOUR

Whilst there is wide variation in the duration of labour, most multiparous patients will deliver in about 8 hours whilst primiparous patients take 12–14 hours. It is now recognized that the fetal skull is probably the best pelvimeter (indicator of pelvic adequacy). Unless labour is contra-indicated, all primigravidas should be allowed to have a trial of labour.

Once patients are in established labour, their progress is recorded graphically on a labour curve called a partogram (see Fig. 5.17) and regular vaginal and clinical examinations should be performed every 4 hours.

Indication of delay in labour

1. Once the patient is in the active phase of labour (more than 3 cm dilated) if the rate of cervical dilatation fails to exceed 1 cm an hour then the staff should be alerted that a problem may exist.
2. Where there is failure of descent of the presenting part. Like cervical dilatation, the presenting part of the fetus descends into the

pelvis at a gradually increasing rate. Disproportion or poor uterine contractions may cause the presenting part to become delayed in its descent.

Once the alert line (see Fig. 5.17) has been crossed then a further vaginal examination is done after another 2 hours. If the rate of progress has now been satisfactory no further intervention is necessary. If however, no further progress has occurred (i.e. the cervix has not dilated any further) then the action line will be crossed. At this point it is necessary to establish a diagnosis as to why the labour has not progressed and a critical vaginal examination and pelvic assessment should be made by an experienced observer to exclude obvious cephalopelvic disproportion.

Cephalopelvic disproportion

This is one of the commonest causes of obstructed labour and the underlying condition may be due to one of the following:

1. Large baby (Absolute disproportion)
   (a) Hereditary factors. Most babies have a birth weight similar to that of their mother/father. Big babies have large heads. Large mothers tend to have large babies.
   (b) Postmaturity. When the placenta functions normally, the fetus continues to grow at a regular rate. If the pregnancy continues beyond 40 weeks then the fetus will be larger than average.
   (c) Diabetes. The increased maternal levels of glucose pass to the fetus, so stimulating insulin production, deposition of glucose in tissue and initiation of growth hormone-like activity.
   (d) Multiparity. Up to the fifth baby, each succeeding baby tends to be heavier and larger than the preceding infant.
2. Abnormal positions (Relative disproportion)
   Normally a fetus delivers in the occipito-anterior position with the head well flexed so that the suboccipito-bregmatic (9.5 cm) and the biparietal (9.5 cm) diameters will easily pass through a normal pelvis. If, however, the fetus is in an occipito-posterior position then the presenting diameter (occipito-frontal) will be 11.5 cm. If there is a brow presentation (mento-vertical, 13.5 cm) then cephalopelvic disproportion will occur. With the onset of contractions forcing the extended head against the pelvic brim, flexion of the head normally occurs (or in brow presentation, further extension to a face presentation) until a small diameter presents. When this occurs, the

fetal head descends, and with moulding and long internal, rotation, the baby will eventually deliver in the occipito-anterior position. Because of the added mechanisms of flexion and long internal, rotation, fetuses in the occipito-posterior and occipito-lateral positions have a longer labour (Fig. 7.1).

3. Small pelvis

Normal women of 160 cm have a true conjugate diameter of the pelvis of about 11.5 cm. Taller women tend to have larger pelvic diameters whilst shorter women have smaller diameters. The risks of absolute cephalopelvic disproportion increase if the woman is less than 150 cm in height. Approximately 25% of mothers who are 155 cm or smaller have some form of surgical interference (forceps, lower segment Caesarean section) to their labour, whereas mothers of 163 cm and taller have only a 5% chance of surgical interference.

4. Abnormal, shape to pelvic brim

Most women will have either a gynaecoid (45%) or an anthropoid (40%) shape to their pelvic brim and the brim, the cavity and the outlet will be adequate for most fetuses to pass through the pelvis. However, about 15% of women have an android shape to the brim, flattened sacrum, narrow subpubic angle and prominent ischial spines. In these women the pelvic cavity tends to be convergent — the fetus, which often presents in the occipito-lateral or occipito-posterior position may become jammed in the mid-pelvis, unable to undergo internal rotation and unable to descend further. This

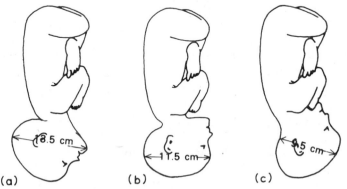

Fig. 7.1 Fetal attitude. (a) Extension to a brow presentation with a mento-vertical diameter (13.5 cm); (b) Extension in the military attitude with an occipito-frontal diameter (11.5 cm); (c) A normal flexed head with an sub-occipito-bregmatic diameter (9.5 cm).

arrest of internal rotation occurs at the level of the ischial spines and is called deep transverse arrest of the fetal head. This may be managed by rotating the head to an occipito-anterior position, either manually, with Kielland's forceps or, by means of a vacuum extractor. If this is not possible it may be necessary to perform a Caesarean section. Another abnormal pelvic shape is associated with a platypelloid pelvic brim, where there is general flattening of the brim in an antero-posterior diameter. The true conjugate diameter is about 10.5 cm with a wider (12.5 cm) transverse diameter. Because the pelvic cavity is usually divergent, the fetus will deliver easily, once it has negotiated the brim (usually by the process of asynclitism) *OBLIQUE PRESENTATION of HEAD – ANT PARIETAL BONE or POST*

5. Abnormality of the genital tract
Cervix: Obstruction can be due to congenital rigidity or postsurgical scarring.
Vagina: Can be due to congenital abnormalities such as septum.
Pelvic tumours very rarely cause obstruction to labour. Ovarian cysts or uterine fibroids only obstruct labour if situated in the Pouch of Douglas.

✱ + FULL BLADDER ✱

(2) Abnormal uterine action

If the labour fails to progress then careful observation should be made of the uterine contractions. The contractions can be monitored by means of external tocodynamometry or by means of an intrauterine catheter to measure the intrauterine pressure directly. Note should be taken of the pressure, the frequency and the duration of each contraction. Care should also be taken to ensure that the uterus is relaxed between contractions.

An accurate diagnosis should be made as to the precise type of abnormal uterine action present and appropriate steps taken to deal with it. It is most important to exclude cephalopelvic disproportion.

7.5 TYPES OF ABNORMAL UTERINE ACTIVITY

Overactive hypertonic

HYPERTONIC INCO-ORDINATE OR IRREGULAR UTERINE ACTIVITY

This generally occurs in primigravid patients and may be associated with occipito-posterior positions. The contractions are inco-ordinate,

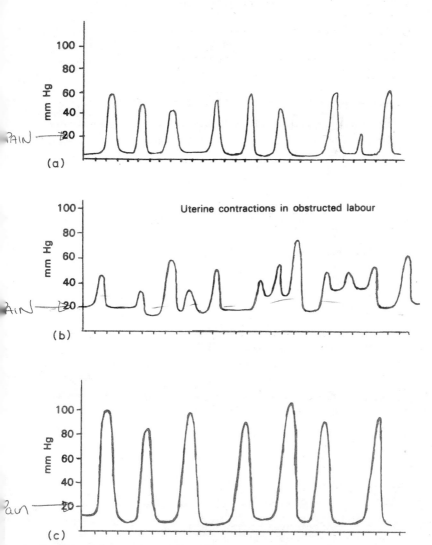

Fig. 7.2 Uterine contractions. (a) Uterine contractions during the first stage of a normal labour. Low resting tone, good amplitude, lasting for 50–70 seconds every 3–5 minutes; (b) Uterine contractions in a primigravid in the first stage of labour, who is responding poorly to obstruction. High resting tone, poor amplitude, irregular time and amplitude. A non-productive uterine action; (c) Obstructed labour in a multigravid. Regular contractions with high amplitude. May cause ruptured uterus.

irregular and ineffectual. There is an absence of fundal dominance and an increased uterine tone in between contractions. Because of the elevated resting tone patients experience pain between contractions (Fig. 7.2).

Management

1. Adequate analgesia usually in the form of an epidural anaesthetic. If this is not available, then adequate dosage of narcotics such as meperidine (pethidine) will suffice.
2. Reassurance it is important to reassure the patient and husband that the problem can be dealt with as maternal anxiety may play a role in the aetiology of this condition.
3. Beta-adrenergic agents a small bolus dose can be used to inhibit uterine activity. When contractions restart 15–20 minutes later, they are often more regular. This treatment is indicated if epidural analgesia fails or is contra-indicated.

RETRACTION RING

This condition occurs late in obstructed babies after the membranes have ruptured. As a consequence of the progressive permanent shortening (retraction) of the muscle fibres with each contraction, the upper segment becomes thickened and the lower segment progressively thinner. This ring and thickening progressively rises up the uterus as the lower segment becomes thinner. When it rises to an abnormally high level, it is termed a Bandl's ring and is an indication of impending uterine rupture.

Management

This is by Caesarean section.

Underactive or hypotonic uterine activity

The uterine contractions are weak and infrequent and the intrauterine pressure will be below 30 mmHg.

PRIMARY HYPOTONIA (INERTIA)

Causes

- Overdistension of the uterus, due to multiple pregnancies, polyhydramnios or fibromyomata.

- Multiple pregnancies.
- Congenital uterine abnormalities such as bicornuate uterus.
- In association with antepartum haemorrhage and marked anaemia.
- As a result of cephalopelvic disproportion.

SECONDARY HYPOTONIC INERTIA

This is where the uterus has been contracting adequately and then the contractions become inefficient later in labour.

Causes

- Cephalopelvic disproportion.
- Overdistension of the uterus in association with multiple pregnancy or polyhydramnios.
- A rigid cervix or perineum.
- Malpresentations.
- Oversedation.

Management

1. Exclude cephalopelvic disproportion, obstruction.
2. Oxytocin stimulation.
3. Adequate analgesia.

[handwritten: Causes: Cephalopelvic disp^s, Inefficient Uterine activity]

7.6 PROLONGED LABOUR

Definition

The definition of prolonged labour has changed over the years and it is believed now that any labour which lasts more than 24 hours is prolonged. However, there is good reason to believe that no patient should be in the active phase of labour (commences at 3 cm of dilatation) for more than 12 hours. This is because of the trend towards preventive obstetrics and because of the consequences of prolonged labour.

Consequences of prolonged labour

[handwritten table: CONSEQUENCES — maternal | fetal]

MATERNAL

- Maternal metabolic abnormalities.
- Potential infection.
- Psychological disappointment.

[handwritten: maternal: Metabolic, Potential Infn, Psychological Anxiety, Mechanical Exhaustion | fetal: Distress/hypc, Infection, Brain damage/hypoxia, IUDeath, Neonatal death]

- Anxiety.
- Mechanical complications such as a rupture of the uterus and fistulae.
- Exhaustion.

FETAL

- Fetal distress.
- Fetal infection.
- Fetal brain damage.
- Intrauterine death — stillbirth.
- Neonatal death.

Abnormal → Passenger (fetus)
→ Passage (birth cana)
→ Powers (uterine actun

Management of prolonged labour

The most important part of the management of prolonged labour is prevention and to recognize potential causes. If patients are correctly managed using a partogram and appropriate attention paid to the alert and action lines, prolonged labour should not occur. The possible causes may be:

1. Abnormalities of the passenger
   (a) Malpresentation.
   (b) Fetal malformation.
   (c) Large fetus (Fig. 7.3).
2. Abnormalities in the passage
   (a) Contracted pelvis.

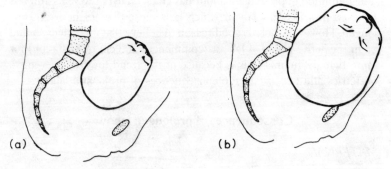

Fig. 7.3 (a) Non-engaged head without disproportion. The skull does not overlap the symphysis pubis; (b) Non-engaged head. The skull overlaps the symphysis pubis.

(b) Abnormalities of the uterus and lower genital tract as well as pelvic tumours.
3. Abnormalities in the power
    (a) Abnormal uterine contractions.

Procedure

1. Establish an intravenous line, adequate fluids and nutrients.
2. Reassure mother that you are aware of the problem of her needs and anxiety, and that you are taking appropriate steps to manage the problem. *3ª Pass a catheter to ensure empty bladder*
3. Judicious use of oxytocin if the contractions are inadequate. *ie augmentation of labour*
4. Use of epidural anaesthesia for pain relief.
5. Monitoring of fetal well-being by the use of a cardiotocograph.
6. Ensuring that the membranes are ruptured.
7. Chemoprophylaxis by using the appropriate antibiotic should the patient be pyrexial or there be any suspicion of intrauterine infection.
8. Instrumental delivery to manipulate the fetus when indicated.
9. Perform a Caesarean section if no progress is made.

Fetal distress

During any labour, but particularly during the labour of an at risk pregnant mother, the signs of fetal distress may develop. These signs imply metabolic abnormalities and may reflect fetal hypoxia and acidosis. These abnormalities can arise as acute events (prolapsed cord, placental abruption), subacute (hypertonic uterine activity) or chronic (as result of placental insufficiency).

Fetal distress is a term applied to a set of signs indicating that if the fetus is not delivered, it will be born dead, or will suffer some brain damage as a result of the hypoxia. Fetal distress needs to be separated from signs of fetal stress which do not have such ominous implications.

2 Chronic.

SIGNS OF FETAL STRESS

1. Meconium staining of the amniotic fluid. Meconium staining of infants who are term or post-term in gestational age is less sinister in its incidence in pre-term infants. The major danger of meconium-stained amniotic fluid is aspiration at the time of delivery.
2. Intrauterine growth retardation.

SIGNS OF FETAL DISTRESS

1. Rapid fetal heart rate (tachycardia), greater than 160 beats/min.
2. Slow fetal heart rate (bradycardia), less than 100 beats/min.
3. Heart rate deceleration (particularly late decelerations).
4. Loss of fetal heart reactivity (beat to beat variability).
5. Low fetal scalp pH and increased base deficit. = acidosis
6. Fetal gasping or absence of fetal respiratory movements *in utero*.

Although many of these signs often indicate fetal distress, all of these may be found in a fetus that is born healthy and active with an excellent chance of normal growth after delivery. The art in obstetric management is to decide what is abnormal, when to intervene and how to interfere with the normal processes of labour.

Fetal heart rate patterns

For a normal fetal heart rate to be maintained, the fetus requires an adequate supply of nutriment (glucose and glycogen) and oxygen. Placental inadequacy or reduced placental blood flow (occurring in conditions such as maternal hypertension, excessive maternal smoking or poor maternal nutrition) reduce the amount of glucose that can be actively or passively transferred to the fetus, so that it is born small for gestational age and with poor glycogen reserves. If such a fetus has a labour which is prolonged or overstimulated, there is added hypoxia, and the fetus will become acidotic. All fetuses that are at risk should be observed in labour by continuous fetal heart rate monitoring.

Fetal heart rate changes

NON-PERIODIC

The normal fetal heart rate varies between 110 and 160 beats/minute. Should the fetal heart rate rise above 160 beats/minute and be sustained for more than 10 minutes, this is regarded as tachycardia. If the fetal heart rate slows to less than 100 beats/minute for the same duration, this is regarded as bradycardia.

PERIODIC CHANGES

These are slowing changes in the fetal heart rate that are associated with uterine contractions. These are classified as:

Uterine contractions

H Rate   Early   Late

1. Early decelerations. This slowing of the fetal heart rate usually occurs in association with contractions and is probably due to vagal nerve stimulation due to head or trunk compression.
2. Late decelerations. Here the slowing of the fetal heart rate starts after the apex of the contraction and may be a sign of fetal hypoxia.
3. Variable decelerations. These are a combination of early and late decelerations and usually are associated with cord compression.

Fetal heart rate variability

When measured directly from a scalp electrode it gives a measure of the R–R wave interval and true beat to beat variability. Reduced beat to beat variability may indicate alterations in the fetal sleep state which either occur spontaneously or as a result of maternal sedation or it may indicate fetal distress.

Relative risks of fetal distress:

1. Approximately 5% of patients who have a normal intrapartum cardiotocograph will be born with low Apgar Scores.
2. Meconium-stained amniotic fluid alone carries a risk of about 5% that the fetus will have a low Apgar Score. The greater the number of abnormal features present in the cardiotocographic tracing, the greater the chances are of the fetus being compromised. The risk depends upon the underlying baseline heart rate, the degree of beat to beat variability plus the extent of the decelerations (if any are present).

To help differentiate true fetal distress in labour from any abnormal heart rate pattern found due to other reasons, fetal scalp blood analysis can be undertaken. A small sample is taken from the fetal scalp and analysed for pH, pCO_2 and base deficit. A normal fetal pH level in the first stage of labour is usually greater than 7.25. During the second stage the fetal scalp pH may drop to 7.15. It may be necessary to assess the maternal acid–base status as alterations in the maternal acid–base balance can affect the fetal acid–base status.

Management of an abnormal heart rate pattern

When any abnormal pattern is present, a cause for it should be sought. Maternal blood pressure should be checked and the patient turned to the lateral position (to avoid the supine hypotensive syndrome) and also to try to exclude cord compression. If an oxytocin drip is running, this should be stopped in case the abnormal heart rate pattern is a result of hyperstimulation. If the fetal heart rate abnormality persists, then a fetal scalp blood sample should be taken. Preliminary evidence with vibroacoustic stimulation suggests that if the fetus is stimulated in labour and responds with a heart rate increase, then the risks of the scalp pH being less than 7.25 is small. If the fetal scalp sample is abnormal or the facilities are not available to do this test and the fetal heart rate abnormality persists, then delivery should be expedited by whichever means is safest to both mother and fetus. If the cervix is fully dilated and the head already engaged it may be delivered by forceps delivery or if this is not possible an emergency Caesarean section should be performed.

Intrauterine resuscitation

In the presence of a severely abnormal fetal heart rate, whilst preparations for Caesarean section are being made a small bolus dose of beta-adrenergic drug (salbutamol, retodrine) or magnesium sulphate can be given to inhibit uterine activity and improve placental perfusion.

7.7 TRANSVERSE AND OBLIQUE LIE

An unstable lie is one in which the presenting part alters from week to week. It may be either a transverse or oblique lie or possibly a breech presentation. These are relatively uncommon events but are found in association with the following conditions:

1. Grand multipara. This is by far the commonest factor, due to the lax uterine and abdominal walls, which prevent the splinting effect found in women with lesser parity.
2. Polyhydramnios. The volume of fluid distends the uterus and allows the fetus to swim like a goldfish in a bowl — often taking up an oblique or transverse lie.
3. Prematurity. Here there is a relative excess of fluid to the fetus. If pre-term labour occurs, the fetus may be found to have a transverse lie.
4. Subseptate uterus. The septum prevents the fetus from turning *in utero*.
5. Pelvic tumours such as fibroids and ovarian cysts may not only prevent the lower pole from engaging, but cause it to take up a transverse lie.

6. Placenta praevia. This usually prevents engagement of the presenting part. Because of this it may present with the fetus in an oblique or transverse lie.
7. Multiple pregnancies may present with a transverse lie. If this does occur, it is more common in the second twin.

Management of transverse and oblique lie

It is not uncommon for the fetus to have a transverse lie until about the 32nd week of pregnancy. If the transverse lie persists after this time a cause should be determined. An ultrasound examination should be done to exclude placenta praevia, ovarian tumour or fibroid and if either of these conditions are present an elective Caesarean section should be performed at 38–39 weeks of gestation. The ultrasound is also used for identifying twins and a subseptate uterus, whilst a vaginal examination will confirm a pelvic tumour.

The main risk of a transverse or oblique lie is in association with pre-term ruture of the membranes and cord prolapse. When diagnosed the state of the cervix should be checked. If the cervix is dilated, the patient should be admitted to hospital. If, however, the cervix is closed and the membranes are intact the patient may be reviewed on a regular basis. If no easily identifiable cause is found, attempted external cephalic version can be made after 34 weeks. In grand multipara patients, the fetus will usually turn easily but will often swing back to an abnormal lie. If the abnormal lie persists or constantly reoccurs, the woman should be admitted to hospital by the 38th week. If external version is successful at this stage and the patient's cervix is favourable then artificial rupture of the membrane can be performed with the head held over the pelvic brim and an oxytocin drip commenced to augment uterine activity. If the cephalic presentation is maintained, labour may be allowed to continue. If the transverse or oblique lie reoccurs in labour then a Caesarean section must be performed.

Complications of a transverse lie

If a mother goes into labour with a transverse or oblique lie, several catastrophes may occur. Because this occurs more commonly in multiparous women and their uterine activity is often much stronger, rupture of the uterus is more likely. When the membranes rupture there is a greatly increased danger of cord prolapse.

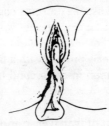

Fig. 7.4 Cord prolapse leads to drying and cooling of the cord causing spasm of vessels or the cord may be compressed at the pelvic brim by the fetal presenting part.

7.8 CORD PROLAPSE

Cord prolapse is that condition when the membranes rupture, allowing a loop of cord to prolapse through the cervical os. The cord is found either in the vagina or protruding outside the labia. This complication has a high fetal mortality rate because the cord is compressed either by the presenting part or the vessels go into spasm due to drying effects and a change in temperature (Fig. 7.4).

Factors associated with cord prolapse

1. Transverse and oblique lie.
2. Breech presentation.
3. Disproportion.
4. Multiple pregnancy.
5. Polyhydramnios.
6. Pre-term rupture of the membranes.
7. Pelvic tumours.
8. Placenta praevia (not type 4).

Management of cord prolapse

A cord prolapse is an accute obstetrical emergency, and is often first seen by those people who are least experienced to cope with it. Steps in the acute management:

1. Determine if the cord is still pulsating.
2. If pulsating, push any exposed loop of cord back into the vagina to keep it warm and moist.
3. Determine the dilatation of the cervix. If fully dilated the patient

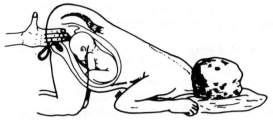

Fig. 7.5 Prolapsed cord. Demonstrating the maternal position and a hand in the vagina in an attempt to replace the cord into the vagina and to keep the presenting part away from the pelvic brim.

can be encouraged to bear down or a forceps delivery can be performed.

If it is not possible to deliver the patient safely vaginally then:

4. The patient is placed in the knee–chest position to allow gravity to keep the presenting part from compressing the cord at the pelvic brim (Fig. 7.5).
5. The operator's hand is inserted into the vagina with the fingers apart so that the cord is kept in the vagina and the presenting part can be pushed up from the pelvic brim.
6. An alternative to this is to insert a number 16 Foley catheter into the patient's bladder which in turn is inflated with 500–700 ml of normal saline. This will distend the bladder and elevate the presenting part off the cord, thereby reducing the need for the operator to elevate the presenting part. This makes the anaesthetic management of the patient less complicated as she can then be anaethetized on her back without great jeopardy to the fetus.
7. Arrange an emergency Caesarean section. When the patient is anaesthetized and the obstetrician is ready to carry out this procedure, then the bladder can be deflated and/or the operator can remove his hand from the patient's vagina.

7.9 TWIN PREGNANCY AND UNSUSPECTED SECOND TWIN

Occasionally, a woman will deliver an apparently normal small infant but before the placenta is delivered, the attendant may notice that the uterus is still sufficiently enlarged and contains a second fetus. The first twin will be managed as for all normal pregnancies but special care must be taken for the second twin. Under ideal circumstances all twin deliveries should take place in an operating theatre, however this may not be possible when the second twin is undiagnosed.

1. Make sure that no oxytocic drugs are given to contract the uterus.
2. Palpate the lie of the fetus. If it is transverse or oblique, an external cephalic version is attempted.
3. Insert an intravenous line, with a side drip containing oxytocin which should be administered unless an external version is attempted.
4. Arrange for an anaesthetist and a paediatrician to be available. Ideally a mother delivering a twin pregnancy should have an epidural anaesthetic in labour.
5. If the lie is longitudinal, wait 5–10 minutes for uterine contractions to return so that the effort will push the presenting part into the pelvis.
6. The fetal heart rate should be continuously monitored. A clamp should be put on the umbilical cord of the first twin and blood should not be allowed to run out from the cord.
7. If after 10 minutes there are no contractions start an oxytocic drip.
8. When the contractions are sufficiently strong to push the presenting part into the pelvis, the membranes are ruptured and a normal spontaneous delivery will follow.
9. If the fetus persists in an oblique or transverse lie after the return of uterine contractions, then should it prove impossible to do an external cephalic version a Caesarean section should be performed.
10. Following the delivery of the second twin and the placenta, an ergot derivative, oxytocin, should be given.

7.10 INDICATIONS FOR CAESAREAN SECTION

In the absence of complications it is safer to allow a normal vaginal delivery than to perform a Caesarean section. However, in those circumstances where difficulty may occur in labour, the risks attached to a Caesarean section may be less than those of a complicated instrumental delivery. The indications for Caesarean section are variable and may include:

1. Absolute disproportion.
2. Relative disproportion.
3. Fetal distress, where the continuation of a vaginal delivery increases the risk of fetal mortality or morbidity.

4. Maternal disease (such as pre-eclampsia) that increase the risk to the fetus and mother.
5. Prolonged labour.
6. Previous Caesarean section for disproportion.
7. Breech presentation.
8. Unstable fetal lie at the onset of labour.
9. Placenta praevia.
10. Prolapsed cord.
11. Obstructed labour.

7.11 APPLICATION OF OBSTETRIC FORCEPS

Forceps fall into two major groups:

1. Traction
   Neville-Barnes, Simpson and Wrigley forceps, which are used to deliver the fetus when sagittal suture is in the occipito-anterior position and the fetus presents in either an occipito-anterior or as a direct occipito-posterior position.
2. Rotational forceps
   Kielland's forceps, which are used to rotate the occiput either from an occipito-transverse or an occipito-posterior position.

Indications for forceps

1. When the delivery process needs to be expedited for maternal reasons (hypertension, maternal distress, cardiac disease, delay in the second stage, epidural anaesthesia, maternal exhaustion).
2. When the delivery needs to be expedited for fetal reasons (fetal distress, prolonged delivery, prolonged labour or failure to progress to the second stage).
3. When the fetus has an abnormal position (occipito-posterior/occipito-transverse) which is delaying the progress of labour (this is the major use for Kielland's forceps).

Conditions that must exist prior to application of forceps

1. The cervix must be fully dilated.
2. The fetal head must present (except for forceps to the aftercoming head of breech).
3. The sagittal suture should be antero-posterior in diameter (except when applying Kielland's forceps).

4. The fetal head must be engaged in the pelvis.
5. The bladder and rectum must be empty.
6. The membranes must be ruptured.
7. The operator should be sufficiently experienced.

Before applying forceps, it must be ascertained that there is a reasonable chance of a normal vaginal delivery. Should there be any doubt in the mind of the operator as to the chance of success of the forceps delivery, then the patient should be taken to theatre, preparations made for a Caesarean section and a trial of forceps may be undertaken in the operating theatre with all facilities available for an immediate Caesarean section should any complications arise.

7.12 POSPARTUM HAEMORRHAGE

Postpartum haemorrhage is the loss of more than 500 ml of blood following the delivery of the infant. If this occurs within the first 24 hours, it is called primary postpartum haemorrhage. The causes of primary postpartum haemorrhage are:

1. Atonic uterus, which may follow:
   (a) Retained placental tissue.
   (b) Full bladder.
   (c) Prolonged labour.
   (d) Forceps or other traumatic delivery.
   (e) Grand multiparity.
   (f) Twins and polyhydramnios (causing overdistension of the uterus).
   (g) Antepartum haemorrhage.
   (h) Anaesthesia.
   (i) Relaxant drugs.
2. Trauma. Bleeding may occur from:
   (a) Episiotomy.
   (b) Perineal, vaginal or cervical tears.
   (c) Ruptured uterus.
3. Coagulation failure may follow:
   (a) Accidental haemorrhage.
   (b) Amniotic fluid embolus.
   (c) Intrauterine death.

Management of primary postpartum haemorrhage

1. Give ergometrine (0.25 mg) ergotrate or methergine by intramuscular or intravenous injection, except in cases of hypertension.

2. Set up an intravenous line and add 40 units Syntocinon or Pitocin to 1 litre Hartman's solution or Ringer's lactate.
3. Arrange for blood to be cross-matched.
4. Examine the patient for signs of uterine atony (bulky, soft uterus). If present, massage the fundus of the uterus (rubbing up the uterus).
5. Inspect the perineum and vagina for tears and lacerations that may be bleeding.
6. Determine whether the placenta has been removed, and if it has then inspect if for completeness — looking particularly for missing cotyledons, succenturiate lobes and possible fragmented membranes.
7. Ensure that the bladder is empty. A full bladder may inhibit uterine contractions.
8. If it is suspected that some or all of the placenta is retained *in utero*, arrange for an anaesthetic. Once the patient has been fully resuscitated a manual exploration and removal of the placenta is done. If no placental tissue is retained, the bladder is empty and the uterus is well contracted and the bleeding persists then a local cause for the bleeding should be determined.
9. If no apparent cause is found, then blood clotting should be checked.
10. If the uterus does not contract adequately, uterine rupture or retained products of conception should be suspected.
11. Finally, make sure that the vaginal and perineal lacerations are resutured. Care should be taken to reach the apex of any vaginal laceration when suturing, as it is a common site for continuing postpartum haemorrhage.

Secondary postpartum haemorrhage

This is dealt with in Chapter 9.

7.13 INTRAPARTUM HAEMORRHAGE

1. Placenta praevia.
2. A heavy show caused by the chorionic membrane shearing off from the decidua.
3. Tears and lacerations to the uterus, cervix and vagina.
4. Vasa praevia. In all placenta praevias the trophoblast obtains poor attachment to the lower segment decidua — the placenta is therefore often membranous in type, with fetal vessels coursing over the

chorionic membrane. Because these vessels may run across the cervical os, they may tear open when the membranes rupture, producing antepartum haemorrhage of fetal origin.

Management

Should bleeding occur during labour, a sample of the blood should be tested to ensure that it is maternal and not fetal blood. Blood taken is tested by means of the Kleihauer Betke test or its resistance to denaturing in the presence of an alkali solution.

7.14 SHOCK IN LABOUR

Any woman who has spent some hours in labour may develop shock, collapse or die. It is important to recognize that certain conditions and problems predispose to these catastrophes. However, a woman in prolonged labour who is poorly managed, becomes dehydrated, ketoacidotic and infected will also be a prime target for some hypotensive condition to occur. The causes of shock may be:

1. Blood loss.
2. Rupture of the uterus.
3. Endotoxic shock from gram-negative organisms.
4. Amniotic fluid embolus.
5. Intracranial haemorrhage (severe hypertension, rupture of a berry aneurysm during straining in the second stage).
6. Uterine inversion.
7. Cardiac failure (valvular heart disease and severe anaemia).
8. Pulmonary embolism.
9. Myocardial infarction
10. Adrenal crises.
11. Hypoglycaemia.

Management

This is related to avoiding the cause and making certain that the mother enters labour in a physically fit condition. By preventing the complications of labour, most of the causes can be prevented.

7.15 PRE-TERM LABOUR

Any labour that occurs before 38 weeks is regarded as pre-term. Approximately 7–10% of women will begin their labour between the

20th and 38th week of pregnancy and the perinatal loss in these labours is proportionate to the degree of prematurity. The survival rate for preterm infants at 28 weeks (1000 g) is 80%, 90% for infants born between 29 and 32 weeks (1200–1500 g), 95% for infants born between 32 and 34 weeks (1500–2000 g) and 99.5% over 34 weeks (2 kg).

Women may go into pre-term labour for many reasons:

1. Cervical incompetence.
2. Amnionitis (beta-haemolytic streptococcus or other pathogens).
3. Multiple pregnancy.
4. Polyhydramnios.
5. Any severe infection.
6. Pyelonephritis.
7. Congenital uterine abnormalities.

General management of pre-term patients

If the fetus is more than 34 weeks, the labour is allowed to continue. Should the patient be less pregnant than this, an attempt should be made to stop the labour to allow the fetus to gain a few vital weeks of maturity. Patients are:

1. Admitted to hospital for bed rest.
2. They are given a mild sedative such as diazepam.
3. If experiencing contractions they can be given Omnopon (papaveratum)/morphine or meperidine (pethidine).
4. Set up an intravenous drip.
5. A gentle vaginal examination should be done to assess cervical dilatation, but care must be taken not to stimulate further release of prostaglandins from the cervix. A digital examination is never done in the presence of ruptured membranes unless delivery is planned. After hydration, magnesium sulphate may be administered: 4–6 g as a bolus over several minutes followed by an infusion of 2 g/hour. A tocolytic such as salbutamol (Ventolin) or ritodrine may also be given. This has a specific stimulant effect on the beta-adrenergic receptors and thus relaxes smooth muscle.
6. If the membranes are ruptured a cervical swab should be taken after passing a sterile bivalve speculum under aseptic conditions.
7. Alert the paediatric staff that a pre-term infant may require special nursery care.
8. If the fetus has a gestational age of less than 34 weeks, it may be

advisable to give steroids intramuscularly to the mother to try and accelerate fetal lung maturity and thus prevent hyaline membrane disease.

9. Should the patient still persist with uterine contractions, consideration can be given to the judicious use of antiprostaglandin agents such as indomethacin (Indocid). This can be given as a suppository but care should be taken as there is a danger that prolonged use may lead to closure of the ductus arteriosus *in utero* and thus pulmonary hypertension.

There is also some evidence that beta-adrenergic agents themselves play some role in developing fetal lung maturity. Oral beta-adrenergic agents suffer from the problem of tachyphylaxis and this leads to down regulation of the receptors and the drug becoming less effective.

Prophylactic antibiotics are not given unless the cervical swab indicates infection. In the presence of ruptured membranes regular checks should be made to exclude infection and to monitor fetal well-being.

Analgesia and anaesthesia in obstetrics

C. R. Climie
Revised by *Stephen P. Gatt*

8.1 GENERAL INSTRUCTIONAL OBJECTIVE

The students should understand the principles of cardiorespiratory function and comprehend the use of analgesia and anaesthesia in obstetric patients to enable them to choose the most appropriate technique for each of their patients during labour and delivery, and, where necessary, to resuscitate such a patient.

8.2 SPECIFIC BEHAVIOURAL OBJECTIVES

1. Describe the pain felt by a labouring woman and indicate the physical and psychological factors that may influence it.
2. Know the clinical pharmacology of the sedative and analgesic drugs given by injection to the woman in labour, and appreciate the limitations and hazards associated with their use.
3. Know the basic clinical pharmacology of nitrous oxide and methoxyflurane as used for intermittent inhalation analgesia.
4. Demonstrate ability to employ Midogas nitrous oxide apparatus and Cardiff vaporizers for inhalation analgesia during labour and normal delivery.
5. Know the anatomy of the pudendal nerve and describe the techniques of pudendal nerve block.
6. Know the basic pharmacology and maximum allowable dosage of lignocaine and bupivacaine.
7. Describe the sensory nerve supply to the uterus and birth canal.
8. Describe the technique of lumbar and caudal epidural blockade, and exhibit knowledge of dangers and limitations of this procedure.

9. Demonstrate ability to perform local infiltrations of perineum with local anaesthetic agent.
10. Describe the indications for and hazards of general anaesthesia in obstetrics.
11. Demonstrate ability to assist anaesthetist at induction of general anaesthetic in obstetric patients.
12. Know causes of cardiac arrest.
13. Demonstrate ability to perform closed chest cardiac compression and expired air ventilation on training mannikin.
14. Demonstrate ability to diagnose and treat acute respiratory insufficiency.
15. Demonstrate knowledge of correct treatment of acute hypovolaemia.

8.3 THE PAIN OF LABOUR

Introduction

The only constant feature of the pain suffered by women in labour is its extreme variability. In any group of 100 labouring women, about 10 of them will have a rapid normal delivery with relatively little discomfort. Most of this group will have had previous confinements. Another 20 or 30 will be less fortunate. They will have a much longer labour and will suffer severe pain for many hours. Unless they are helped effectively, they will always remember their labour as a dreadful ordeal. The remaining 60 or 70 patients will experience something between these two extremes. Their contractions will be most uncomfortable and painful at certain stages and they will have a lot of pain during the actual delivery. However, with competent medical and nursing care, their degree of discomfort can be reduced to a tolerable level.

As with any other field of pain relief, an assessment of the severity of pain being experienced by a patient depends on observation of the patient's reaction and on her own description of the pain. Any complaint of pain must be given sympathetic consideration and relate both to the clinical situation and to the patient's personality.

The pattern of labour pain

In an average normal labour, contractions usually become painful when the cervix is dilated 3–4 cm, and the intensity of the pain increases as cervical dilatation proceeds. The last quarter of the first stage may be accompanied by severe pain.

After full dilatation of the cervix has been reached, the pain will change in character. As the presenting part descends onto the pelvic floor, the distension, stretching and tearing of the perineal tissues causes sensations of pressure and pain and an intense urge to bear down with the contractions.

The patient feels the pain of intense contractions not in the uterus but as a colicky pain across the lower abdomen. It is also frequently referred to the back and sometimes radiates down the thighs. It starts soon after each contraction begins, rises to a peak as the intrauterine pressure increases and dies away completely between contractions.

Factors that influence severity of pain of childbirth:

1. Physical factors
   (a) The intensity and duration of uterine contractions.
   (b) The resistance of the cervix to dilatation.
   (c) The resistance to distension of perineal tissues.
   (d) The presence of any degree of cephalopelvic disproportion.
   (e) Other obstetric conditions prolonging labour, especially occipi-to-posterior position of the fetal head, which produces a most distressing backache
   (f) Fatigue, anaemia, general debility and malnutrition influence the patient's tolerance to the painful experience.
2. Psychological factors
   (a) Cultural patterns and customs. A noisy patient is not neces-sarily having more pain than a silent one.
   (b) Antenatal education and emotional preparedness for labour. Fear, apprehension, ignorance and loneliness lower the tole-rance to discomfort.
   (c) The attitude of the patient's attendants, both medical and nursing. Cheerful, sympathetic and competent management will do a great deal to make pain more tolerable.

Nerve pathways

Pain of the first stage of labour is carried along fine unmyelinated fibres (from the uterus and the cervix) which gather together at the base of the broad ligaments. They pass via various plexuses to reach the lumbar and lower thoracic sympathetic chains, and then via white rami communicantes to the dorsal roots of the 11th and 12th thoracic nerves.

The pain of the second stage and delivery results from distension of the birth canal and stretching of the levatores muscles and perineum. Sensory nerve supply is provided by the pudendal nerve, which is a somatic nerve made up from the 2nd, 3rd and 4th sacral roots.

Anatomy of the pudendal nerve

The pudendal nerve is formed by branches of the 2nd, 3rd and 4th sacral nerves in the sacral plexus. It lies behind the ischial spine on each side medial to the pudendal artery, where it begins to divide into several branches. As it curves forward to the medial aspect of the ischial tuberosity, it gives off the inferior haemorrhoidal nerves, perineal nerves, the dorsal nerve of the clitoris, and the nerve to the labia majora.

8.4 PAIN RELIEF IN LABOUR

As far as the patient is concerned the desire for a healthy infant and adequate relief of pain are the most important aspects of her labour. The aim of any pain relief programme should be to reduce pain and distress to a degree that is tolerable and to ensure that the patient's recollection of her labour is reasonably pleasant. At the same time, there should be no added risk to mother or child.

Pain relief is not easily accomplished in all patients. It depends on a combination of three factors:

1. Education (antenatal classes);
2. Sympathetic and competent nursing care; and
3. Analgesia (by the intelligent use of drugs).

Natural childbirth

Various schools of antenatal preparation are followed by a large number of women who earnestly desire to have their baby by their own unaided efforts and without the need for drugs. Various forms of exercises are taught, and the belief that childbirth can be a pleasurable experience is promoted. The psychological preparation for labour involved in these regimens will result in a valuable reduction in the total amount of pain experienced by a considerable proportion of the women practising them. But many will not be able to carry on in labour without assistance, and it is most important that they should not feel that they have failed. Painless labour should never be promised to any patient who undertakes to study and practise a method of psychological preparation for labour. All obstetricians should have a general knowledge of the various methods that may be used by their patients, and, even if not themselves enthusiasts, should do nothing to destroy the patient's faith in her chosen regimen.

Hypnosis and acupuncture

These are two other methods of pain relief that have been employed. Unfortunately, the results have not been impressive.

Pharmacological analgesia

Analgesia may be systemic (by injections or inhalation), or regional (by the use of local anaesthetics and narcotics). Systemic analgesia raises the patient's pain threshold — the level of awareness at which any sensation becomes painful.

MILD SEDATIVES AND TRANQUILLIZERS

1. Diazepam (Valium)
   * Mode of action: Acts on central nervous system to reduce anxiety and apprehension. Anticonvulsant.
   * Dose: 10–20 mg orally. 5–10 mg intravenously.
   * Onset of action: Orally — 30 minutes.
   * Not effective when given intramuscularly.
   * Duration of action: 0.5–4 hours.
   * Advantages: Safe, few side effects.
   * Disadvantages: No analgesic effect. Hypotonia of the neonate.
2. Promethazine (Phenergan)
   * Mode of action: An antihistamine with a marked tranquillizing effect. Anti-emetic.
   * Dose: 25–50 mg intramuscularly.
   * Onset of action: 15 minutes.
   * Duration of action: 6–8 hours.
   * Advantages: The anti-emetic effects are useful in view of the emetic effects of narcotics.
   * Disadvantages: No analgesic action. Prolonged drowsiness.
3. Promazine
   * Similar in mode of action and use to promethazine.
4. Hyoscine (Scopolamine)

- Mode of action: Acts on the central nervous system, producing sedation and amnesia. Atropinic effects — drying of secretions.
- Dose: 0.4 mg intramuscularly.
- Onset of action: 15 minutes.
- Duration of action: 2–4 hours.
- Disadvantages: Causes disorientation. Rarely used in current practice.

NARCOTIC ANALGESICS

1. Pethidine (meperidine; Demerol)
   - Mode of action: Central nervous system depressant.
   - Dose: 50–150 mg intramuscularly.
   - Onset of action: 15 minutes.
   - Duration of action: 2–4 hours.
   - Side effects: Dizziness, nausea.
   - Disadvantages: Poor sedative action. Respiratory depression of the infant.
   - Pethidine may be combined with a tranquillizing agent (e.g. Scopolamine, 0.4 mg; or promazine, 25–50 mg) to improve sedation.   (Pamergan)
2. Morphine
   - Mode of action: Central nervous system depressant.
   - Dose: 10–15 mg intramuscularly.
   - Onset of action: 10–15 minutes.
   - Duration of action: 3–4 hours.
   - Side efects: Nausea.
   - Disadvantages: Respiratory depression of the infant.
3. Omnopon
   - Mode of action: Similar to morphine.
   - Dose: 15–20 mg intramuscularly.
   - Onset of action ⎫
   - Duration of action ⎬ Similar to morphine.
   - Side effects ⎪
   - Disadvantages ⎭

   Note: Narcotic antagonists are used to prevent or reverse respiratory depression of the infant. To achieve this they must be given either intravenously to the mother at least 20 minutes before delivery, or to the infant (either via the umbilical vein or intramuscularly).
   Naloxone (two preparations: Narcan, Narcan Neonatal).
   Dose: 0.4 mg to the mother, or 0.01–0.04 mg to the infant.

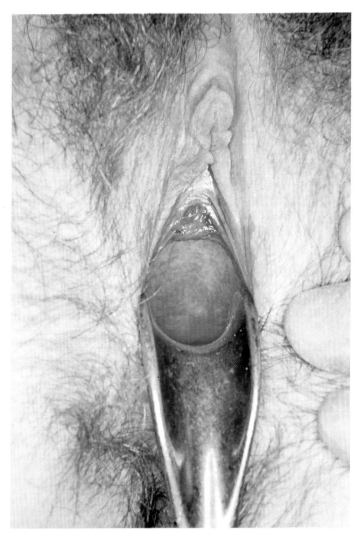

Colour plate 1 Senile vaginitis. Demonstrating senile vaginitis in a post-menopausal woman. Note the orange-red colour of the epithelium (the capillary network is close to the surface) whilst there is shrinking and loss of fascial support around the urethral opening.

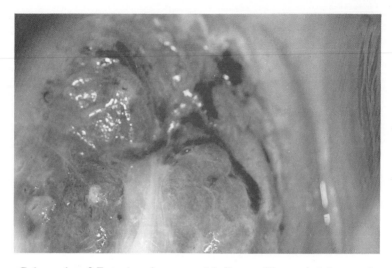

Colour plate 2 Ectopic columnar epithelium. The cervix is large and there is an old laceration of the os. Surrounding the os is a large area of columnar epithelium which has a 'velvety' appearance and is a deep pink colour. A cascade of mucus secretion can be seen running over the posterior lip of the cervix. Peripherally on the cervix the flat squamous epithelium has a pink-grey colour whilst there is evidence of metaplasia at the squamo-columnar junction.

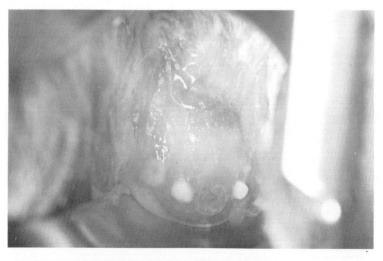

Colour plate 3 Monilial cervicitis. The cervix is covered with squamous epithelium of a mid-pink colour on which can be seen several white plaques of monilia and an increased amount of mucus secretion.

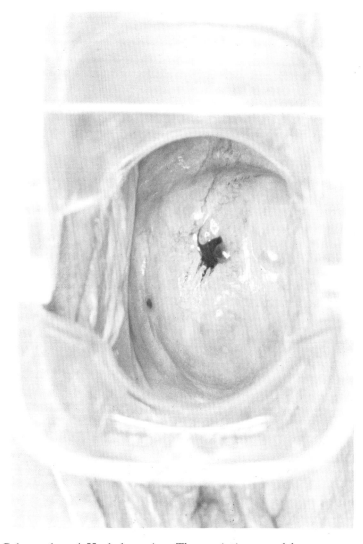

Colour plate 4 Healed cervix. The cervix is covered by squamous epithelium which gives the appearance of old scarring. This has occurred when ectopic columnar epithelium had undergone metaplastic change to squamous epithelium.

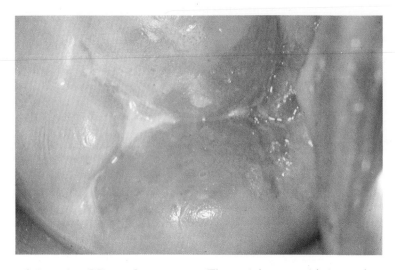

Colour plate 5 Signs of pregnancy. The cervix has a mauvish tinge to the squamous epithelium indicating an increase in blood supply to the cervix. There are previous lacerations to the os in an 'H' shape whilst from the endocervical canal, ectopic columnar epithelium is beginning to replace squamous epithelium. A thin grey physiological discharge is seen in the lacerated os.

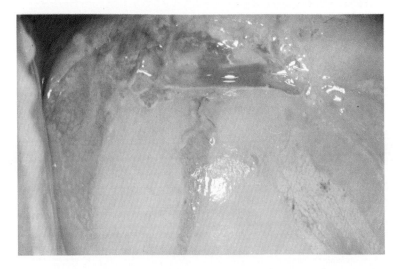

Colour plate 6 Dysplasia of cervix. An area of ectopic columnar epithelium surrounding the os has undergone partial metaplasia to squamous epithelium. However, at 4 o'clock, 6 o'clock and 7 o'clock there are areas of dysplasia on the cervix. The area of dysplasia at 4 o'clock has undergone a 'mosaic' change which is regarded as pre-malignant.

INHALATION ANALGESIA

This is administered via a mask held by the patient. It alleviates the peaks of pain. Inhalation analgesia may be necessary during the last quarter of the first stage and during the second stage, especially at the time of delivery.

It take 15–30 seconds for these agents to build up in the brain, so inhalation should be started at the onset of a contraction, rather than when the pain becomes severe.

Agents in popular use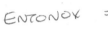

1. Nitrous oxide. This gas is contained under pressure in cylinders. Its release from the Midogas apparatus is activated by the patient inhaling from a closely fitting mask. The patient should be asked to hold the mask herself, so that if she becomes unconscious it will fall away from her face.
   - Action: Central nervous system action, producing first analgesia and, later, anaesthesia (if a high concentration is inhaled continuously).
   - Dose: The Midogas apparatus allows a maximum concentration of 70% nitrous oxide (N_2O) with 30% oxygen (O_2). At this concentration, provided that maternal respiration and circulation are adequate, maternal or fetal hypoxia should not occur.
   - Onset of action: May take up to 30 seconds, especially if concentration is less than 70%.
   - Duration of action: 60 seconds after cessation of inhalation.
   - Advantages: Quick action; safe with adequate O_2; no interference with uterine action; no fetal depression; does not build up in the body — can be used intermittently for several hours; suitable for patients with cardiac or pulmonary pathology.
   - Disadvantages: Mixture requires adjustment according to individual tolerance; expensive, complicated equipment which must be checked often.
2. Methoxyflurane (Penthrane)
   - Action: Used in a Cardiff vaporizer, 0.35% in air. Central nervous system effect, producing analgesia. If the concentration is high enough, or inhaled for a prolonged period, anaesthesia may result.
   - Advantages: Very potent analgesic.
   - Disadvantages: Pungent odour. Renal dysfunction is possible following prolonged continuous use.

Note: Points to remember in administering inhalation analgesia:

1. Antenatal education in use of apparatus, with revision when admitted to labour ward, is advisable.
2. Check that:
   (a) N_2O and O_2 taps are turned on.
   (b) Machine is turned on.
   (c) For methoxyflurane (Penthrane), check the contents of the vaporizer.
3. Check the fit of the mask on the face. If the face mask does not form a good seal on the face, ambient air will leak in around the mask and reduce the effectiveness of the gas.
4. Ensure that inhalation starts as soon as the contraction is felt.
5. Check the expiratory valve (it may stick).

LOCAL ANAESTHESIA

Local anaesthesia occurs when a drug produces a reversible blockade of conduction in nerves.

Conduction in all types of axons is blocked, but fibres of small diameter are usually (though not always) more susceptible to local anaesthetics and are slower to recover than fibres of larger diameter.

Action: Probably inhibits the transient increase in permeability of excitable membranes to sodium ions.

Metabolism: Esters (chloroprocaine, procaine) are hydrolysed by pseudocholinesterase. The products then undergo biotransformation in the liver. The amides (lignocaine, bupivacaine, mepivacaine) are metabolized by hepatic cyclo-oxygenase microsomal enzymes.

1. Lignocaine (Xylocaine, lidocaine)
   - Dose: Maximum safe dose is <u>3 mg/kg</u> (about 180 mg) — this may be raised to 7 mg/kg (450 mg) if the lignocaine is combined with 1/200 000 adrenaline. For example, if 2.0% (2.0 g in 100 ml) lignocaine with 1/200 000 adrenaline is used, the maximum safe dose for an adult is 27 ml. Lignocaine is available in concentrations of 0.5, 1 and 2%.
   - Onset of action: 5–15 minutes.
   - Duration of action: About 45–60 minutes following local infiltration and regional block and about 90 minutes following epidural block.
   - Advantages: Potent local anaesthetic.
2. Bupivacaine (Marcaine)

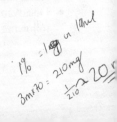

- Dose: Maximum safe dose is 2–3 mg/kg (120 mg)
- Concentration: 0.25, 0.375 and 0.5%.
- Onset of action: 15–30 minutes.
- Duration of action: Addition of vasoconstrictor does not seem to markedly attenuate duration of action. Prolonged (but variable) duration of action.

Complications of regional blockade (including spinal subarachnoid and lumbar epidural blockade)

1. Local nerve injury as a result of:
   (a) Adrenaline ischaemia.
   (b) Intraneural injection of local anaesthetic, or
   (c) Direct needle trauma.
2. Toxic reaction: Caused by the effects of a high plasma level on the CNS and CVS. Characteristics of a mild reaction include pallor, anxiety, nausea and restlessness, which may be difficult to distinguish from simple nervousness. In its more severe forms, CNS stimulation leads to convulsions, followed by drowsiness, unconsciousness, medullary depression, apnoea, and vasomotor collapse. Often the first observed indication of any overdosage is a sudden convulsion.

Hypotension and cardiac arrest may either be due to direct myocardial depression or due to effects on the medullary vasomotor control network.

Allergy or sensitivity to local anaesthetics is very rare; reactions are nearly always caused by overdosage.

Prevention of systemic reaction

1. Use the minimum effective concentration and do not exceed the maximum safe dosage. Check the dose and concentration before injecting.
2. Vasoconstrictors (e.g. adrenaline 1/200 000) prolong the action and result in lower plasma levels. Vasoconstrictors may, however, reduce placental blood flow.
3. Avoid intravascular injection by:
   (a) Aspirating the syringe before injecting.
   (b) Using a small, adrenaline-containing test dose.
   (c) Dividing the total bolus into several smaller incremental doses.

Local infiltration of perineum

Advantages

1. Maternal and fetal mortality and morbidity resulting directly from use of this technique is negligible.
2. Simplicity of administration.
3. Uterine contractions are not impaired.
4. No interference with the desire to bear down during labour.
5. Toxic effects are minimal provided safe dosages are not exceeded and the agent is not injected intravascularly.

Technique

The patient is placed in the lithotomy position. The fourchette and the adjoining area are first infiltrated using a 5-cm, 23-gauge needle. The infiltration is then extended in a fan-shaped manner.

Alternatively, if analgesia is required simply to perform an episiotomy, only the area to be incised need be infiltrated — with 0.5% lignocaine, the maximum amount being 40 ml (200 mg).

Pudendal block

1. Transperineal. First a small skin wheal is raised by injecting local anaesthetic into subcutaneous tissue on each side, midway between the anus and the ischial tuberosity. The index finger of the left hand is inserted into the vagina and the left ischial spine is palpated. A 10-cm, 20-gauge needle is guided to a point just below and beyond the spine. After drawing back (to exclude the possibility of intravascular location), 10 ml of 1% lignocaine are injected to anaesthetize the pudendal nerve. Repeat on the right side. Wait 10 minutes.
2. Transvaginal. A transvaginal guarded needle is guided to the ischial spine. It is held with the point just posterior and medial to the tip of the spine. The needle is then advanced until it touches the sacrospinous ligament, which is infiltrated with 2 or 3 ml of 1% lignocaine. It is then advanced through the ligament, and about 10 ml of 1% lignocaine are injected. Repeated on the other side. Wait 10 minutes.

Advantages of pudendal block

1. Relatively simple and painless procedure.
2. Anaesthetizes large area of vagina and perineum.

Disadvantages of pudendal block

1. Considerable failure rate; constant practice is necessary.
2. Inadequate for anything except the simplest outlet forceps.

Epidural anaesthesia

Is achieved by the introduction of local anaesthetic solution into the epidural space (outside the dura). A needle is inserted into this space in the lumbar or sacral (caudal) region.

There is diminished or absent perception of pain from the waist down with variable degree of motor paralysis. Uterine contractions continue, but the patient is not aware of them.

Attempts have been made to use this form of anaesthesia in surgery and obstetrics since the beginning of this century, but its major development has taken place since 1950.

Indications

1. Maternal distress caused by painful uterine contractions not adequately relieved by simpler forms of analgesia (pethidine, nitrous oxide).
2. To provide anaesthesia for a forceps delivery or vacuum (ventouse) extraction.
3. Pregnancy-induced and associated hypertension. Epidural anaesthesia is useful in reducing the amount of sedation required and also is helpful in lowering the blood pressure.
4. Caesarean section. The majority of Caesarean sections are performed under epidural anaesthesia.

Technique

Patient is positioned in left lateral position and flexed as much as possible to open up the intervertebral spaces.

After infiltrating skin with local anaesthetic, a large-bore (Tuohy) needle is introduced at right angles to the back in the midline at the L 2–3 or L 3–4 intervertebral spaces. It is advanced through the ligaments until the epidural space is identified by a sudden loss of resistance to injection through the needle. The anaesthetic solution is injected through the Tuohy needle, and an epidural catheter (a fine plastic tube) can be inserted through the needle and left *in situ* for subsequent injections. The needle is withdrawn.

Disadvantages

1. Instrumental delivery rate may be increased.
2. Maternal hypotension.
3. Accidental dural puncture.
4. Epidural haematoma secondary to bloody tap.
5. Post-dural puncture headache.

8.5 GENERAL ANAESTHESIA FOR OBSTETRICS

Indications

1. Caesarean section, when a regional technique is contra-indicated.
2. Need for full uterine relaxation (e.g. breech extraction; correction of transverse lie by intrauterine manipulation).
3. Manual extraction of the placenta.
4. When it is desirable for humane reasons that the patient should remain unconscious (e.g delivery of deformed infant).

Advantages

1. Fast.
2. Reliable and reproducible.

Disadvantages

1. Fetal depression.
   (a) Directly due to anaesthetic agents passing the placental barrier.
   (b) Secondary to maternal hypoxaemia or hypotension.
2. Danger of aspiration. Labour ward patients often have a full stomach — it is best to assume that all labour ward patients will have a full stomach. Although a stomach tube may be passed to remove stomach contents, it must never be relied upon. Cricoid pressure (Sellick's manoeuvre) should be maintained by an assistant, from the time of induction until an endotracheal tube has been inserted and the cuff inflated. Pressure on the cricoid cartilage will compress the oesophagus and prevent passive regurgitation of gastric contents. This method is only to be used on a paralysed patient.
   As a prophylactic measure, no solid foods or hypertonic fluids should be administered during labour. If aspiration does occur, one or both of the following problems may result:
   (a) Obstruction of the airway with large particles of food. Treat with suction, posture (head dependent), oxygen administration under pressure. Bronchoscopy may be necessary.
   (b) Mendelson's syndrome. After the inhalation of a small volume of highly-acid gastric contents, acute inhalation pneumonitis occurs. After a latent period of about one hour cyanosis, tachycardia, dyspnoea and pulmonary oedema supervene. Treat with

oxygen administration; 200 mg of hydrocortisone intravenously; intubation; intermittent positive-pressure ventilation; bronchial lavage.

3. Hypoxaemia from blood loss which can lead to acute renal failure and Sheehan's postpartum pituitary necrosis.

Emergency Caesarean section — an anaesthetic plan

PRE-ANAESTHETIC PHASE

1. Full pre-anaesthetic evaluation.
2. Ensure an intravenous (14–16 gauge venous cannula) infusion is running.
3. Ensure that blood is cross-matched.

IMMEDIATE PRE-OPERATIVE PHASE

1. Obtain adequate intravenous access — at least one 14–16 gauge venous cannula.
2. Displace uterus to the left — with a right pelvic wedge or by placing the patient in the left lateral position.
3. Adminster oxygen by facemask.
4. Start basic monitoring — blood pressure cuff, ECG, urinary indwelling catheter.

PRE-INDUCTION PHASE

1. Prepare and check equipment — including anaesthesia machine, suction apparatus and intubation and resuscitation equipment.
2. Monitoring — precordial stethoscope, CVP line, automated blood pressure cuff, intra-arterial line as needed.
3. Ensure that left uterine displacement is maintained — by inserting a right hip wedge.
4. Administer 100% oxygen by anaesthesia circle absorber system.

INDUCTION PHASE

1. Induce anaesthesia: 2–4 mg/kg thiopentone (thiopental) intravenously (IV), or 0.5 mg/kg ketamine + 2 mg/kg thiopentone IV.
2. Administer suxamethonium (succinylcholine) 1.5 mg/kg IV — do not pretreat fasciculations with a non-depolarizing muscle relaxant (as Caesarean section patients do not get muscle pain from

depolarizing muscle relaxants, because the fasciculations give a suitable end-point for intubation and because an increased dose of suxamethonium will be needed to guarantee intubating conditions).
3. Apply cricoid pressure (Sellick's manoeuvre).
4. Confirm tube placement. Start surgery. Start 50:50 $N_2O : O_2 \pm$ 0.75% isoflurane, 0.5% halothane, or 1% enflurane.
5. Improve monitoring — temperature probe, oesophageal stethoscope, twitch monitor. When suxamethonium wears off start non-depolarizing muscle relanant (e.g. 20 mg atracurium, 6 mg vecuronium, 2–4 mg pancuronium, or suxamethonium infusion).
6. At delivery, administer midazolam (Hypnovel) 0.05 mg/kg and fentanyl 0.5–1.0 µg/kg. Start infusing 20–40 iu Syntocinon per 1000 ml crystalloid. Change over to $70 : 30 \ N_2O : O_2$. Remove the uterus displacing wedge.

REVERSAL-EXTUBATION PHASE

1. Aspirate stomach contents using an orogastric tube.
2. Cease the suxamethonium infusion or reverse the non-depolarizer when neuromuscular twitch returns, using neostigmine (Prostigmine) and glycopyrrolate or atropine.
3. Extubate when ventilatory exchange is appropriate and patient is cardiovascularly stable and able to guard her airway.

General anaesthesia for forceps delivery

Usually epidural or other forms of local anaesthesia will be used, but general anaesthesia may be desirable, especially where speed or uterine relaxation is required.

REQUIREMENTS

1. Maximal oxygenation.
2. Minimal narcosis.
3. Relaxation of the pelvic floor.
4. Uterine relaxation if requested (uncommon).

TECHNIQUE

1. Mother breathes 100% oxygen via a face mask from a circle absorber system. Check the suction, laryngoscope and all connections.

2. Insert a cannula into hand or arm vein. Inject atropine (0.6 mg intravenously), followed by thiopentone (5 mg/kg) and succinyl choline (75–100 mg). Assistant applies cricoid pressure until the endotracheal tube is inserted and the cuff inflated. The patient is ventilated with nitrous oxide (50% in oxygen).

3. Paralysis is then maintained by intermittent injections of succinyl choline in doses of 20 mg. Once delivery is completed, spontaneous respiration is allowed to return, and anaesthesia may be deepened with an inhalational agent during the repair of the episiotomy. The endotracheal tube should not be removed until the patient is on her side and showing signs of consciousness.

4. Syntometrine or ergometrine is administered after delivery.

General anaesthesia for manual removal of the retained placenta

If severe blood loss has been experienced but has abated, the loss should be replaced before the anaesthetic is begun. Proceed as for the forceps delivery. Isoflurane, enflurane or halothane may be required to relax the uterus if oxytocics have been given.

DRUG USED

Inhalational agents.

ADVANTAGES

Good skeletal and uterine muscle relaxants. Rapid action. Non-irritant. Little tendency to cause nausea and vomiting.

DISADVANTAGES

Cardio/respiratory depression. Uterine relaxation may predispose to postpartum haemorrhage.

8.6 CARDIAC ARREST

This is failure of the heart to maintain an adequate cerebral circulation in any situation other than that caused by progressive and irreversible disease.

Causes

1. Central nervous system
   (a) Hypoxia from any cause.
   (b) Effect of analgesic or anaesthetic agents on cardiac and respiratory centres of the medulla.
   (c) Cerebrovascular accident (e.g. in eclampsia).
2. Cardiovascular system
   (a) Depressant effect of drugs on myocardium.
   (b) Heart failure due to increased peripheral vascular resistance and/or reduced venous return.
   (c) Acute cor pulmonale following pulmonary oedema.
   (d) Myocardial infarction.
   (e) Acute hypovolaemia due to blood loss or endotoxic shock.
3. Respiratory failure
   This is usually secondary to pulmonary oedema or depression of the medullary respiratory centre.
4. Electrolytic disturbance, especially hypo- or hyperkalemia.

Management

1. Make the diagnosis. Absent carotid pulse, unconsciousness and widely dilated pupils within 6–8 seconds, cessation of respiration within 10–20 seconds. At this stage cerebral circulation is inadequate and irreversible brain damage will occur if arrest continues for 3–4 minutes.
2. Ventilation
   (a) Place patient on her back on a firm surface — the floor if necessary.
   (b) Clear the airway — turn head to one side, remove false teeth, food, mucus, etc.
   (c) Mouth-to-mouth breathing — with head tilted back, nose pinched closed and jaw held forward. The chest should rise visibly. Repeat rapidly at first, but then continue at about 15 breaths per minute.
   (d) Hand-held resuscitators may be used instead of mouth-to-mouth breathing. Ensure:
       (i)   Firm fit of face mask.
       (ii) Clear airway (head tilted well back, jaw held forward).
       (iii) Good chest expansion with each bag inflation.
       (iv) Abrupt bag release for exhalation.

(v) Oxygen flow is set at 6 litres/min.

(e) Endotracheal intubation — when a skilled operator arrives.

3. External cardiac compression

(a) Elevate legs at an angle of 30° to improve venous return. Patient must remain on a hard surface.

(b) Using the heel of one hand, with the other hand on top of it, depress the lower third of the sternum sharply for up to 5 cm, hold briefly in compression and then release. Compression phase should occupy 60% of cycle. Repeat this compression about 60 times/min without pausing for ventilation which should proceed simultaneously. (If acting alone, 2 inflations to 12 chest compressions.) The cardiac output produced by cardiopulmonary resuscitation is up to 40% of normal.

4. Attach electrocardiograph (ECG) monitor and set up defibrillator. Begin drug therapy:

(a) For ventricular fibrillation. Apply generous amounts of paste to the electrodes, and massage paste over the skin. Place one electrode just below the right clavicle and the second just over the apex of the heart. Apply firm pressure. Contact must be avoided with the patient and the bed. Charge the defibrillator to 200 J or more, then discharge the countershock by the switch. If unsuccessful, give adrenaline (5 ml of 1/10 000 intravenously) and repeat shock.

(b) For ventricular asystole. Give calcium chloride or gluconate (5 ml of 10% intravenously) and adrenaline (5 ml of 1/10 000 intravenously). Both drugs may be repeated in 5–10 minutes.

(c) For electrolytic disturbance.

(i) Low potassium. Give potassium (10 mmol slowly intravenously) and propranolol (2 mg slowly) with atropine (1.2 mg).

(ii) High potassium. Give calcium chloride or gluconate (5 ml of 10% intravenously) and give insulin with glucose (3 g glucose for each unit of insulin).

5. Transfer patient to intensive care unit when spontaneous heart beat and adequate circulation have been restored. Controlled ventilation via an endotracheal tube may be necessary during the journey. The patient should be monitored continuously and accompanied by a competent medical officer.

Sequelae of successful resuscitation:

(a) Cerebral oedema and prolonged unconsciousness is very common.

(b) Renal damage (acute tubular necrosis).
(c) Trauma to ribs, lung, liver.

8.7 ACUTE HYPOVOLAEMIA

1. Administer oxygen by face mask.
2. Restore blood volume rapidly. While blood is being cross-matched infuse SPPS (if not available, use Macrodex, Haemaccel or normal saline). In extreme emergency, use group-specific or O Rh-negative uncross-matched blood.
3. Warm all intravenous infusions.
4. Use two or three infusion sites, with pump drip sets and large cannulae, if heavy blood loss is continuing.
5. When using large volumes of banked blood, coagulopathy may occur. Check clotting time and arrange for fresh blood.
6. Central venous pressure measurement will assist in preventing over-transfusion. This is most likely in elderly or toxic patients.
7. Monitor urine output. Oliguria persisting after restoration of blood volume may respond to intravenous frusemide (40 mg).

8.8 SUMMARY

This chapter looks at analgesia in labour and methods of anaesthesia available to obstetric patients. It gives a typical plan of action for a Caesarean section under general anaesthesia. Acute resuscitation in the event of cardiac arrest or acute hypovolaemia supervening is summarized.

Puerperal pyrexia. - Temp 38° + within 4/

Causes ① Genital tract infection
② Urinary tract infxn
③ DVT
④ Mastitis
⑤ Respiratory infxn
⑥ Unrelated cause

9

The puerperium

Leo R. Leader

9.1 GENERAL INSTRUCTIONAL OBJECTIVE

The students should understand the normal physiology and psychology as well as the pathological changes that occur in the puerperium so that assistance can be given to the normal mother and baby, as well as recognizing deviations so that appropriate management can be initiated.

9.2 SPECIFIC BEHAVIOURAL OBJECTIVES

1. Define the puerperium and explain the anatomical and physiological changes that occur during normal involution.
2. Identify by history and examination the normal progress of the mother and baby in the puerperium.
3. Discuss the emotional changes and needs in the normal puerperium.
4. Communicate with the mother and baby to provide them with physical and emotional support.
5. Explain the anatómical and physiological changes occuring during lactation.
6. Instruct the mother, and assist in the care and feeding of the normal baby in the puerperium.
7. Discuss appropriate advice on sexual relations and family planning for the normal puerperal mother.

9.3 REASONS FOR LEARNING ABOUT THE PUERPERIUM

The puerperium is the time during which the mother's altered anatomy, physiology and biochemistry returns to the normal non-pregnant state. By definition, it commences at the completion of the third stage of labour and is completed six weeks later. There are some variations within each organ system and complications of labour or delivery, exogenous drugs or hormones may alter the normal process.

9.4 NORMAL ANATOMICAL AND PHYSIOLOGICAL CHANGES DURING THE PUERPERIUM

Reproductive tract

UTERINE INVOLUTION

During pregnancy, the uterus increases in size and weight due to the effect of oestrogen, progesterone and chronic stretching on the myometrium by the enlarging fetus. The withdrawal of the sex hormones leads to tissue breakdown (catabolism) due to the increased activity of uterine collagenase and the release of proteolytic enzymes. There is an immigration of macrophages into the endometrium and myometrium. Involution of the uterus occurs as a result of a decrease in the size of myometrial cells and not as a decrease in their number. Following delivery, the uterus weighs about 1 kg and the uterine fundus is at the level of the umbilicus the day after birth. By 10–14 days the fundus should no longer be palpable abdominally. By six weeks the weight of the uterus has dropped to 50–60 g.

The net result of pregnancy is a slightly enlarged uterus due to the permanent increase in the number of cells, elastin in the myometrium, blood vessels and connective tissue.

Following completion of the third stage, uterine activity continues. For the first 12 hours contractions are well co-ordinated, strong and regular; but they decrease over succeeding days as involution occurs. Contractions of 150 mm or more have been recorded in the early puerperium and are accentuated during breast feeding (afterpains).

PLACENTAL SITE INVOLUTION

The placenta separates in the decidual layer. Following its delivery, the placental site contracts to 50% of its original area. This contraction and retraction results in the occlusion of the spiral arterioles (the so-called living ligatures). These processes are more important in the prevention of postpartum haemorrhage than the normal coagulation mechanisms. The placental bed becomes infiltrated by inflammatory cells and the layers superficial to this are shed.

Re-epithelization occurs from the glands and stroma in the decidua basalis. By 7–10 days, the uterine cavity has been re-epithelized except for the placental bed which does not completely regenerate until six weeks postpartum. The trophoblast and decidua are shed over this time and the uterine discharge is termed lochia. Usually it is blood tinged (lochia rubra) during the first 2–3 days but then becomes serous and pale (lochia serosa) consisting of some red blood cells, inflammatory cells, decidua plus bacteria and lasts for up to 20 days. After this the loss become thicker, more mucoid and yellowish-white in colour (lochia alba) and may last 4–8 weeks. The lochial discharge usually ceases about the sixth week as healing nears completion.

The lochia provides a good culture medium for bacterial infection but because of the cellular barrier, infection rarely occurs. Persistence of red lochia for more than ten days or the persistent passage of blood clots may indicate that placental site involution is not occurring properly.

CERVICAL AND VAGINAL INVOLUTION

Immediately after delivery, the cervix is patulous and haemorrhagic. It gradually closes down over the first week of the puerperium to a little more than 1–2 cm in dilatation. By the end of the second week the cervical os has closed. Most cervical lacerations will heal spontaneously. The external os is converted into a transverse slit.

The vagina, which as a result of overdistension by the fetus is bruised and swollen, regains its tonicity and rugal pattern and by the end of the third week has almost returned to its antepartum condition. The torn hymenal remnants are termed carunculae myrtiformes.

The perineum, whether torn, incised (episiotomy) or stretched, heals rapidly so that by 5–7 days it has healed.

Pelvic floor muscles

Voluntary muscles of the pelvic floor gradually regain their tone. Tearing or overstretching of these muscles at the time of delivery predisposes to prolapse. This effect is aggravated by interference with neuromuscular function as a result of nerve compression from the presenting part during the latter stages of pregnancy. It may take up to six months before the pelvic floor muscles return to their original state. Overdistension of abdominal skin may result in persistent striae (striae gravidarum) and divarication of the rectus abdominis muscles.

Urinary tract involution

During a normal delivery trauma to the bladder base leads to bruising, oedema and some detrusor hypotonia which may lead to difficulty with voiding. Care should therefore be taken to ensure that the bladder does not become overdistended as retention of urine further compounds the loss of tone. These problems may be increased by the use of epidural blockade and forceps delivery. It may be necessary to catheterize the patient to prevent this from occurring. During the first few days, due to a transfer of fluids from cellular to vascular compartments, a marked diuresis occurs. Dilatation of the ureters may remain for up to three months after pregnancy.

Cardiovascular changes

1. Coagulation. During pregnancy, concentrations of Factors I, II, VII, VIII, IX and X increase gradually. Following placental separation, consumption of coagulation factors and platelets occur at the placental site with a local intravascular coagulation. There are usually no major systemic changes due to coagulation factors but this predisposes to thrombosis during the puerperium, particularly if the delivery is complicated by trauma, sepsis or immobility.
2. Blood volume changes
   (a) Plasma volume. After delivery, the plasma volume decreases by approximately 1000 ml, most of this being due to blood loss during the third stage. Some patients may show a gradual increase in plasma volume, reaching a maximum of 900–1200 ml above the immediate postpartum values on the 3rd day of the puerperium, suggesting a transfer of extravascular fluid to the intravascular spaces. Plasma volumes have usually returned to the normal non-pregnant state by 6–8 weeks.
   (b) Red cell volume. The average red cell loss at delivery is about 14%. The sudden loss of blood leads to reticulocytosis with an increased erythropoietin level for about 1 week. The red cell volume returns to the normal pre-pregnancy level at about 8 weeks.
   (c) White cell count. A neutrophil leucocytosis occurs during labour and extends into the puerperium. The white blood cell

count may be as high as 25 000/μl with an increased percentage of granulocytes.

(d) Haemodynamic changes

   (i) Cardiac output. Immediately following delivery, cardiac output and stroke volume remain elevated or may even rise for at least 30–60 minutes. (This obviously depends on the duration of the labour and the method of delivery and varies from patient to patient.) These haemodynamic changes have usually returned to normal by approximately 6 weeks postpartum.

   (ii) Heart rate. The heart rate which normally increases in pregnancy returns to normal by about 6 weeks.

   (iii) Heart sounds. The physiological changes in heart sounds include increasing intensity of first heart sound with splitting, loud third heart sound, split second heart sound after 30 weeks and systolic flow murmur. These sounds usually disappear early in the puerperium.

   (iv) Blood pressure. Blood pressure returns to normal early in the puerperium.

Hormonal changes

1. Human placental lactogen (HPL) has a half-life of 20 minutes, and reaches undetectable levels during the 1st postpartum day.
2. Human chorionic gonadotrophin (HCG) has a mean half-life of 9 hours and falls below 100 iu/ml by the 7th day.
3. Oestradiol-17β falls to 10% of the antepartum level within 3 hours, and the lowest levels are reached by the 7th day. Follicular levels are reached by the 21st day in non-lactating women, although it is delayed in lactating women. The onset of breast engorgement at 3–4 days coincides with a significant fall in oestrogens.
4. Progesterone has a very rapid half-life, and is below luteal phase levels by the 3rd day.
5. Prolactin rises throughout pregnancy and reaches levels of 250 ng/ml or more. Postpartum, there is a gradual decline over 2 weeks in non-lactating women. Nipple stimulation causes increased prolactin secretion, although levels are diminished after several months of lactation. Increased levels of prolactin have been associated with the relative refractoriness of the puerperal ovary. This would appear to be an anti-gonadotrophic effect of prolactin at the suprasellar or pituitary levels (rather than a direct effect on the

ovary), causing a disturbance in the cyclical release of luteinizing hormone (LH).

6. Thyroid-stimulation hormone (TSH) levels are very low in all women during the first 2 weeks postpartum. Levels increase slowly, and reach the follicular phase during the 3rd week. The onset of menstruation varies in lactating and non-lactating women. Usually the first menses follows an anovulatory cycle, and most non-lactating mothers will ovulate by 90 days.

Gastrointestinal tract

The gastrointestinal tract gradually regains its normal absorptive and contractile function. Constipation is common for 3–4 days and the result of dehydration, low oral intake, lack of tone and sometimes reflex inhibition of defaecation as a result of a painful perineum.

Psychological state

About 80% of patients experience some emotional lability (mood swings) in the puerperium, especially in the first week. Many patients experience depression or melancholia with bouts of crying (postpartum blues). This is regarded as a reaction of the physical and mental stress of childbirth together with the marked physiological changes that occur as a result of tissue breakdown and alteration of the hormonal level. A deep depression is seen in approximately 5% of patients and a frank psychosis in about 0.3%.

9.5 MANAGEMENT OF THE PUERPERIUM

Management in the first 24 hours

MANAGEMENT DURING THE FIRST HOUR

1. Prevention and control of postpartum haemorrhage. Five units of Syntocinon are usually give intramuscularly with the delivery of the anterior shoulder of the fetus. As the effects of Syntocinon wear off after a few minutes, ergometrine 0.25–0.5 mg is given intramuscularly after the delivery of the placenta unless there are maternal complications such as hypertension or cardiac disease.
2. Repair of any perineal trauma that has occurred during the delivery.
3. The parents are both encouraged to handle and touch their baby. This encourages bonding of the newborn infant after which it is

carefully examined and the parents are reassured that the baby is structurally normal.

4. The bedding is changed and the mother is given clean, dry clothing and made more comfortable.
5. Provided no complications have occurred, mother may feel like having something to eat or drink.

MANAGEMENT OVER THE NEXT 23 HOURS

1. Haemorrhage. Regular observation should be made of the maternal abdomen to ensure that the uterus remains well contracted and that an excess amount of bleeding does not occur.
2. Analgesia. The mother should receive adequate analgesia, particularly if she has had a Caesarean section or has had an episiotomy or perineal tear. Analgesia may also be required for postpartum contractions (afterpains).
3. Rest. It is essential that the mother has an opportunity to have adequate rest — particularly if she has had a long labour.
4. Urinary tract. Regular observation should be made of the patient's abdomen to ensure that she is passing adequate amounts of urine and that urinary retention does not occur. Should the patient be unable to void then the bladder should be catheterized before overdistension develops.
5. Maternal nutrition. The mother should be given adequate amounts of calories and fluid, particularly if she plans to breast-feed her infant.
6. Breast-feeding. Over the next 24 hours the mother is shown how to put the baby to her breast and encouraged to establish lactation.

Management over the next 6 days

1. Detection and prevention of sepsis.
2. Establishment of breast-feeding.
3. Prevention of deep vein thrombosis.
4. Rest — ensure that the mother gets adequate rest, particularly if the baby is restless at night or she is being plagued by visitors.
5. Psychological support.
6. Physiotherapy — this is necessary if the mother has had an operative delivery.
7. Contraceptive advice — this is usually given prior to the patient being discharged from hospital.

Conduct of the puerperium

Following their discharge from hospital most patients are encouraged to maintain close contact with nursing staff at their community centre until lactation is successfully established. Rising hospital costs have led to a reduced duration of the traditional lying-in period, but even patients delivered by means of Caesarean section are discharged after 5–7 days, if there are no complications.

IMMEDIATE LABOUR WARD MANAGEMENT

Patients are kept in the labour ward until their vital signs (pulse and blood pressure) are stable, following which they are transferred from the labour ward provided there are no abnormalities which require close observation. During this time women should be encouraged to hold and cuddle their newborn infant. Should the mother so desire, she should be helped to suckle the baby for a short period of time. Provided the labour has been uncomplicated, a free choice of fluids is provided. If she has had an epidural anaesthetic then she is kept in the labour ward until she has voided at which time an intravenous infusion will be removed.

IN THE POSTNATAL WARD

Blood pressure, temperature and pulse are taken 4-hourly for the first 24–48 hours. Thereafter twice-daily observations are sufficient provided all readings are in the normal range. Each day the patient's breasts are checked, her uterine fundus is palpated to ensure that it is involuting appropriately. Her perineum is checked for evidence of infection and her calves are palpated to ensure that there is no evidence of deep vein thrombosis. The mother's psychological state should be observed, looking for signs of depression and instability.

Prevention of postpartum haemorrhage

Postpartum haemorrhage (PPH) is prevented by the judicious use of oxytocic agents in most pregnancies. Under normal circumstances 5 units of Syntocinon are given intramuscularly with the delivery of the anterior shoulder of the infant. Once the placenta is delivered, unless there are contra-indications, she is given Ergometrine 0.25–0.5 mg intramuscularly. Particular attention is paid to ensure that the uterus remains well contracted. Should any bleeding persist, the placenta should be examined for completeness and the fundus may be rubbed up manually to stimulate a contraction. A Syntocinon infusion of 40 units in 1 litre of Hartman's solution may be used to maintain uterine contraction.

Bladder care

Many patients are unable to void postpartum because of bruising to the urethra and the loss of reflex detrusor activity. They may not be able to relax due to perineal or abdominal pain or because of interference of bladder function due to an epidural anaesthetic. If the patient is unable to void, she should be catheterized under aseptic conditions as overdistension of the bladder must be prevented. If the residual urine is more than 500 ml, an indwelling catheter should be retained for 24 hours. Most women have a diuresis postpartum and therefore have associated frequency. Frequency may also, however indicate overdistension of the bladder. Should the residual volume be more than 100 ml after the patient has emptied her bladder, then an indwelling catheter should be left *in situ* for a period of 24 hours. If symptoms suggest a urinary tract infection a mid-stream or catheter specimen of urine should be taken for culture and sensitivity. If the discomfort is due to local trauma, then alkalizing the urine will improve these symptoms.

Psychological state

Soon after the infant is born, a physical examination should be made and the mother reassured that baby has no major structural abnormality. Even though the parents have seen and handled the baby they find this positive observation very reassuring. The sensation of touch, holding and cuddling their baby strengthens maternal ties as does early suckling of the baby. Observations should be made during this early postpartum period to ensure that there is normal parent to infant interaction or bonding. Mothers frequently experience quite marked emotional lability (mood swings) in the first week of the puerperium. Immediate elation of the postpartum period is often followed in a few days by bouts of crying (postpartum blues). This is usually seen as a reaction to the physical and mental stress of labour as well as being related to alterations in hormone levels, together with other marked physiological readjustments that are occurring. These emotional symptoms may be aggravated should the mother be experiencing physical discomfort from operative trauma, breast discomfort or lack of rest. The patient should be encouraged to breast-feed and many new mothers have negative feelings as to whether they will be able to cope with the awesome responsibility of taking care of their newborn child. They often fear that they will be unable to feed their infant appropriately and require a great deal of emotional and physical support from the staff. Postpartum depression is seen in approximately 25% of patients but a frank psychosis develops in less than 0.3%.

Patients who have had a history of postpartum mental illness should be referred for psychiatric assessment during the antenatal period as there is a high recurrence rate in the postpartum period.

Analgesia

Patients who have had an operative delivery require adequate analgesia. This may take the form of intramuscular opiates such as Omnopon 10–15 mg or pethidine 75–125 mg intramuscularly, 4–6-hourly. Perineal pain following an episiotomy usually requires either paracetamol or dextro-propoxyphene compounds which are more potent. A further source of discomfort are afterpains due to uterine contraction, particularly during breast-feeding. These require reassurance and mild analgesics.

Diet

Once the effects of sedation and anaesthesia have worn off, the patients may have a normal diet. Patients are encouraged to increase their fluid intake to overcome the lack of fluid intake and increased fluid losses which occur during labour and the postpartum diuresis.

Perineal care

Patients are encouraged to have perineal showers and sitz baths regularly throughout the day, particularly after defaecation. The use of infra-red lamps help relieve local discomfort and promotes healing. Episiotomy wounds rarely become infected unless haematoma formation occurs.

Bowels

Patients very rarely experience a desire to defaecate due to the mild ileus and decreased fluid intake that occurs during labour. The postpartum perineal discomfort and fluid shifts also predispose to constipation. Patients may be given oral senna (Senakot) or a rectal suppository on the 3rd or 4th postpartum day.

Rest

Early mobilization after delivery is encouraged even if the patient has had an operative delivery. This lessens the incidence of venous thrombosis and respiratory complications. Women often have difficulty sleeping as a result of the strangeness of the surroundings, concerns about her home and family or due to physical discomfort from surgical trauma. Appropriate measures should be taken to deal with all of these aspects. A mild hypnotic may be prescribed to ensure that the mother has adequate rest. Rooming-in is encouraged whereby the infant is in a cot beside the mother's bed for most of the day. This has the advantage of improving mother–infant relationships. However, should this proximity exacerbate the lack of sleep then the infant should be removed to the nursery to ensure the mother gets adequate rest. Some restriction may need to be placed on visitors if they interfere with maternal rest.

Postpartum immunization

1. If the mother's blood group is Rh-negative and she has no antibodies, and the baby is Rh-positive, she should be given 100 µg of anti-D immunoglobulin. Should there be any suspicion of a larger transplacental haemorrhage then the amount of fetal blood in the maternal circulation can be estimated and an increased amount of anti-D immunoglobulin can be given.
2. If the mother does not have an appropriate immunity to rubella then vaccination with a live attenuated rubella virus can be undertaken in the puerperium.

Physiotherapy and postnatal exercises

These are usually a continuation of the antenatal exercises designed to improve involution and restore tone to the abdominal and pelvic muscles. Deep breathing and leg exercises help to prevent venous thrombosis and chest complications. These are usually supervised by the physiotherapist and should be carried out on a daily basis.

Puerperal infection

DETECTION AND PREVENTION OF POSTPARTUM INFECTION

Puerperal pyrexia is defined as a rise of temperature to 38 °C on two or more occasions after the first 24 hours of labour. This may be due to a number of different causes so careful physical examination and investigations are required.

Puerperal infection is usually due to an infection of the genital tract. The commonest sites are:

1. Genital tract infection.
2. Urinary tract infection.
3. Breast infection.
4. Respiratory infection.
5. Thrombophlebitis and venous thrombosis.
6. Other causes of pyrexia.

Due to shorter labours, better labour ward techniques and the availability of potent antibiotics genital tract infections occur in only about 1–3% of patients.

The commonest pathogens are:

1. Streptococci, both anaerobic and on occasion the β-haemolytic streptococcus.
2. Coliform organisms.
3. Staphylococci.
4. Anaerobic organisms such as bacteroides.
5. Chlamydia.
6. Mycoplasma.
7. Very rarely, *Clostridium welchii* can cause serious genital tract infection.

MODE OF INFECTION

In most cases infection arises as a result of invasion by normal bacterial flora. If the uterus contains some placental fragments, the growth of these organisms is enhanced. Spread may also occur from the blood stream or gastrointestinal tract.

In the remaining cases the cause may be exogenous — from the attendants or the patient herself.

CLINICAL FEATURES

Infection may be localized in the following sites:

Lower genital tract

Vulva and vagina. The commonest site is the episiotomy which becomes infected usually as the result of haematoma formation. It becomes red and swollen and painful. Treatment usually consists of local cleaning and appropriate antibiotics. Infected wounds usually heal extremely well, but occasionally superficial dyspareunia may result.

Upper genital tract

Endometritis/parametritis/salpingitis. Most patients with puerperal infections have endometritis. This usually occurs at the placental site as this area takes longer to re-epithelialize. The myometrium is also relatively more resistant to bacterial infection. The infection usually occurs between 36 and 72 hours postpartum, and the clinical picture depends on the virulism of the organism. Usually some or all of the following features occur:

1. Pyrexia
2. Offensive lochia
3. Malaise
4. Tachycardia
5. Uterine tenderness

In puerperal infection due to group (A) or β-haemolytic streptococci, the lochia may be scanty and odourless, but rapid lymphatic spread and bacteraemia may occur.

COMPLICATIONS

Delayed complications of puerperal infection are:

1. Pelvic abscess formation
2. Pelvic thrombophlebitis
3. Paralytic ileus
4. Disseminated intravascular coagulation
5. Septic shock
6. Subsequent infertility

Salpingitis, pelvic cellulitis and pelvic peritonitis are seen less frequently now that antibiotics are usually administered much earlier.

MANAGEMENT

This usually consists of obtaining appropriate bacteriological specimens such as endocervical swabs and blood culture for bacterial identification and antibiotic sensitivity. Should chlamydia or mycoplasmic infection be suspected, then appropriate swabs should be taken for these. An intravenous infusion may be necessary, both for hydration and administering parenteral antibiotics. Until the organism and its sensitivity are known, a broad-spectrum antibiotic such as amoxicillin, either alone or in combination with metronidazole can be given. If there is excessive uterine bleeding and retained products of conception are suspected then digital evacuation of the uterus under general anaesthetic may be required.

9.6 LACTATION

Anatomical structure of the breast (Figs 9.1–9.3)

The mammary glands are specialized skin appendages which have probably developed from sweat glands. Their role is to provide nourishment for the new baby and to transfer antibodies from mother to infant.

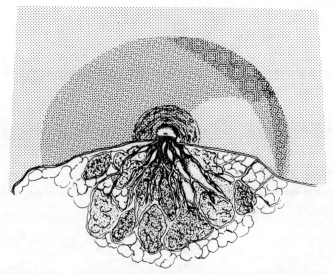

Fig. 9.1 Showing a schematic representation of the alveolar system and the collecting ducts draining to the nipple.

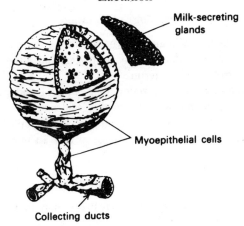

Fig. 9.2 Lactating alveolus.

Each gland is divided into 15–20 lobes, each of which is further subdivided into a number of lobules. Each of these are made up of masses of milk-secreting units known as alveoli. These cells take up the substance they require to form breast milk from the maternal blood. Intralobular ducts lead from the alveoli and unite to form lactiferous ducts which are the main duct of each lobe. Under the areola each duct expands to form a lactiferous sinus which opens directly upon the surface of the nipple. The number of these openings varies from 6 to 15. The alveoli and main ducts are surrounded by contractile myoepithelial cells. The remainder of the breast consists of fat and fibrous septa.

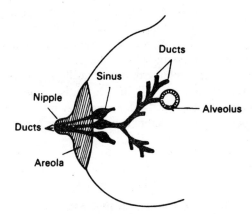

Fig. 9.3 The anatomy of the lactating breast.

Physiology of lactation

Mammary development begins just before the onset of puberty. The duct development is influenced by oestrogen and alveolar cells are under the control of progesterone.

During pregnancy, the secretion of oestradiol and progesterone stimulates both duct and alveolar growth. Besides these two hormones, prolactin, growth hormone, insulin, cortisol and an epithelial growth factor as well as human placental lactogen play an important role.

Breast changes in pregnancy

1. Enlargement of both breasts. Each breast may increase by up to 750 g in weight.
2. Increased blood supply. There is an enlargement of the veins over both breasts.
3. Montgomery's glands in the areola become more prominent.
4. The areola becomes more prominent and there is an increase in pigmentation.
5. Colostrum can be expressed. Striae may develop during pregnancy.

Colostrum

The pre-milk (colostrum) is an alkaline yellowish secretion that may be present in the last few months of pregnancy, and for the first 2–3 days after delivery. It has a higher specific gravity, higher protein, vitamin A, sodium and chloride content as well as a lower potassium, carbohydrate and fat content than breast milk. Colostrum contains antibodies which play a part in the immune mechanism of the newborn.

Milk is a complex fluid; it is a suspension of protein and fat in a solution of lactose and sodium salts. Human milk contains 87% water, the acqueous phase resembling dilute intracellular fluid, although the potassium levels are higher. Milk production is a monocrine process. Milk passes through the apical cell membranes into the acinar lumen (a similar process to the secretory activity of the pancreas and salivary glands).

Onset of lactation

Many physiological and behavioural processes are involved in lactation. At a local level in the breast it consists of three stages: the production of milk in the alveoli, the flow of milk along the ducts to the nipple and the withdrawal of milk by the baby.

Secretion of milk occurs after delivery (even as prematurely as 16 weeks of gestation) as a result of falling oestradiol, progesterone and human placental lactogen levels as well as the increase in prolactin levels. The milk usually comes in by the 3rd or 4th postpartum day. This may be associated with the breasts becoming full, tense and uncomfortable. Often the baby becomes unsettled for approximately 24 hours when the milk comes in due to the increased volume of milk produced. If suckling is delayed for any reason the onset of lactation may be inhibited. As local nipple stimulation leads to increased prolactin stimulation, the pain and fullness associated with the coming in of the milk needs to be differentiated from the pain that occurs early in the puerperium due to vascular congestion.

For milk secretion, the breast must elaborate specific milk components (lactose, fat, protein) from the plasma, concentrate and exclude

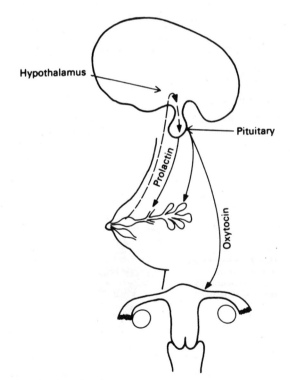

Fig. 9.4 The 'let down' reflex.

plasma substrates. Regular removal of milk prolongs secretion and some women have nursed for as long as 4 years. Should conception occur, lactation only continues until late in pregnancy.

Nipple stimulation following suckling leads to stimulation of the paraventricular nucleus of the hypothalamus and release of oxytocin from the posterior pituitary gland (Fig. 9.4). This leads to the let down reflex whereby oxytocin stimulates the myoepithelial cells to contract, which in turn assist to express the milk from the alveoli and ducts into the lactiferous sinuses where they are accessible to the infant. Therefore the baby obtains most of the available milk in the first few minutes of suckling.

Oxytocin release also stimulates uterine contractions, encouraging uterine involution and causing afterpains.

Mechanism of sucking (Figs 9.5–9.7)

Sucking produces a negative pressure, which draws the nipple and areola into the mouth of the baby and holds these structures in this position. By compression of the areola, and also the lactiferous sinuses, between the tip of the baby's tongue and the roof of its mouth milk is expressed from the sinuses. At the same time, the let down reflex is initiated and this helps to express the milk from the alveoli and ducts into the lactiferous sinuses.

Pain, fear, discomfort, anxiety, lack of privacy and many other psychological influences may inhibit the milk ejection reflex at the hypothalamic level.

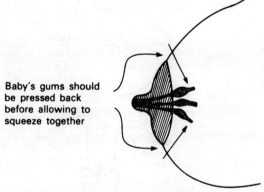

Baby's gums should be pressed back before allowing to squeeze together

Fig. 9.5 Demonstrating the technique which allows the baby to express milk from the breast.

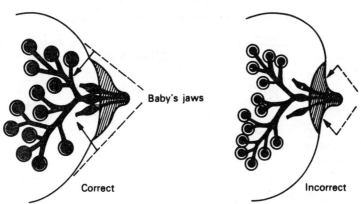

Fig. 9.6 The lactating breast, showing the correct and incorrect positions of the baby's jaws.

Because of the action of the milk ejection reflex, the baby will obtain most of the available milk in the first 5–7 minutes of sucking. Leaving the baby on the breast for periods longer than 10 minutes results only in the baby swallowing additional air, and may lead to colic.

With prolonged or excessive sucking, the nipples may crack, and so lead to considerable maternal discomfort.

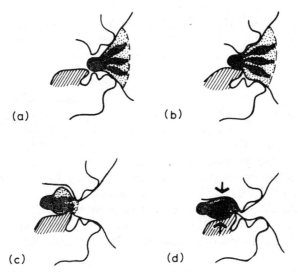

Fig. 9.7 Lactation. Demonstrating: (a) How the whole nipple is drawn into the mouth; (b) The gums close behind the nipple: (c) To squeeze milk from the sinuses and then; (d) The tongue compresses the nipple to obtain the milk.

Antenatal preparation for breast-feeding

During the antenatal period, instruction should be given about breast-feeding to avoid anxiety and fear of failure during the first few days of feeding when the milk production may not be adequate. The advantages and disadvantages of breast-feeding should be discussed with parents, but the ultimate decision should be made by the couple. The advantages of breast-feeding are:

1. Convenience.
2. Economy.
3. Emotionally satisfying to most women and may improve mother–baby relationship.
4. Helps contract the uterus and accelerate involution.
5. Sterile natural food which is easily available.
6. Passive antibody transfer.
7. Breast food is easily digestible and always at the correct temperature.
8. Errors in formula do not occur.

Disadvantages of breast-feeding are:

1. Disrupts activities.
2. Mastitis may develop.
3. Breast-feeding may not be possible if the infant is pre-term or has difficulty with sucking. However, the mother may express her milk which may be used until the infant is well enough to feed.

There is no convincing evidence that antenatal breast preparation increases the number of mothers who are successfully able to breast-feed. It is doubtful whether the skin of the nipples can be toughened by the application of any particular cream or lotion. Many patients find that exposure of the breast to direct sunlight prenatally and whilst breast-feeding has a positive beneficial effect on the skin.

Flat or inverted nipples may be gently regularly massaged and with gentle traction the patient may elevate the nipples during the latter part of pregnancy. Some people believe that nipple shields worn under the brassière for inverted nipples are of value. Patients require a firm, well-fitting and supporting brassière during pregnancy and lactation to support their enlarged breasts.

There is no evidence that regular manual expression of colostrum during the last few weeks of pregnancy is of any value in the initiation of lactation.

Breast-feeding technique and timing

Breast-feeding usually starts 8–12 hours after delivery, although suckling the baby after delivery may shorten the third stage and give the parents a greater sense of pleasure. The milk usually does not come in until 3–4 days postpartum. The newborn infant should be fed when hungry (demand feeding) if possible. This is not always practical in a busy nursery, therefore rooming-in is encouraged.

Both breasts should be emptied at each feed to avoid engorgement and milk stasis and promote milk production. As soon as the breast is empty feeding should cease so to avoid nipple problems — 5–10 minutes of suckling on each side is usually sufficient.

Prior to breast feeding the mother should:

1. Wash her hands with soap and water.
2. Cleanse the nipples with fresh water.
3. Assume a comfortable position for her and her baby.

Demand feeding or 3–4-hourly feeding is the usual aim, but each baby nurses differently so the guidelines need to be varied.

1. Usually 5 minutes at each breast is sufficient, initially increasing by a minute each day, not exceeding 10 minutes.
2. Compression of the periareolar area and expression of a small amount of milk, or colostrum into the baby's mouth may provide the stimulation to suck.
3. Place nipple well back in the baby's mouth, so that it rests against its palate where it can be compressed. The breast should be kept away from the baby's nostrils during feeding.
4. The infant can be removed by gently opening the mouth, and lifting the outer border of the upper lip to break the suction.

Diet

The maternal diet should be well balanced, with adequate food and fluid intake. There are no special foods that enhance milk production.

Drugs excreted in breast milk

Most drugs are excreted in small amounts in breast milk. Sedatives and analgesics used in normal therapeautic doses in the postpartum period will not affect the infant to any great extent. Antibiotics which are safe during the pregnancy may also be used if the mother is lactating. Alcohol, nicotine and caffeine all cross into breast milk.

Complications of breast-feeding

1. Inadequate lactation. The commonest problem encountered is inadequate lactation. Its origins are complex and may be due either to lack of milk production by the breast or the inadequacy of the let down milk reflex in response to suckling. The latter may be psychological, or due to pain or inadequate suckling. If the nipples are painful, manual expression or expression by means of a breast pump may be required until the nipples heal. If the nipples are not painful then more frequent feeding will supply extra stimulation. Oxytocin nasal spray may be used to induce milk let down reflex. Failure of milk production is much rarer and may indicate pituitary failure or systemic disease. Patients should be encouraged to increase their fluid intake. Drugs which increase prolactin secretion such as metoclopromide have been used to increase milk production.

2. Engorgement. Tightness and swelling which occur on the 2nd or 3rd day are usually vascular phenomena whilst their occurrence after that is usually due to milk retention within the breast, as well as lymphatic and venous stasis. This is an extremely painful and uncomfortable condition. The pain and swelling inhibit the let down reflex. Tightness of the breast flattens the nipples so that the baby is unable to suck thereby reducing stimulation.

   Management consists of emptying the breast either by manual expression or breast pump. It is also useful to use an oxytocin spray or 10 units of Syntocinon intramuscularly, 20 minutes prior to this. Appropriate analgesia is also necessary.

3. Mastitis. This is now much less common and affects only 1% of obstetric patients. The usual pathogen is *Staphylococcus aureus* which gains entry through the nipple fissures or ducts.
   The symptoms usually occur between 3 and 14 days after delivery.
   Signs and symptoms are:
   (a) Unilateral breast tenderness and induration.
   (b) Spiking fever.
   (c) Malaise.
   (d) The affected breast may be inflamed over the area of infection.
      Management consists of:
   (a) Culturing the breast milk.

(b) Antibiotics. Because the infection usually occurs with a hospital staphylococcus (which is usually penicillin resistant), cloxacillin or methicillin should be the drug of choice. If the infection has been acquired after discharge from hospital, large doses of amoxycillin can be given until the organism's sensitivity becomes available.

(c) Breast support. Prompt treatment may allow even a fulminating mastitis to resolve without abscess formation. Should an abscess form it should be drained. The baby may continue to breast-feed if the breasts are not too tender. It is important to empty the breasts and, if necessary, the baby should be fed from the non-infected breast and the milk expressed from the infected one.

Suppression of lactation

If the mother does not intend to breast-feed or if there has been a stillbirth then lactation can be suppressed. Stimulation of the breast should be avoided and mother should wear a good supporting brassière. Mild analgesic drugs may be necessary should some engorgement occur. This is all that is required in 40% of patients. Should the breasts become uncomfortable then bromocriptine (Parlodel) is the drug of choice. It is given in a dosage of 2.5 mg twice daily for 10 days. Bromocriptine inhibits prolactin synthesis and its release from the anterior lobe of the pituitary gland. Suppression of lactation with bromocriptine leads to an earlier return of fertility, which can occur as early as the 27th day postpartum.

Previously oestrogens were used to inhibit lactation but because of the increased incidence of thromboembolic disease, they have largely been abandoned.

9.7 THROMBOSIS AND EMBOLISM

Fatal pulmonary embolism is the major cause of maternal death, other than abortion. Two-thirds of these deaths occur after delivery, and one-third antenatally. Most emboli occur without any clinical evidence of pre-existing venous thrombosis.

Predisposing factors

Infection, venous stasis and altered coagulation predispose to thrombosis during pregnancy and the puerperium.

Infection may be the result of puerperal pelvic infection. If the external iliac vein is involved, phlegmasia alba dolens (white leg) may occur.

Stasis due to inferior vena caval obstruction is present throughout the pregnancy and may be compounded by enforced rest in bed if there are any obstetrical complications. These factors can be minimized by the use of leg exercises and early mobilization. The increased coagulation has been referred to elsewhere in this chapter.

Other factors are:

1. The delivery. Patients delivered operatively (whether by Caesarean section or forceps) have a higher rate of thrombosis.
2. Trauma to leg veins. From pressure by stirrups when the patient is in the lithotomy position.
3. Age. Older patients are more at risk.
4. Anaemia.

Clinical features

Venous thrombosis presents in several ways:

1. Superficial thrombophlebitis. This is probably the most common — and always occurs in varicose veins. It is probably a misnomer, because infection plays only a very small part in its aetiology. It is usually caused by venous stasis. Clinically, a superficial varicose vein is tender and thrombosed, with an area of redness surrounding it.

   Occasionally the long saphenous vein can be involved. Very rarely the superficial thrombosis may spread and be associated with deep venous thrombosis. This must always be investigated.

   Management consists of analgesia and encouragement of physical activity. Careful bandaging (from toe to groin) may give added support.
2. Deep venous thrombosis. This may affect either the vein of the foot or calf initially, but may spread to the thigh involving the iliofemoral vessel. It may also occur in the pelvic vessels. Clinically it may present with some or all of the following:
   (a) Pain in the calf.
   (b) Swelling.
   (c) Pyrexia.
   (d) Painful and swollen, cold, white leg. (This is due to secondary arterial spasm.)

(e) Swollen, warm, blue leg. (This is due to unimpeded arterial supply, with occluded venous return.)
(f) Thrombosis may present with a sudden pulmonary embolism.

Investigation: It is important to examine all puerperal patients for evidence of deep venous thrombosis. However, all signs and symptoms are most imprecise. Almost half of those patients with a positive Homans' sign will not have a deep venous thrombosis — and a similar number will have a false negative Homans' sign.

To establish a clear diagnosis, special investigations are necessary. The most frequently used ones are:

(a) Venography. This is the most accurate way of diagnosing venous thrombosis up to and including the common iliac veins. Its accuracy does depend on the experience of the operator.
(b) Ultrasound scanning. This utilizes the Doppler effect to detect blood flow in the vein, and is of greatest benefit above the knee.
(c) Radioactive iodine-labelled fibrinogen. The radioactive iodine (^{125}I) is taken up by the developing thrombus, and best defines the calf veins. Radioactivity counts are compared from one leg to the other.

Of these tests, the most widely available and useful is venography.

Management: Prophylaxis is important; early mobilization, avoidance of calf pressure, and regular leg exercises should the patient be confined to bed.

In high-risk patients (those that are obese, elderly, have cardiac disease or have had surgical procedures), prophylactic subcutaneous heparin can be given. This does not affect the whole blood clotting time, so does not need to be monitored. Its action is explained by the antifactor Xa-potentiating effect of heparin.

The use of dextran 70 infusion in surgical patients may also reduce the incidence of deep vein thrombosis, probably by altering the viscosity and platelet function.

Management of the thrombosis is by mean of intravenous heparin. This should be given as a continuous infusion, monitored by whole blood clotting times, thrombin times or partial thrombin times. Treatment is usually continued for 10 days. At present, haematologists advise introduction of oral anticoagulants 3–4 days prior to cessation of heparin. This should be continued for 3 months (for deep vein thrombosis) or 6 months if a pulmonary embolus has occurred. The effects of warfarin are monitored by means of the prothrombin index.

Streptokinase and urokinase have been used in an attempt to

dissolve the clot. Oral anticoagulants should be reduced slowly rather than ceased abruptly, because of the risks of rebound thrombosis.

Pulmonary embolism

The immediate effects of pulmonary embolism vary from subclinical to cardiac arrest and death, and obviously depends on the size of the embolism and the haemodynamic effects.

Symptoms are:

1. Dyspnoea
2. Cough
3. Pleuritic chest pain
4. Central chest pain
5. Haemoptysis

Signs are:

1. Tachypnoea
2. Rhonchi
3. Tachycardia
4. Pleural rub
5. Gallop rhythm
6. Loud pulmonary valve closure
7. Cyanosis
8. Elevated venous pressure
9. Fever
10. Systolic blood pressure less than 80 mmHg

Special investigations include:

1. Ventillation–perfusion scan.
2. Electrocardiogram — showing classical $S_1Q_3T_3$ changes, right axis deviation or right bundle-branch block.
3. Chest radiology — showing reduced vascular markings. A normal chest X-ray does not exclude a pulmonary embolus.
4. Blood gases — showing reduced arterial pO_2 + pCO_2 with an elevated pH.
5. Pulmonary angiography should be performed before pulmonary embolectomy is considered.

MANAGEMENT OF EMBOLISM

This depends on the severity and varies from external cardiac massage with oxygen, heparin, vasopressor agents and correction of acidosis with possible pulmonary embolectomy to heparinization alone and subsequent confirmation of the diagnosis. Streptokinase or urokinase may be therapeutic in massive pulmonary embolism.

The place of surgery (ligation, plication or thrombectomy) on the venous drainage is uncertain. It is certainly indicated for patients who have recurrent embolism from a proven lower limb thrombosis.

9.8 SECONDARY POSTPARTUM HAEMORRHAGE

After the first few days, bright bleeding occurring during the puerperium should be regarded as abnormal. Secondary postpartum haemorrhage can occur from 24 hours to 6 weeks after delivery. The amount of bleeding may vary from light to very heavy. The usual causes are:

1. Retention of placental tissue or membranes.
2. Infection of the placental site.
3. In the case of Caesarean section, the dehiscence of the uterine wound.
4. In later cases, choriocarcinoma is a rare condition which should be considered.

Treatment consists of admission to hospital and if the bleeding is only moderate antibiotics can be given in the first instance and the patient reassessed after 12–24 hours. If the bleeding continues to be heavy then surgical emptying of the uterus can be undertaken under antibiotic cover after appropriate cervical swabs have been taken. Care must be taken during this procedure, because of the risk of uterine perforation.

9.9 DISCHARGE

Before discharge from hospital, the patient should be thoroughly examined. If involution is occurring normally, the patient can be discharged after advice on normal activities and contraception.

Hygiene should be the same as practised in hospital. On discharge, most women find management of a new infant strenuous and require adequate support from their husbands. The usual household activities should be curtailed for the first few weeks until a routine with the infant is established. If possible, the mother should have a few hours sleep during the day. The doctor should be notified immediately of any onset of fever or bright vaginal bleeding.

Intercourse can take place whenever the couple feel so inclined usually after the lochia has subsided and all cuts have healed. Patients are usually advised to return for postnatal check at 6 weeks. At this stage contraception is discussed. Provided the mother is fully breast-feeding it is most unlikely that ovulaton will occur before 20 weeks. However, ovulation may occur as early as the 5th postpartum week if not breast-feeding. If the patient is breast-feeding then the mini-pill (progestogen only) is probably the best form of contraception. It does have the disadvantages that it may be associated with poor cycle control and a slightly higher pregnancy rate. Oestrogens, however, do suppress lactation and this outweighs the use of a combination oral contraceptive. The earliest reported time of ovulation as determined by endometrial biopsies is 33 days postpartum in non-lactating and 49 in lactating women. It appears that provided mother is still doing the early morning feed she will have some protection against ovulation from lactation. Mechanical methods (condoms, foams, diaphragms or IUDs) may be preferred by some nursing mothers.

Some women require permanent contraception. A tubal ligation can be performed easily in the puerperium with minimal disruption to the family, and only minimally increases the length of hospitalization. There is, however, an increased failure rate of sterilization when undertaken following a pregnancy.

Abortion, ectopic pregnancy and trophoblastic diseases

Barry G. Wren
Revised by *Michael J. Bennett*

10.1 GENERAL INSTRUCTIONAL OBJECTIVE

The students should understand the aetiology, pathology and clinical manifestations of abortion, ectopic pregnancy and trophoblastic diseases so that such conditions can be identified and appropriate management instituted.

10.2 SPECIFIC BEHAVIOURAL OBJECTIVES

1. List the types of abortion and discuss how to differentiate one from the other.
2. List the major causes for early abortion and discuss the possible steps in management.
3. List the possible causes of midtrimester abortion and discuss the management.
4. Examine a pregnant patient who is bleeding during the first trimester and make a diagnosis as to the likely cause of the bleeding.
5. Take a history from a patient who has had previous abortion and discuss the most likely causes for that abortion.
6. Discuss the differentiating symptoms and signs of ectopic pregnancy, acute salpingitis, torsion of ovarian cyst and abortion.
7. Discuss the presenting symptoms and signs of hydatidiform mole.
8. Discuss the complications and management of trophoblastic tumours.
9. List the steps necessary for the emergency management of a woman who presents with vaginal haemorrhage and signs of shock during the first half of pregnancy.

10. Counsel a woman, who has lost an early pregnancy, on the possibility for future normal pregnancies.
11. Discuss the aetiology and pathology of ectopic pregnancy.
12. Differentiate by description of clinical and pathological process how ruptured ectopic pregnancy varies in presentation to unruptured ectopic pregnancy.
13. Discuss the general management of women who have an ectopic pregnancy.

10.3 REASONS FOR LEARNING ABOUT ABORTIONS

Often a woman will present with a history that suggests pregnancy is present but may be in the process of being lost. This may be due to the expulsion of a normally implanted conception from within the uterus (abortion or miscarriage), from an abnormal site (ectopic pregnancy) or because the conception itself is grossly abnormal (hydatidiform mole). The understanding of the pathophysiology, the diagnosis and the management of these problems requires knowledge, skill and personal involvement on the part of the attending physician, otherwise the woman may suffer severe morbidity or even die if the appropriate management is not given at the right time.

Medical practitioners must be able to diagnose and manage women who present with abortion states, ectopic pregnancy or even a rare neoplasia of pregnancy. They will certainly see women presenting for the first time for assistance because of some abnormal pregnancy condition — and it is important to remember that the loss of a pregnancy can have very serious physical and emotional consequences.

Students of obstetrics and gynaecology who are given lectures and tutorials related to abortion, will see women in the outpatient clinics and the wards and will observe and assist in operations on women who are suffering from one or more complications of an early pregnancy. The students thus have the opportunity to observe and note the presenting history and signs, and can then become involved in the practical management of these conditions.

10.4 ABORTION (MISCARRIAGE)

When discussing abortions, nomenclature may give rise to some confusion, because the lay public tend to associate abortion with a criminal procedure, and miscarriage with spontaneous onset of the expulsion of the products of conception. The two terms are in fact synonymous and the definition for both is: 'the expulsion of the products of conception before the 28th week of amenorrhoea'.

A Threatened Abortion is said to occur when a pregnant patient bleeds vaginally. About 75% of women who threaten to abort carry on to a normal delivery.

An inevitable abortion occurs when a pregnant patient not only bleeds, but has uterine contractions sufficiently strong and painful enough to dilate the cervix, so that the products of conception will eventually be passed through the cervix.

An Incomplete Abortion occurs when a portion of the products of conception has been expelled through the dilated cervix but some products still remain in the uterus.

A Complete Abortion has occurred when the products of conception have been completely expelled from the uterus.

A Missed Abortion occurs when the fetus dies but the products of conception are retained within the uterus, and either become surrounded with layers of inspissated blood or are gradually absorbed.

A Termination of Pregnancy (commonly incorrectly called an 'abortion') is caused by some interference to the implantation of the trophoblast or the decidua, is usually achieved by applying a negative pressure via a hollow plastic catheter and is more safely done in the first trimester.

A Septic Abortion occurs when organisms invade any retained products of conception. This condition may be life threatening.

1. A Threatened Abortion typically has the following symptoms and signs: There is amenorrhoea for 5 or more weeks, followed by a vaginal bleed. The bleeding may be slight as a faint brown discharge or as profuse as a heavy red loss with clotting. Pain is generally not present but there may be a dull ache or discomfort due to congestion of the pelvic organs. Unless the abortion is proceeding, the bleeding subsides and over 75% of cases continue to a normal delivery of a normal infant. The risk of pre-term labour and delivery, however, is three times higher than in women who do not bleed in the first trimester, i.e. 18% versus 6%.

2. Inevitable abortion. About 25% of women with a threatened abortion proceed to colicky uterine contractions, leading to cervical dilatation. Almost all of these women will lose their pregnancy. The

uterine contractions which are normally present from the beginning of any conception become vigorous and painful, the cervix dilates, bleeding continues and the pregnancy separates from its attachment to the decidua.

3. The next phase in the process is that of *Incomplete Abortion* in which the uterine contractions have continued the process of inevitable abortion. The cervix is dilated, there is continuing haemorrhage, uterine contractions persist and on inspection of the material that has been expelled, fetal and placental debris may be recognized. However, some products of conception are still present in the uterus, which is enlarged and soft. During the phase of inevitable and incomplete abortion, the patient may be found to suffer from shock with a low blood pressure and thin, thready pulse. She will be pale, cold and sweating and the degree of shock will be out of proportion to the observed blood loss. One of the rare causes of such a shock-like picture is the vaso-vagal effect of the products of conception passing through the dilating cervix. A vaginal speculum should be passed and, using a sponge-holding forceps, the material should be removed from the endocervical canal. This simple procedure will alleviate the features of shock if dilatation of the cervix is the cause. If despite this manoeuvre the patient remains shocked, then a search for the cause should be made elsewhere, i.e. hypovolaemia or septicaemia.

4. The final phase in the sequence is that of *complete abortion*, in which all the products of conception have been expelled. Bleeding slows and ceases, the cervix closes and the uterus becomes smaller and firm.

5. A missed abortion differs from the other stages of abortion in that although bleeding and possibly some dull lower abdominal pain may be present, the cervix does not dilate. Because the trophoblast separates from the decidua, the pregnancy dies but remains within the uterus. Layers of blood and clot usually form around the dead material to produce a hard mass of tissue, which may remain *in utero* for weeks, months or even years. When it is expelled, heavy bleeding may occur, which may be difficult to control.

Epidemiology of abortion

There are a number of facts known about spontaneous abortion and these are important in the management of this condition.

Recent work indicates that as many as 50% of all conceptions come to grief. With the advent of radioimmunoassay of the beta sub-unit of HCG, it has been shown that approximately 30% of fertilized ova failed to survive long enough to cause a missed menstrual period. Since these very early losses have no specific clinical implications, it is best to concentrate upon the estimated 20% of recognized conceptions which terminate as spontaneous abortions.

The majority of intrauterine deaths occur during the first trimester and are primarily caused be serious genetic abnormalities. Chromosomal abnormalities have been observed in approximately 60% and 23% of spontaneous abortions ocurring during the first 7 and 8–12 weeks of gestation respectively. The majority of chromosomally-abnormal pregnancies lost are anembryonic (old term —blighted ovum) and are triploid. Chromosomal abnormalities continue to contribute to fetal mortality during the second the third trimesters but their importance relative to other factors diminishes. It is clear that a large majority of fetal losses are unavoidable, especially those which occur early in the pregnancy. However, current data indicates that the risk of loss is associated with a number of demographic and behavioural factors, several of which can be either directly or indirectly influenced by couples contemplating childbearing.

1. Maternal age. Many studies have shown that women under the age of 20 and over the age of 35 have a disproportionate number of fetal losses (including late fetal and neonatal deaths). Recent studies have shown that if an ultrasound examination is performed at or after 7 weeks of amenorrhoea (when a live fetus of 10 mm should be seen) and a normal continuing pregnancy is found, the risk of subsequent loss is very low, but appears to be related to maternal age. Under the age of 30, the incidence of loss of an ultrasonographically normal pregnancy is under 2% (1.8%) whereas over the age of 35 the incidence is more than doubled at 4.5%. In summary, the general risk of loss of an ultrasonographically normal pregnancy is approximately 3% but maternal age is an independent variable. Paternal age is not believed to play a role.

2. Parity. There is evidence that higher order pregnancies are at increased risk of loss and this increased risk is independent of age. This increase in loss rate is applicable throughout the fetal period.

3. Pregnancy spacing. Pregnancies preceded by either short or prolonged intervals suffer higher rates of fetal mortality. Current data suggest that the optimal interval appears to be approximately 12–36 months and that the most extreme rate of early loss occurs when

the interval from previous loss to next conception is less than 6 months.

4. Previous fetal loss. A woman who has had a previous spontaneous abortion is at an elevated risk of aborting her next pregnancy. The most straightforward explanation of this association is that some women are inherently at higher risk of loss, owing either to genetic or physical factors.

Causes of abortion

The simplest method of categorizing the various causes of pregnancy loss is to divide them into maternal, fetal and paternal.

Before doing so it is important to point out the error of a commonly held belief. For the last four decades many studies have been mounted to evaluate the role of various female hormones in cases of spontaneous abortion. To date, no normal pregnancy has ever been shown to have been lost as a result of abnormal hormone production. In addition, no study has been able to demonstrate any beneficial effect of the adminstration of either oestrogenic or progestational agents. Indeed there is clear evidence of teratogenic effects of such compounds as diethylstillboestrol and the synthetic 19−nor group of steroids. An expert writing in an English textbook in 1972 said, 'The idea of giving progestational agents for recurrent or threatened abortion is as illogical as the giving of hydrochloric acid to correct the achlorhydria of pernicious anaemia'. In 1980, two American authors wrote: 'The use of hormones in pregnancy without substantial evidence of benefit is no longer admissible. The evidence that prenatal exposure to female sex hormones may be teratogenic is strong enough to prohibit the use of such drugs.' Recently, an Australian author wrote: 'No normal clinical pregnancy has ever been shown to have been lost as a result of abnormal hormone production. The giving of powerful female sex steroids to pregnant women has absolutely no scientific foundation, is potentially teratogenic and cannot be condemned too strongly'.

MATERNAL CAUSES

General

1. Chromosome abnormalities. Balanced translocations may result in gametes with abnormal chromosome complements and therefore chromosomally abnormal conceptuses.

2. Hypertension. Women with chronic untreated hypertension have an increased risk of pregnancy loss when compared to normotensive women. Treatment may result in reduction of this risk.
3. Systemic lupus erythematosus. Women with this condition have an incidence of pregnancy loss as high as 40%. There is no evidence that treatment of the condition will reduce the rate of pregnancy wastage.
4. Thyroid dysfunction. Severe thyroid dysfunction is much more likely to be associated with abnormal ovarian function and resultant infertility. Occasionally spontaneous abortions occur in women with such dysfunction; appropriate treatment reduces the risk of subsequent loss.
5. Infections. Bacterial and viral infections producing systemic effects, specifically a pyrexia, may be associated with the demise of a fetus in the early part of the first trimester and subsequent abortion. Syphilis has a specific effect upon the pregnancy and in untreated cases results in early loss, then stillbirth and the subsequent birth of an infant with the stigmata of congenital syphilis.
6. Smoking. Although the regular consumption of more than 10 cigarettes daily is more often associated with intrauterine growth retardation, smoking women abort more frequently then non-smokers.
7. Alcohol. Heavy drinking (more than 100 g of alcohol per week) may be associated with the birth of a baby with the fetal alcohol syndrome; there is clear evidence that even moderate consumption of alcohol may be associated with spontaneous abortion. The combined effects of smoking and drinking (social habits often associated with each other) are graphically shown in Fig. 10.1.

Local

1. Cervical. Cervical incompetence is either of a functional or an anatomical nature. In this condition cervical dilatation usually occurs in the second trimester in the absence of overt uterine contractions — the so-called silent dilatation. With the support for the membranes at the level of the internal os lost, rupture occurs and is typically followed by a few contractions and expulsion of the fetus.

Cervical incompetence may be congenital (present in 30% of uteri with a congenital fundal abnormality) or acquired. The latter form is usually traumatic as a result of over-vigorous mechanical dilatation, e.g. lateral cervical tears at the time of delivery or

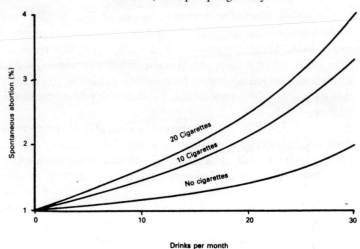

Drinks per month

Fig. 10.1 The effects of drinking and cigarette smoking on spontaneous abortion.

dilatation beyond 8–10 mm as is necessary for a second trimester dilatation and evacuation.
2. Uterine. Uterine anomalies are believed to be quite common but most do not result in reproductive difficulties. Nevertheless they are found in some 15% of women who abort more than once and are to blame for both first and second trimester abortions equally. Surgical correction of only some of these congenital abnormalities is possible but should only be attempted by those with expertise in this field since the literature shows that even in expert hands, 30% of such operations are followed by sterility.

Acquired uterine abnormalities such as submucous fibromyomata may also be associated with spontaneous abortion, and the judicious use of myomectomy may effect a cure.

FETAL CAUSES

For practical purposes this is a mixed group of fetal anomalies. Some 60% of spontaneous abortions are chromosomally abnormal. As many as 20% more are structurally abnormal, e.g. anencephaly, etc. The majority of spontaneous abortions are anembryonic (blighted ovum) and in these instances the fate of the fetus remains conjectural.

PATERNAL CAUSES

Chromosomal translocations in the father may also result in abnormal gametes and therefore abnormal conceptuses, as described for the mother. Approximately one couple in ten with a history of recurrent abortion will have one of its members exhibit a chromosome abnormality.

Over the last decade increasing interest in the immunology of reproduction has developed. Recent studies have revealed the possibility of an immunological cause for spontaneous abortion. Research has shown that women who recurrently abort, and in whom no other cause can be found, have a significantly different response to their husband's tissue antigens when compared to women who reproduce successfully. The foreign genetic material contributed by the father usually provokes the formation of a series of maternal blocking antibodies. In an apparently paradoxical fashion these antibodies seem essential to the normal continuation of a pregnancy and absence thereof is associated with the loss of an otherwise normal fetus. Studies in progress reveal that this form of rejection may be prevented by the intradermal injection of the husband's lymphocytes. This form of immunotherapy is still best regarded as experimental, although its use is being studied in some centres, because of the inherent potential risks attendant upon such manoeuvres.

Management

The management depends entirely on the stage at which the abortion presents. A woman with a threatened abortion should be reassured that three-quarters of such cases will carry on to deliver a perfectly normal baby, albeit with an increased risk of pre-term delivery. She should have an ultrasound examination performed which will confirm or refute the diagnosis of a continuing pregnancy. In the event that the ultrasound reveals evidence of a continuing pregnancy she should be advised to take it easy for the next few days until the bleeding ceases. The visualization of a fetal heart beat will almost always allay the anxiety associated with vaginal bleeding in early pregnancy. There is seldom an indication for admission to hospital under these circumstances. The ultrasonic evidence of a non-continuing pregnancy indicates the need for admission and evacuation of the uterus. When an inevitable or incomplete abortion is diagnosed, admission to hospital is indicated. Evacuation of the placental and fetal tissues is performed under a general anaesthetic. Blood transfusion may be required if haemorrhage is severe. When the risk of infection is high, antibiotics should be administered to reduce the risk of post-abortal sepsis. If sepsis is already present when the patient is first seen it is wise to treat with broad-spectrum antibiotics both before and after evacuation of the uterus.

Complete abortion needs no active management when diagnosed. However, a missed abortion should be evacuated under general anaesthesia. Care should be exercised when using a curette for a missed abortion, because bleeding may be heavy and transfusion may be required.

TERMINATION OF PREGNANCY

Termination of pregnancy by interference before the 20th week of pregnancy is commonly, though incorrectly referred to as an abortion. The termination of a pregnancy in New South Wales is still illegal, but the ruling given in 1971 by Judge Levine in the *Heatherbrae* case now allows a doctor to perform an abortion if, in his or her opinion, the continuation of the pregnancy is likely to cause harm to the mother or the fetus. Similar legal judgments in the UK and the USA have also liberalized the laws regarding the availability of termination in these countries. The earlier in pregnancy the termination is performed, the safer is the operation. If performed before 12 weeks the risk of major morbidity is only 1% whereas when a termination is performed after 12 weeks the major morbidity rate rises to 4%. The safest time to perform a termination is between 6 and 8 weeks of amenorrhoea; the safest person is a doctor who has an extensive experience in termination procedures; and the safest place is in a large institution such as a teaching hospital which has developed the special skills to handle the abortion procedures and the associated complications.

Complications of abortion (spontaneous or induced)

HAEMORRHAGE

This may be immediate and require blood transfusion, or may occur several days or weeks later due to retained placental tissue. In the latter case, the patient should be readmitted to hospital, transfused if necessary and then thoroughly curetted to remove any tissue. All such tissue should be examined in a pathology department to confirm that the debris is indeed innocent.

INFECTION

The commonest organisms that may be associated with all types of abortion are the coliform anaerobes: *Escherichia coli, Klebsiella* and *Streptococcus faecalis.*

Coliform organisms release endotoxins that cause endotoxic shock. The endotoxin is a lipid released (as a lipopolysaccharide) from the cell wall of a gram-negative organism, after the death or lysis of that organism. The lipid endotoxin acts as an antigen, in a complex reaction in which complement is utilized, histamine is produced, and lysosomes and kinins are released. This reaction results in increased vascular permeability and capillary dilatation, leading to a peripheral pooling and loss of intravascular fluid, as well as activation of the plasmin enzymes to produce hypofibrinogenaemia. The end result of such a reaction is stagnation and pooling of blood in the periphery, poor return of blood to the heart and eventual cardiac output failure. Shock (and often death) follows.

Because of the cellular reaction to infection, there is also an increase in leucocytosis. This causes cellular phagocytosis and release of lysosomal enzymes, which further increase tissue damage. This combination of hypofibrinogenaemia, capillary damage and phagocytosis leads to haemolysis, shock, cardiac failure, renal failure, bleeding disorders, cellular anoxia, acidosis and death. It is a serious complication and requires urgent and adequate management. The steps in management of endotoxic shock are:

1. Insert an intravenous line and begin transfusion with a volume expander such as blood, dextran or even saline/dextrose.
2. Insert a central venous pressure manometer to ensure that the circulatory blood volume is not increased to the extent where cardiac failure ensues.
3. Improve capillary tone and activity by agents such as cortisone or dexamethasone.
4. Use digitalis/digoxin as indicated.
5. Measure hourly urine output after inserting an indwelling catheter.
6. Take blood, cervical and vaginal, urethral and other appropriate culture material to identify the organism and obtain the antibiotic sensitivity.
7. Only after taking the appropriate swabs for culture should antibiotics be given. It is usual to begin with crystalline penicillin (2 million units every 4–6 hours) and an aminoglycoside such as

streptomycin, kanamycin or gentamicin. Care must be taken to ensure that the urine output is adequate when using these drugs.

8. Take blood for analysis of electrolytes and blood gas. Metabolic acidosis produces a very poor prognosis.
9. Remove surgically any focus of dead and infected tissue by D and C or hysterectomy if necessary.
10. Avoid using vasoconstrictors, as these are more likely to do more harm than good to the patient.
11. Check the haemoglobin and bilirubin, and transfuse blood as required.
12. Check the blood urea and creatinine levels. Renal failure may require dialysis.

TRAUMA

Another major complication of abortion is trauma, and is almost always associated with clinical abortions. The types of trauma may include vaginal lacerations, cervical tears, uterine perforations, avulsion of loops of bowel, and gas or fluid in the abdominal cavity.

In addition to the acute emergency procedures, it is important to remember the likelihood of long-term sequelae that increase morbidity and mortality. For instance, tubal occlusion and cervical incompetence may occur. Cervical incompetence is present when the internal os is forcibly dilated and torn. Future pregnancies may be lost between the 16th and 25th weeks of amenorrhoea.

Recurrent abortion

Formerly a patient was regarded as suffering from recurrent abortions when three or more successive pregnancies had been lost. Once this definition had been satisfied it was suggested that investigations be instituted. To-day, however, the expectations of couples intent upon having children is such that this definition should be modified and it is recommended that investigations should begin after two first trimester abortions or one second trimester abortion. A general practitioner may perform some of the more standard tests before referral to a specialist or may choose to effect referral immediately.

The basic investigations are indicated by the causes listed previously and are summarized as follows:

1. Karyotype both parents.
2. Hysterogram. (hysterosalpingogram)

3. Maternal blood for the presence of the lupus anticoagulant.
4. Serological test for syphilis.

It is wise to remember that many couples who experience spontaneous abortions develop profound emotional problems of which guilt is the commonest. They need careful patient handling and counselling, and need to be told that pregnancies are rarely lost because of what they might have done or not done.

10.5 ECTOPIC PREGNANCY

Ectopic pregnancy is the implantation of a pregnancy in a site outside the normal uterodecidual area (Fig. 10.2). It occurs in about 1 in 300 pregnancies. The common site is the tube, but a pregnancy may implant in the ovary, the abdominal cavity or the uterus, and may produce some bizarre symptoms and signs.

Like abortion, an ectopic pregnancy is usually associated with a period of amenorrhoea followed by bleeding and then pain.

The pathophysiological process of tubal ectopic pregnancy is as follows.

1. A normal ovum is fertilized near the site of ovulation and usually passes into the fimbrial end of the tube.
2. The zygote becomes blocked in the tube either by adhesions and agglutination of the endosalpingeal processes, or there is narrowing or spasm of the tube (isthmial implantation), or loss of the cilial processes of the endosalpinx. The zygote then develops into a blastocyst, which implants into the endosalpinx at about the 6th day after ovulation.
3. Following implantation, the trophoblast produces chorionic gonadotrophin. This maintains the corpus luteum.

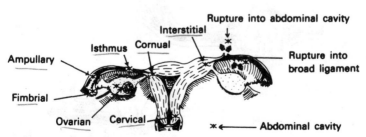

Fig. 10.2 Sites of ectopic pregnancy.

4. The corpus luteum produces oestrogen and progesterone, which changes the secretory endometrium of the uterus into decidua.

5. The trophoblast produces bleeding and necrosis within the tube at its implantation site, and the ectopic pregnancy begins to degenerate. The levels of chorionic gonadotrophin, oestrogen and progesterone fall, and the corpus luteum regresses.

6. The decreased level of progesterone induces a withdrawal bleed as the decidua breaks up and is shed. This withdrawal bleed from the decidua is the most common presenting symptom in ectopic pregnancy.

7. Occasionally the whole decidua is shed as a cast and the expulsion of this may resemble an incomplete abortion.

8. The trophoblast in the tube usually results in one of three processes occurring:

   (a) The trophoblast may die and be reabsorbed without any further management required.

   (b) It may be disrupted in the same way that an abortion separates from the decidua of the uterus. This leads to bleeding from the fimbrial end of the tube, peritonism and tubal abortion. Like an incomplete abortion, removal, or evacuation, is required. This type of ectopic pregnancy is by far the most common (80% of cases), and it is rarely associated with sudden shock from heavy blood loss.

   (c) The trophoblast may continue to erode into the endosalpinx until it passes right into the muscle surrounding the tube. If the pregnancy is still growing and enlarging, then rupture of the tube is likely to occur (Fig. 10.3). This type of case presents with acute pain and shock, requiring urgent operation and transfusion.

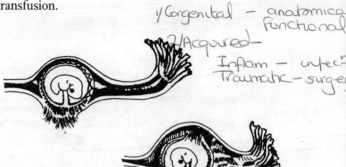

Fig. 10.3 Ectopic pregnancy. The trophoblast may invade the wall of the tube or pressure may rupture the tube into the abdominal cavity.

Symptoms and signs

An ectopic pregnancy usually presents with vaginal bleeding for several days, accompanied by vague lower abdominal pain. The bleeding is caused by decidua breaking down and the pain is caused by the tube distending and leaking blood (usually through the fimbrial end of the tube) onto the peritoneum. Patients presenting at this stage will be found to have amenorrhoea of up to 6–8 weeks and some symptoms of pregnancy. Examination discloses the cervix to be closed but soft and blood oozing through the os. The uterus may be slightly enlarged and softer. Movement of the cervix or uterus usually elicits an exquisite pain in the pelvis; this is due to the involvement of the serosal surface of the uterus with the peritonism that is associated with the free blood irritating the peritoneum. A small tender mass may be palpated in the tube. Difficulty may be experienced in differentiating these cases from those women who present with a threatened abortion. It may be some days before positive symptoms or signs develop.

If the ectopic pregnancy continues to grow in the tube, it may suddenly rupture. Blood striking the peritoneum then causes severe pain accompanied by shock. Hypovolaemic shock may follow if the intra-abdominal bleeding persists. Although only 15–20% of ectopic pregnancies present in this manner, it is the dramatic picture that most clinicians remember. The woman suddenly collapses with severe abdominal pain and, on recovering from the initial vasovagal shock, develops shoulder-tip pain and eventual hypovolaemic shock. This is a relatively uncommon manifestation of ectopic pregnancy, but one which is easy to diagnose.

Diagnostic procedures

There are several procedures that may assist in diagnosing an ectopic pregnancy:

1. A pregnancy test may be helpful in differentiating between ectopic pregnancy and follicular cysts, but is of no value in diffentiating threatened abortion from ectopic pregnancy.
2. A laparoscopy is of immense value before the tube ruptures or bleeds, but is of little help when blood fills the peritoneal cavity.
3. Where free blood is present, an aspiration (using a large-bore needle) through the posterior fornix of the vagina into the pouch of Douglas may be of immense help.
4. Ultrasound, with enhanced resolution, has become an invaluable diagnostic aid.

Management

1. Admit to hospital.
2. Cross-match blood.
3. Transfuse if necessary.
4. Order relevant investigations if indicated.
5. When the diagnosis is confirmed, perform a laparotomy to remove the ectopic pregnancy. This usually involves removal of the tube and may often include an oophorectomy as well.

Sequelae

Following removal of an ectopic pregnancy, there is an increased incidence of infertility and subsequent ectopic pregnancies. Approximately 50% of women who have had an ectopic pregnancy find difficulty in conceiving again, and about 10% of those who do conceive suffer a further ectopic pregnancy in the other tube.

10.6 HYDATIDIFORM MOLE AND CHORIOCARCINOMA

Hydatidiform moles are neoplastic tumours that arise from the placenta. The villi become grossly hydropic and distend to form masses of vesicles resembling bunches of grapes. The trophoblastic tissue is highly active, having invasive properties and high hormonal activity.

The incidence of hydatidiform mole varies geographically. It is 1:600 in Hong Kong and Singapore, 1:2000 in the USA and about 1:800 in Australia. It follows from fertilization of an ova, so will only be found in reproductive women.

Although hydatidiform mole is considered to be a benign tumour of the placenta, it is pseudo-malignant due to its activity. The mole may invade the uterine myometrium or the parametria or be carried by the blood stream to deposit in a metastatic manner in tissue far removed from the pelvis.

Clinical features

1. The most common presenting symptom is uterine bleeding occurring between the 6th and 12th weeks of amenorrhoea. Other symptoms and signs of pregnancy are also present, so it is often first diagnosed as a threatened abortion.

2. The uterus is enlarged to a size greater than expected in 50% of cases, and may be confused with a multiple pregnancy. However, in 25% of cases the uterus is the size expected, and in the remaining 25% the uterus is smaller.
3. Because of the increased trophoblastic activity, there is an increase in hormonal levels. Nausea and breast changes are thus more marked, the incidence of pre-eclampsia is higher and occurs early in the pregnancy, and uterine contractions are more pronounced.

Diagnosis

This is usually made when a woman presents with amenorrhoea followed by persistent bleeding, usually after the 8th week of amenorrhoea. A search should be made for hydropic villi in the vaginal blood, chorionic gonadotrophin estimations should be ordered (these are usually increased) and an ultrasonic echogram should be performed (this usually gives a typical snow-storm picture pathognomonic of hydatid moles). Radiology and fetal doppler will give negative results.

Management

Admit to hospital, cross-match blood, and arrange for an evacuation of the uterus under general anaesthesia. A drip containing high doses of syntocinon must be kept running throughout the procedure, during which sponge forceps, suction curettes and blunt curettes are used to remove all the products of conception.

Following the initial evacuation, beta chorionic gonadotrophin tests (βHCG) are performed twice weekly for 4 weeks and then every two to four weeks for twelve months. A recurrence of a positive βHCG during the year is an indication to perform a further curette.

Moles that appear to be invasive or to show metastasis should be treated with a course of methotrexate. A hysterectomy is rarely indicated.

Choriocarcinoma

This is a rare malignant condition derived from trophoblastic tissue. In 50% of cases it follows hydatidiform moles, but only about 2% of moles ever develop in this manner. Choriocarcinoma is an anaplastic, invasive, highly mortal tumour. The use of methotrexate and surgery has reduced the previously high mortality rate to under 40%.

Any woman who has had a pregnancy that has terminated (whether by abortion, ectopic, hydatidiform mole or a normal pregnancy) and has persistent uterine bleeding should have a curettage and a βHCG to exclude the possibility of a choriocarcinoma arising in trophoblastic material.

Infertility and contraception

Barry G. Wren and Graeme J. Hughes

11.1 GENERAL INSTRUCTIONAL OBJECTIVE

The students should understand the physiology of conception and the factors that can prevent pregnancy so that they can initiate management of patients with infertility and advise patients about contraception.

11.2 SPECIFIC BEHAVIOURAL OBJECTIVES

1. Describe the structure and function of the human reproductive organs.
2. Describe the physiology of the menstrual cycle.
3. Describe the actions of the female sex hormones.
4. Outline the factors necessary for fertilization and implantation.
5. Outline the factors that may interfere with fertilization and implantation.
6. Discuss variations in the levels of human fertility and the factors that may influence it.
7. Discuss the investigation of an infertile couple.
8. Discuss those factors identifiable by history taking that are relevant to infertility.
9. Discuss the psychological factors and the emotional sequelae of infertility.
10. Describe the methods of contraception, their modes of action and their efficiency.
11. Discuss the implications of sterilization and its medicolegal aspects.
12. Discuss the complications of and the contra-indications to various methods of fertility control.
13. Discuss counselling of an individual and a couple in the selection of a contraceptive technique.

14. Discuss the problems of counselling a woman with a pregnancy following failure of her method of conception control.
15. Outline the management of common causes of infertility.

11.3 REASONS FOR LEARNING ABOUT INFERTILITY AND CONTRACEPTION

Approximately one couple in every six who wish to have a baby find that they cannot conceive after two years of trying, whilst almost every sexually active woman at some stage wishes to avoid becoming pregnant. It is because of the needs of these two groups of women that doctors must have the knowledge and the counselling skills to advise and manage these women.

11.4 NORMAL MENSTRUATION (FIG. 11.1)

The hormonal control of normal menstruation is fully covered in Chapter 13 but will be summarized here.

The anterior pituitary of a normal young woman will begin to produce follicular-stimulating hormone (FSH) at about the age of 11–12 years. This acts on the maturing ovaries to stimulate the growth of one or more Graafian follicles (Fig. 11.2), which in turn produce oestrogen from granulosa cells and theca interna. The oestrogen has effects on the physical, hormonal and psychological characteristics of maturing women. Breasts, hips, vagina, uterus and supporting pelvic tissue all develop and together give rise to the physical characteristics of young adult females. Concomitant with this physical development are the

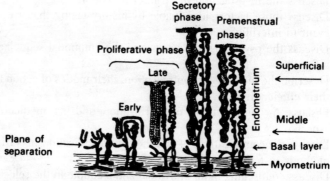

Fig. 11.1 The endometrial cycle.

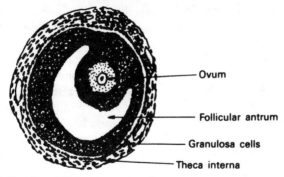

Ovum

Follicular antrum

Granulosa cells

Theca interna

Fig. 11.2 Graafian follicle near maturation.

psychological changes of femininity and sexuality. Oestrogen also plays an important role in the interaction with other hormone-secreting areas (by feedback on the pituitary and hypothalamus), as well as effecting bone epiphyseal closure and limitation of growth.

The effect of oestrogen on the endometrium and the anterior pituitary is discussed in this chapter.

Briefly, menstruation occurs in the following manner:

1. At the end of a normal menstrual cycle, the plasma level of oestradiol reaches its lowest concentration. The plasma progesterone concentration has also fallen to a low level.
2. Under these circumstances the arcuate nucleus in the hypothalamus produces pulses of gonadotrophin-releasing hormone (GnRH) every 90 minutes.
3. This releasing hormone activates the basophil cells of the anterior pituitary to secrete FSH and luteinizing hormone (LH).
4. FSH stimulates the growth of follicles in the ovary and increases the protein that binds sex steroids in the ovary.
5. By attachment to cell membrane receptors LH causes the release of adenyl cyclase. This enzyme controls the reaction in which adenosine triphosphate (ATP) forms cyclic adenosine monophosphate (AMP) which stimulates the theca interna cells of the ovary to produce oestradiol. While the follicles are small, they secrete only small amounts of oestradiol. As the follicles increase in size, the production of oestradiol increases.
6. These increasing levels of oestradiol act on the pituitary to modulate the level of FSH and LH being produced (negative feedback loop). Eventually however the level of oestradiol exceeds 150 pg/ml

for at least 36 hours. At this level the positive feedback mechanism overrides the negative effect and a surge of gonadotrophin is released from the pituitary.

7. The Graafian follicle responds to this surge of gonadotrophins by full maturation, massive oestradiol secretion, follicular rupture, ovulation, corpus luteum formation and progesterone production. Because progesterone inhibits any new follicular development, a new cycle is not begun (even though gonadotrophins are still being produced in quantity) until the corpus luteum undergoes regression. This normally takes 14 days and at this stage a new ovulatory cycle begins again.

8. Whilst this whole system can continue to function in a regular cyclic manner every 28 days, there is no doubt that the midbrain can be profoundly influenced by higher centres as well as by other endocrine systems and hormones. These changes are probably initiated by changing the pulsatile release of GnRH by the arcuate nucleus.

Suckling, prolactin secretion and progesterone production act to inhibit or change the frequency of the pulses of GnRH and so interfere with the production of gonadotrophins by the pituitary. This ultimately interferes with the maturation of follicles within the ovary.

11.5 MODE OF ACTION OF ORAL CONTRACEPTIVES

Progestogens

– Progesterone not absorbed

Progestogens are thought to act by two main mechanisms:

1. They are inhibitors to the development and maturation of new follicles in the ovary.
2. They act either directly, or through other midbrain centres, on the arcuate nucleus of the medial basal hypothalamus. In this manner they interfere with the pulsatile release of GnRH and thus reduce the amount of FSH and LH being produced by the anterior pituitary. In this manner progestogens inhibit the development and maturation of follicles and thus prevent ovulation.

Ethinyl oestradiol

1. Ethinyl oestradiol given from the start of the cycle (i.e. commenced on the first day of menstruation) depresses both FSH and LH.

Ovulation will usually occur 10–14 days after stopping the ethinyl oestradiol.

2. Ethinyl oestradiol (0.1 mg daily) commenced on days 7–9 of a normal cycle produces an initial elevation in FSH concentration, followed by a marked decline. Following the cessation of oestrogen administration, there is a prominent rebound in FSH levels. Ethinyl oestradiol (0.05 mg daily) produces raised levels of LH in the plasma. Peak levels of LH will not produce ovulation unless the follicle is mature. However, the gonadotrophin luteinizes the follicle, with the consequence that a new cycle is commenced and ovulation occurs about 14 days later.

3. When ethinyl oestradiol is used to suppress ovulation, its effectiveness can be determined by measuring the total urinary oestrogen excretion per 24 hours. When follicular development is depressed, there will be no increase in total urinary oestrogens. When the dose of ethinyl oestradiol absorbed is only just sufficient to inhibit ovulation, there may be some follicular development and a rise in total urinary oestrogen. However, the rise in oestrogen concentration may not be sufficient to stimulate the surge of FSH and LH from the pituitary needed for ovulation. The rise in oestrogen under these circumstances occurs towards the end of the cycle.

11.6 TYPES OF ORAL CONTRACEPTIVES

In commercially available preparations, the two oestrogens used are ethinyl oestradiol and its 3-methyl ether, mestranol. On a weight-for-weight basis, ethinyl oestradiol is nearly twice as active as mestranol and has a slightly better therapeutic-to-toxic ratio. In order to produce consistent ovulatory suppression 0.05 mg daily of ethinyl oestradiol has to be given for 7–14 days prior to ovulation. The effectiveness of suppression of ovulation is highest when tablets are begun on the first day of the cycle (beginning of menstruation). However, oestrogens used alone may produce irregular, prolonged and unpredictable menstrual bleeding patterns. For this reason it is necessary to use a progestogen with the oestrogen.

Synthetic steroids that are capable of producing a secretory change in the endometrium are known as progestogens. A progestogen alone (in a dose equivalent to 0.4 mg of norethisterone) will suppress ovulation if given for a week prior to the expected date of ovulation. However, it is not commonly used because irregular bleeding, breakthrough bleeding and amenorrhoea may occur in 25% of patients. When the progestogen is used for more than 7 days, there is an increased frequency of breakthrough bleeding. To overcome these problems, an oestrogen is combined with the progestogen.

The combined type of oral contraceptive is the most common one on the market and includes all brands apart from the progestogen-only pills, such as Noriday and Micronor (see Table 11.1).

Table 11.1 Types of commercially available oral contraceptive (Dosages in micrograms)

Brand Name	Ethinyl Oestradiol	Progesterone			
		Norgestrel	N.E	N.E.A	E.D.A
Loestrin 1/20	20			1000	
Nordette	30	150			
Microgynon 30	30	150			
Brevinor/Brevicon	35		500		
Brevinor −1	35		1000		
Modicon	35		500		
Demulen 1/35	35				1000
Ovral	50	500			
Ovulen	50				500
Ortho-novum 1/50	50 (mestranol)		1000		
Biphasil	50	50 (11 tabs)			
	50	125 (10 tabs)			
Triphasil	30	50 (6 tabs)			
(Logynon)	40	75 (5 tabs)			
	30	125 (10 tabs)			
Tri-Norinyl	35	50 (7 tabs)			
	35	100 (9 tabs)			
	35	50 (5 tabs)			
Noriday			350		
Micronor			350		
Microval	30				
Microlut	30				

Marvelon	30 ethinyl oestradiol with 150 micrograms of desogestrel

N.E.   Norethisterone/Norethindrone
N.E.A.   Norethisterone acetate
E.D.A.   Ethynodiol acetate

11.7 SIDE EFFECTS OF ORAL CONTRACEPTIVES

Some women who are taking one of the many oral contraceptive preparations suffer from some of the side effects of either the oestrogen or the progestogen component. Table 11.2 summarizes the side effects and the best management of these problems.

Table 11.2 Side effects of oral contraceptives

Side effect	Cause	Management
Fluid retention	Excess oestrogen	Reduce oestrogen
Full, bloated feeling	Excess progestogen	Reduce progestogen
Nausea, vomiting	Excess oestrogen	Reduce oestrogen
Breast engorgement and tenderness	Oestrogen and progestogen	Reduce oestrogen and progestogen or give progestogen alone
Increased mucous discharge	Excess oestrogen	Reduce oestrogen or increase progestogen
Irritability	Excess progestogen	Reduce progestogen
Headaches, migraine	Excess oestrogen or progestogen	Reduce oestrogen and progestogen
Ectopic columnar epithelium	Excess oestrogen	Reduce oestrogen or increase progestogen
Menorrhagia	Excess oestrogen	Reduce oestrogen or increase progestogen
Weight gain	Progestogen	Reduce progestogen
Skin pigmentation	Oestrogen	Reduce oestrogen
Blood pressure	Oestrogen and progestogen	Reduce oestrogen and progestogen
Thrombophlebitis	Oestrogen	Reduce oestrogen, or cease the pill
Growth of fibroids	Oestrogen	Reduce oestrogen or cease the pill
Uterine or breast cancer		Cease the pill
Heart attack		Cease the pill
Liver disease		Cease the pill
Diabetes worsening		Cease the pill
Scanty menses	Excess progestogen, deficient oestrogen	Increase oestrogen
Loss of libido	Excess progestogen	Increase oestrogen, reduce progestogen

Table 11.2 cont'd

Side effect	Cause	Management
Breakthrough bleeding	Excess progestogen, deficient oestrogen	Increase oestrogen, reduce progestogen
Depression	Excess progestogen, deficient oestrogen	Increase oestrogen, reduce progestogen
Dry vagina	Deficient oestrogen	Increase oestrogen
Reduced breast size	Decreased oestrogen	Increase oestrogen
Acne	Increased progestogen	Reduce progestogen, increase oestrogen
Hirsutism	Increased progestogen	Reduce progestogen, increase oestrogen
Moniliasis	Increased progestogen	Reduce progestogen

The combined oral contraceptive depends on progestogen for suppression of ovulation. The oestrogen is added to prevent breakthrough bleeding and to promote a predictable and satisfactory menstrual flow 2 days after finishing the hormonally active tablets. The numerous commercially available preparations vary in their content of oestrogens and progestogens. Thus a patient who is sensitive either to progestogen or oestrogen may be placed on a preparation containing a lower amount of that particular hormone. However, lowering the dose of either hormone will give slightly reduced reliability.

It is not simply the weight but rather the activity and the amount of the hormone that needs to be taken into account when comparing the relative potency of the various available brands.

The sequential oral contraceptive is made of a sequence of oestrogen and combined oestrogen and progestogen tablets, commencing on the 3rd or the 5th day of the cycle (depending on the preparation used). Because it is begun so late in the cycle, a comparatively high amount of ethinyl oestradiol is used to ensure suppression. Progestogen is added on days 18–25 to produce a predictable withdrawal bleed. A serial formulation differs from a sequential one only in that placebo tablets, usually lactose, are used on the days when active tablets are not taken. This minimizes failure from forgetting to take the tablet.

Other hormonal preparations

Progestogen injections and implants act in the same way as the mini pill, or progesterone-only pill.

Postcoital pills contain high doses of oestrogens and progestogens and are taken within 72 hours of intercourse. This interrupts implantation of the ovum. Hormonal side effects are very common — 25% of women experience nausea and vomiting.

Coital pills are single doses of progestogen taken 5 hours prior to coitus. This gives protection from fertilization until 18 hours after ingestion. If coitus occurs 12 or more hours after ingestion, sperm may survive, causing fertilization.

Prostaglandins in effective doses can be used to produce an early abortion. They are thus abortifacients and not contraceptives. Their side effects of diarrhoea and nausea make them unacceptable generally.

Effect on plasma proteins

The steroid contraceptives act on the liver to alter the metabolism of protein synthesis and thus most plasma proteins are altered. This fact must be taken into consideration when interpreting the results of investigations carried out on women taking the pill.

The levels of the plasma proteins alter:

Albumin   — decreased
Ceruloplasmin — increased
Transferrin   — increased
Transcortin   — increased
Thyroxine   — increased

There is also an increased liver production of the substrate angiotensinogen. This results in an alteration in the renin–angiotensin–aldosterone balance, which may lead to hypertension in some women. Fortunately, these hypertensive changes are usually reversed when the pill is ceased. Other adverse effects include an increase in the coagulation proteins, with an associated increased risk of thromboembolism.

Oestrogen steroids also increase the production rate of certain lipids, particularly the triglycerides and the lipoproteins. Progestogen steroids appear to be involved in producing an elevation in the blood glucose levels.

All these metabolic changes are significant in relation to the following clinical conditions:

1. Monilial vaginitis is increased.
2. Diabetes may develop or be unmasked.
3. Existing diabetes may become less easy to control.
4. Heart disease and thrombosis appear to be slightly increased in cigarette smokers.
5. Existing liver and gall bladder disease may be aggravated. (When known liver or gall bladder problems exist, the pill should not be prescribed.)
6. Blood pressure may be increased and is probably related to the amount of progestogen in the combined pill. Fortunately, only about 3–5% of women develop an increase in blood pressure, and in most cases this is reversible when the pill is ceased.
7. Increase in the incidence of migraine headaches, particularly the premenstrual type. This is probably due to the fall in levels of progestogens prior to the onset of menstruation, and the resultant increase in aldosterone levels.

Side effects of the pill

1. Nausea. Due to too much oestrogen in the preparation being used.
2. Spotting (or breakthrough bleeding). Commonly occurs with low-dosage combined or progestogen-only pills. In these instances, there is not sufficient oestrogen to maintain the endometrium.
3. Absence of withdrawal bleed. When this occurs, it is usually due to the oestrogen level being too low to produce any proliferation of the endometrium.
4. Non-compliance. Some women find it difficult to comply with the usually accepted regimen of pill-taking. Their unanswered problems and fears require counselling and explanation, so that they may accept the regime.

Summary

The combined oestrogen/progestogen pills are probably the best and safest to use for the majority of women.

In prescribing any combination of hormones to provide contraception, the risks and complications of the therapy must be balanced against the benefits to be derived. In reaching such a decision, the following factors must be taken into consideration:

1. History of any medical disorders.
2. Prior menstrual history.

3. Feelings and fears expressed by the patient.
4. Symptoms or signs that develop whilst on the pill.
5. Development of complications whilst on the pill.
6. Risk factors due to the pill.
7. Side effects of the pill.

Oral contraceptives, besides providing adequate protection against pregnancy, also have the advantage that they regulate the menstrual cycle, can be used to prevent intermenstrual bleeding of hormonal origin, and can be used to ameliorate dysmenorrhoea due to increased uterine muscle activity. Preparations that contain high levels of oestrogens may also assist in management of acne conditions. Those that contain small quantities of oestrogen and relatively more progestogen may be of great benefit in treating women with endometriosis.

The risks of taking oral contraceptives include the possible suppression of hypothalamic activity, producing amenorrhoea, oligomenorrhoea and anovulation, with the associated increase in subfertility. Also there are the risks of an increase in hypertension, glucose intolerance and thrombosis, but these are rare.

11.8 OTHER FORMS OF CONTRACEPTION

1. Methods used by both partners
   (a) Continence.
   (b) Rhythm method. This is the avoidance of coitus around the time of ovulation. In a woman with a regular 28-day cycle, ovulation takes place on about the 14th day. Allowing for slight irregularities and sperm survival, intercourse should *not* take place from day 9 to day 19 of the cycle — or, to be safer still, from day 7 to day 21.

   Advantages: Acceptable to the Roman Catholic Church. Relatively simple procedure.

   Disadvantages: Cycles must be regular. Requires an intelligent patient. Requires continence during part of each cycle. High failure rate.
   (c) Billings method. Ovulation can be anticipated in regularly ovulating women when cervical mucus becomes thinner, and more elastic. This is usually accompanied by a cascade of mucous secretions and indicates ovulation is impending or has just occurred. Whilst it is reasonably reliable when used by intelligent women in conjunction with a temperature chart, it has a high failure rate and is not acceptable for most women.

2. Methods used by the male
    (a) Condom (Sheath, protective, French letter).
        Advantages: Simple to use. Male's responsibility. Mechanical barrier to infection.
        Disadvantages: Expensive. Diminished sensation. Lack of spontaneity. Failure rate, mostly due to faulty technique (defect rate 0.25–0.89). Danger of rupture (1 in 150–300 times).
    (b) Coitus interruptus (withdrawal method). This is probably the most common method used. Related to it are coitus interfemora and coitus reservatus.
        Advantages: Simple and easy to understand.
        Disadvantages: Much self-control needed by both partners. Often unsatisfying. High failure rate.
    (c) Vasectomy. Surgical removal of a section of the vas deferens, the remaining ends being turned back on themselves. The patient should be warned that sterility is not effective for at least 3 months, in which three seminal analyses, 1 month apart, must show complete absence of sperm.
        Advantages: Simple technique that can be done on an 'out-patient' basis under local anaesthesia. Little morbidity. Very effective.
        Disadvantages: Surgery is necessary. Male (and female) attitudes towards the procedure often prevent its acceptance. Not totally reversible (only in 30–40% of cases), so reversibility must not be expected. The possible death of a couple's children, or of a couple's possible divorce must be taken into consideration. Long post-vasectomy time before 'safe' period is reached. Theoretical possibility of late autoimmune effect to sperm.
3. Methods used by the female
    (a) The diaphragm. Once inserted, the diaphragm must be left in place for at lease 6 hours after intercourse and no longer than 16 hours, as the rubber and prolonged retention can cause an unpleasant discharge. The safest technique is to insert the diaphragm nightly. A spermicide should also be used.
        Advantages: Relatively simple to use. Woman's responsibility. Inexpensive.
        Disadvantages: Doctor is required to instruct the patient how to fit the device (Fig. 11.3). Must be used regularly. Anatomical variations may make fitting impossible. Psychological fear of touching the genitalia and general patient unwillingness may prevent use. Lack of spontaneity unless fitted nightly.

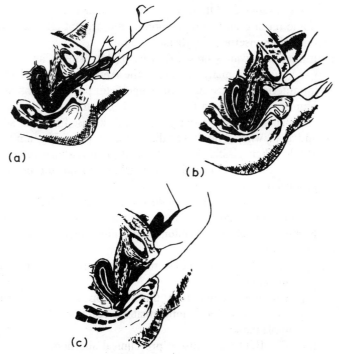

Fig. 11.3 Insertion of the diaphragm.

(b) Cervical cap. A plastic or metal cap fitting over the cervix and left in place for several days. A spermicide must also be used.

Advantages: May be left in place for days. Cheap and will last. Woman's responsibility.

Disadvantages: Doctor required to instruct patient and to fit the device. Not effecive for abnormal cervices. Technique difficult to learn. Psychological fear of touching the genitalia and general patient unwillingness may prevent use.

(c) Douches (postcoital). Water or chemical douching is very unreliable, and often induces pathological infestation of vagina by washing out the normal vaginal flora.

(d) Chemical. The types of preparations are:
   (i) Gels, creams and pressure-pack vaginal foams.
   (ii) Vaginal foam tablets.
   (iii) Vaginal pessaries.
   (iv) Sponge and foam.
   (v) Sponges and tampons with spermicides.
   Advantages: Simple to use. Most are inexpensive.

Disadvantages: Often messy. Equipment must be at hand. Some require much preparation. A few are not effective for a time after insertion. High failure rate.

(e) Intrauterine contraceptive devices (IUD). This is an age-old technique. For many centuries, the Arabs have placed small intrauterine stones in their camels to prevent pregnancy. Human experience in this century dates back to Grafenberg's first paper in 1928 (a ten-year series); he used rings of silver and gold wire. The IUDs did not gain popularity until the 1960s, when plastic devices (with flexibility, shape retention, ease of introduction and non-irritability to the uterus) were produced.

Mode of action: The mode of action of the IUDs is uncertain. They do not cause obstruction to sperm ascent, hormone imbalance or endometritis. Three theories have been put forward:

(i)   The IUD accelerates tubal peristalsis, so hindering implantation.

(ii) The encroachment of the IUD on the endometrium produces a local inflammatory reaction so inhibiting implantation.

(iii) The IUD may cause a pre-clinical abortion.
      The inert plastic IUDs do not cause cancer or fetal injury (if accidental pregnancy occurs).

Advantages: Usually easily inserted. Acts immediately after insertion. Complete return to normal after removal. Does not irritate either partner. Very good in those patients with little motivation. Effective contraceptive.

Disadvantages: Must be inserted by a doctor or trained technician. Expulsion may occur (in 10% of cases). Uterine perforation (1 in 2500 cases). Pelvic infection may occur (in 1% of cases). Side effects may be seen (40% of cases), such as:

(i)   Bleeding. Usually after insertion.

(ii) Pain. Abdominal cramps.

(iii) Discharge. Increased normal discharge.

(f) Intrauterine contraceptive device plus copper. Metallic copper is thought to greatly enhance the biological effect of the IUD (Fig. 11.4).

(g) Surgical sterilization.

(i)   Tubal laparoscopic cautery. The Fallopian tubes are cauterized in the isthmic region by using a laparoscope.

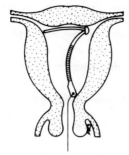

Fig. 11.4 Intrauterine contraceptive device 'Copper 7' in situ.

Advantages: Relatively simple. Little disturbance to the patient, as compared with the formal tubal ligation.

Disadvantages: Requires a general anaesthetic. Peritoneal cavity is entered. Possibility of damage to other organs. Expensive.

(ii) Tubal ligation, partial excision or excision.

Advantages: Relatively simple. Effective.

Disadvantages: Requires a general or regional anaesthetic. The peritoneal cavity is opened (abdominally or vaginally). There is an associated morbidity and mortality. Expensive.

(h) Hormonal contraception. Ovulation may be suppressed either with oestrogens or progestogens. These act at the level of the hypothalamic centres, suppressing the output of FSH and LH releasing factors.

SUMMARY

Table 11.3 Use and failure rates of methods of contraception

Contraceptive technique	Usage by at-risk population (%)	Failure rate, pregnancies/100 woman-years (%)
Combined pill	25	0.5–2.0
IUD	10	2–3
Condom	10	5
Diaphragm and spermicides	10	5
Coitus interruptus	20	30
Rhythm	5	30–40
None	15	60–70

11.9 INFERTILITY AND SUBFERTILITY

Infertility is the inability to conceive. Subfertility is defined as failure to conceive after one year of normal coitus. Of women desiring to become pregnant, 70% do so within twelve months and 85% within two years.

About 10% of all married couples will seek advice about fertility.

There are only four main questions that need be answered when investigating fertility:

1. Are there enough sperm? Subfertility in men accounts for at least 30% of infertility problems.
2. Is ovulation occurring? Endocrine factors causing anovulation account for about 15% of infertility problems.
3. Can the egg and sperm meet? Barriers to fertilization account for 40% of infertility.
4. Are there other, more subtle factors, preventing fertility? Unexplained infertility accounts for 15% or more of infertility.

Male infertility

INCIDENCE

About 1 out of 25 men has a problem with the reproductive tract.

TERMINOLOGY

- Oligospermia — decreased number of sperm.
- Azoospermia — total lack of sperm.
- Aspermia — absence of semen.
- Motility — ability of sperm to move.

CAUSES OF MALE INFERTILITY

1. Testicular atrophy (e.g. mumps orchitis, trauma).
2. Undescended testes.
3. Chromosomal abnormalities (e.g. Klinefelter's syndrome).
4. Epididymal block (e.g. from previous infection or herniorrhaphy).
5. Raised temperature of the testes (e.g. varicocele).
6. Sperm antibodies.
7. Unexplained or idiopathic is probably the commonest cause for male infertility.

INVESTIGATIONS

Two semen analyses should be performed. The first one (specimen A) is to test the man at his best. The count is done after four or five days' abstinence from intercourse. The second test (specimen B), to test the man at his worst, is performed within 48 hours of intercourse.

WHAT IS A NORMAL COUNT?

Volume: 2–5 ml
Density: 20–100 million sperms per ml of semen.
Motility: At least 50% should still move after 4 hours.
Morphology: At least 60% of sperm should appear microscopically
          normal.

Values lower than these do not preclude a normal pregnancy occurring, but if an abnormality is found, then a full urological examination should be performed.

TREATMENT

1. Donor insemination (DI)

This is a most successful form of treatment of male subfertility. Fresh DI has a 70% success rate over 12 months, but frozen sperm have a lower pregnancy potential. Sperm donors are usually anonymous to the female recipient, and are screened to ensure that there is no significant family history of genetic disease. Tests are done to exclude venereal disease. Sperm donations are frozen for at least six months so that AIDS screening can be performed before the donation is used.

The recipient has her time of ovulation assessed using temperature charts, cervical mucus and daily LH estimations. At her peak ovulatory time a small sample of sperm (usually 0.5 ml) is injected high into the vagina and occasionally through the cervix. The donors are carefully matched to some of the husband's physical characteristics including hair colour, eye colour, body build and race.

2. Artificial insemination by husband (AIH)

This treatment is less successful, with reported pregnancy rates of around 10–20%. It is used mainly for couples who find donor insemination ethically unacceptable. Highest success rates occur if the infertility is caused by impotence, hypospadias, retrograde ejaculation or cervical mucus hostility. Concentrating the sperm of men with poor counts does not improve pregnancy rates.

3. Drug treatment

The treatment of male infertility with hormones, anti-oestrogens and zinc has a low success rate unless a hypothalamic–pituitary insufficiency is present and appropriate treatment has been instigated.

4. Surgery

Varicocoele operations and sperm tube reconstruction have varying published success rates, and probably only improve the success rate in selected individuals.

5. Antibiotic therapy

If prostatitis or other genito-urinary infection is present then antibiotic therapy may improve the potential for fertilization.

Ovulation disorders

Ovulation is the physical rupture of one or more follicles within the ovary, allowing the egg to be released. Problems associated with ovulation account for 15% of infertility.

Provided a women has a normal uterus, only two things can happen, after ovulation has occurred:

1. Menstruation no later than 16 days after ovulation, or
2. Pregnancy

CAUSES OF ANOVULATION

1. Physiological
   (a) Before menarche. The hypothalamus has not yet initiated cyclic hormonal release.
   (b) Pregnancy. Amenorrhoea persists due to increasing levels of oestrogen and progesterone.
   (c) Lactation. Ovulation is suppressed due to prolactin inhibition of gonadotrophin production.
   (d) Postmenopausal. The ovary fails to respond to gonadotrophin.
2. Local causes
   (a) Surgical intervention: oophorectomy.
   (b) Excess irradiation: rarely seen now, but previously used in the treatment of menstrual problems.

    (c) Hermaphroditism: in this rare condition, both testes and ovaries coexist.

    (d) Pseudo-hermaphroditism: female genitalia exist with male gonads.

3. Genetic causes

Turner's syndrome: XO genotype, with dwarfism and webbing of the neck.

4. Endocrine causes

    (a) Cerebral. Emotional stress

    (b) Hypothalamic

        (i) Postpill amenorrhoea.

        (ii) Anorexia nervosa.

        (iii) Obesity.

        (iv) Marked or relatively rapid weight changes.

    (c) Pituitary

        (i) Hyperprolactinaemia. Excess prolactin is produced during lactation and from certain types of pituitary tumours. The prolactin depresses the release of the gonadotrophin releasing hormone.

        (ii) Acromegaly.

        (iii) Cushing's disease.

        (iv) Postpartum ischaemic necrosis of the pituitary due to haemorrhage, shock or infection following childbirth and sometimes known as Sheehan's syndrome.

    (d) Ovary

        (i) Premature Menopause. The average age for the menopause is about 52 years. If it occurs when the patient is under the age of 35, it is defined as premature. The diagnosis is made by high levels of FSH and LH and if confirmation is required in doubtful cases, then an ovarian biopsy will demonstrate complete absence of promordial follicles.

        (ii) Polycystic ovary syndrome (Stein–Leventhal syndrome). This involves amenorrhoea or oligomenorrhoea, obesity, hirsutism, infertility and enlarged ovaries.

        (iii) Arrhenoblastoma of the ovary. This is an androgen–producing tumour which inhibits the hypothalamic centre.

        (iv) Granulosa-cell tumour. These tumours produce excess oestrogen and, like arrhenoblastoma, are very rare.

    (e) Adrenal

        (i) Congenital adrenal hyperplasia. This condition is caused

by enzyme defects that prevent cortisol synthesis from progesterone, so leading to raised ACTH levels. This inhibits
ovulation.

(ii) Adrenal tumour, producing excess androgens and cathe-
cholamines.

(f) Thyroid

Both hypo- and hyperthyroidism may lead to abnormal feedback responses to the hypothalamus.

PHYSIOLOGY OF OVULATION

Gonadotrophin releasing hormone is secreted by the arcuate
nucleus and other areas of the hypothalamus and reach their target
organ, the pituitary, via the pituitary portal venous system. Follicle
stimulating hormone (FSH) is released and stimulates the development of follicles (which contain the ova). The maturing follicles produce oestrogen, and this has a positive feedback on the pituitary gland.
When the follicle reaches a critical diameter, usually about 22 mm, the
oestrogen stimulates a luteinizing hormone (LH) surge. This causes
rupture of the follicle and so the egg is released. The remnants of
the follicle develop into the corpus luteum which produces increasing amounts of progesterone. Progesterone causes the development of
a glandular endometrium which becomes ripe to accept the fertilized
egg.

TESTS OF OVULATION

1. Menstrual history
   If a woman consistently has regular menstrual cycles of 21–35 days
   it is almost certain that she ovulates, and that ovulation occurs
   about 14 days before menstruation.
2. Basal temperature chart
   This is a simple and very useful tool for assessing when ovulation
   has occurred. Just before ovulation there is a dip in the temperature
   recording followed by 0.5 °C rise in the temperature. This rise is a
   reflection of progesterone production and indicates ovulation. The
   best time to have intercourse, if a pregnancy is desired, is just after
   the dip in temperature (Fig. 11.5).
3. Hormone assays
   (a) Progesterone. If the progesterone level in the blood is greater
   than 10 nmol/l (3 ng/ml), then ovulation has occurred. For
   fertile cycles the midluteal level should be above 30 nmol/l
   (10 ng/ml).

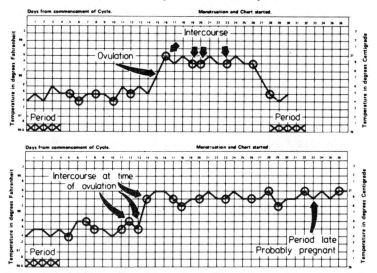

Fig. 11.5 Basal body temperature chart showing a normal cycle and the temperature following fertilization.

  (b) LH. If tested daily the LH surge may be detected. New urinary dip stick methods are now available to help the timing of ovulation. A blue colour change usually corresponds with the LH surge.

4. Endometrial biopsy

The endometrium demonstrates a secretory pattern if ovulation has occurred. While this is unnecessary for documenting the occurrence of ovulation, a well-timed endometrial biopsy is sometimes done to rule out an inadequate luteal phase, an uncommon cause of infertility.

5. Cervical mucus

This is not a precise way of determining the exact time of ovulation but an increase in mucus production and Spinnbarkeit (stretchiness of the mucus), occurs 2 or 3 days before ovulation. If the cervical mucus is put on a slide and dried, ferning will occur if there is no progesterone present.

TREATMENT OF ANOVULATION

1. Clomiphene

This stimulates ovulation in about 80% of cases but only one-half will conceive. This drug is an anti-oestrogen and acts primarily by blocking the effects of oestrogen on the hypothalamus. Therefore more FSH is produced which stimulates follicle growth. It has the disadvantage of drying up the mucus in some patients because of its anti-oestrogenic effect.

2. Gonadotrophins

   FSH in the form of human menopausal gonadotrophin or human pituitary gonadotrophin can be used to bypass the pituitary gland and directly stimulate the ovaries. The treatment is given by injections, and intensive monitoring with daily blood samples and frequent ultrasound examinations is required. Hyperstimulation of the ovaries can occur which may lead to multiple pregnancies and/or huge cystic ovaries.

3. Gonadotrophin-releasing hormones

   This is successful in patients who have a hypothalamic cause for anovulation and the hormone is delivered via a pulsatile pump. This can be strapped to their belt, with the needle inserted either subcutaneously or intravenously. A bolus of hormone is injected, usually every 90 minutes around the clock. The pump is used until ovulation occurs.

4. Bromocriptine

   This drug achieves an excellent pregnancy rate if anovulation is caused by hyperprolactinaemia. The drug lowers the hormone level, even in cases where there is a microadenoma of the pituitary, allowing the return of normal ovulation.

Barriers to fertilization

A. TUBAL DISEASE

Tubal disease accounts for about 35% of infertility problems, despite improvements in prevention and treatment.

Physiology

The Fallopian tubes are amazing organs and have the ability just after ovulation to pick up the ovum and transport it towards the centre of the tube (ampulla). At the same time the sperm swims in the opposite direction towards the egg. Fertilization normally occurs in the ampulla and for about two days the fertilized egg stays in the tube where it is supplied with nutrition by the tubal fluid. Then as the progesterone concentration increases, the direction of cilial movements transports the embryo to the uterus for implantation into the uterine lining. For this process to be carried out efficiently the tube must be patent and the cilia intact.

Damage to the fimbrial end of the tube may result in the surface area of the fimbria being greatly reduced, therefore decreasing the chances of picking up the newly-released egg. Blockage of the tube will prevent the sperm and the ovum from meeting and this may be caused from within or by adhesions around the outside of the tube.

Causes of tubal disease

1. Infection

   This is the most common cause of tubal disease. An active tubal infection is called pelvic inflammatory disease (PID). PID is difficult to diagnose and is often confused with many other conditions including appendicitis, endometriosis, ovarian cysts, inflammatory bowel disease, ectopic pregnancy, and even constipation. Therefore it is sometimes necessary to confirm a diagnosis of PID with a laparoscopy. It is a diagnosis that should never be made on history alone.

   There are several types of PID, the most damaging of which are gonorrhoea and chlamydia. The latter disease process may be silent and atypical. It can be diagnosed by taking a culture from the cervix or from the tubes themselves if laparoscopy is performed. When diagnosed, treatment should be vigorous and prompt. Even with good care, 10% of women having one episode of gonorrhoea can become infertile. Other infections include chlamgdia, mycoplasma, streptococcus and staphylococcus. Tuberculosis these days is rare but devastating, and even if pregnancy does occur, 85% will be ectopic.

2. Intrauterine devices (IUD)

   Pelvic inflammatory disease is five times more common in women with IUDs. The risk is greater if she has a history of PID.

3. Female sterilization

   Between 20 and 30% of women in the reproductive age group use sterilization as a method of contraception. Circumstances change and requests for reversal of sterilization are increasing. Of all the causes of tubal block, reversal of sterilization has the highest pregnancy rate. This depends upon the type of sterilization done initially, but reversal rates as high as 70% are possible with modern methods of sterilization, including clips and rings.

4. Congenital

   Rare; but occasionally women exposed to diethylstilbestrol (DES) *in utero* can have non-functionig tubes.

5. Endometriosis

   Endometrosis of the tube is much less common than endometriosis in other sites, but can cause tubal damage because of the formation of adhesions around the tube.

6. Pelvic surgery

   Any pelvic surgery can lead to adhesion formation. Operations on the ovary should be avoided if at all possible.

Investigations

1. Dye laparoscopy.
2. Hysterosalpingogram.

Treatment

Several surgical procedures are performed on the tubes. If the distal end of the tube is blocked it may be reopened by salpingostomy. If the tube is distorted by adhesions, salpingolysis may improve tubal function. A midtubal block may be removed and both ends reanastomosed if the proximal end of the tube is blocked; the block may be removed and the distal end reimplanted into the uterus.

Results of surgery may be very poor with a pregnancy rate of about 10–20%. However, results depend largely on the extent of disease. Adhesions alone in the presence of otherwise normal tubes may offer a pregnancy rate of 50–60%. Microsurgery, using an operating microscope, improves the accuracy of the procedure, as does prevention of tissue damage by gentle handling. An alternative treatment is *in vitro* fertilization, and this has a pregnancy rate of 15–20% per cycle.

B. CERVICAL FACTOR

The cervix is the first major barrier that the sperm must penetrate in order to achieve fertilization. Problems with the cervix and its mucus account for about 5% of all infertility.

Physiology

Mucus is a normal healthy discharge which is produced by glandular epithelium in the endocervix. The cervix has at least three main functions:

1. Sperm transport
2. Sperm selection
3. Sperm storage

The cervical mucus is a three-dimensional network of linked mucus strands (about 400). Variations in the structure and viscosity of the mucus determine whether the sperm are allowed to penetrate. As the oestradiol secreted from the ovary increases towards the time of ovulation, the water content between the strands of mucus increases, ensuring free movement of the sperm. This allows some to pass through into the uterus and some to be stored in the crypts of the endocervix. The sperm passing through to the uterus take less than 10 minutes to reach the tube whilst those sperm stored in the crypts have a slower migration towards the tube, thus allowing a constant supply of sperm over the next 24 hours. It is thought that the cervical mucus also acts as a sieve for abnormal sperm. For every million sperm deposited in the vagina, only two thousand will be selected to reach the tube.

A knowledge of the normal physiology of cervical mucus production may help the couple decide when the fertile time is near. This is particularly helpful if the female has irregular cycles. If ovulation is delayed the onset of the mucus is usually delayed. If ovulation is going to occcur early, the signs of mucus change may begin immediately after the period.

Causes of cervical hostility

1. Acidity of the cervical mucus

   The pH of the cervical mucus is important for spermatozoal motility. Motility is inhibited if the pH is below 6.3 or above 8.5. The ideal pH of the mucus occurs 2 or 3 days before ovulation and up until the time of ovulation. After ovulation, under the influence of progesterone, an impenetrable plug is formed in the cervix.

2. Trauma

   Trauma from cone biopsy, over-enthusiastic cautery and cervical amputation as part of repair operations can decrease the amount of fertile mucus and this may decrease the pregnancy rate.

3. Antisperm antibodies

   Sperm antibodies are non-sperm specific and form cross-links between the sperm and the glycoproteins of the mucus. This stops forward progression of the sperm. The antibodies can be autoantibodies on the sperm or antibodies within the cervical mucus.

4. Cervicitis

   T-mycoplasma and chlamydia are the most common causes of cervicitis, and although these can be easily treated with doxycycline, it is doubtful whether the treatment improves the pregnancy rates.

Investigations

1. Postcoital test (PCT, Sims–Huhner)

   The aim of this test is to detect whether motile sperm are present in the mucus. Standardization is difficult but very important because the most common cause of an abnormal test is incorrect timing. An easy way to remember one form of a standard test is 2,2,2. The test should be done after 2 days of abstinence from intercourse, within 2 days before ovulation and the mucus should be collected 2 hours after intercourse and examined immediately. A normal postcoital test should disclose at least 5 motile sperms per high power field.

   Poor postcoital test. This occurs when no sperm are seen at all in the cervical mucus. Surprisingly this is associated with a 10% pregnancy rate.

   A non-progressive test. This is associated with one or more immotile sperm present in the mucus. This is associated with a 25% pregnancy rate.

   Progressive test. This occurs when one or more motile sperm are seen in the mucus and it is associated with a 40% pregnancy rate.

2. Hostility test

   Several tests may be used to detect cervical hostility including the sperm cervical mucus contact test (SCMC) or sperm penetration migration test (Kraemer test). They are all dependent on good timing, good mucus pH, the absence of pus cells and the presence of sperm in the mucus. These tests can detect the presence of antisperm antibodies and demonstrate sperm shaking.

Treatment of cervical hostility

Poor mucus quality can be improved with the use of small doses of oestrogen in the early part of the menstrual cycle, but it is doubtful whether this leads to an improved pregnancy rate. Antisperm antibodies in the cervical mucus may be bypassed with intrauterine artificial insemination of the sperm. More recently treatments using high-dose steroids for a short time have been shown to decrease immunity and improve pregnancy rates.

Unexplained infertility

This condition occurs in 10–15% of all infertile patients. It is defined as infertility in a couple who have been trying to become pregnant for at least two years, in whom no abnormaility has been found with the sperm count, ovulation and tubal assessment including a laparoscopy.

These patients usually see many doctors and the constant refrain from doctors and relatives is 'relax'; 'go and have a holiday' or 'it's all psychological'.

Most patients hate to hear from the doctor that all the tests are normal. They often need to find something wrong, something to explain why they are not pregnant.

SOME POSSIBLE CAUSES OF THE UNEXPLAINED

1. Minimal endometriosis

   This is a condition in which the tissue lining of the uterus is found in ectopic sites outside the uterus. If severe, it may cause excruciating dysmenorrhoea and dyspareunia. Even in its mild form it can be associated with infertility. How endometriosis causes infertility is unclear. It is very rare for it to cause tubal block. The diagnosis of minimal endometriosis is usually made at laparoscopy and treatment is controversial.

   (a) Diathermy of the endometriotic spots is often done at the same time as laparoscopy.

   (b) Progestogens used continuously may reduce endometriosis.

   (c) Danazol (Danocrine), a synthetic steroid, is the commonest drug at present used in the treatment of endometriosis. This is a potent androgen and some patients find the side effects unacceptable.

   (d) Luteinizing hormone releasing hormone (LHRH) analogue is given in high doses, suppresses the LH, therefore stopping ovulation and menstruation. The only recorded side effects of this non-steriod are those of oestrogen deficiency. It can be taken as a nasal spray or as a daily injection.

2. Deficient luteal progesterone

   Occasionally in regularly ovulating women, progesterone deficiency can occur and is diagnosed by serial progesterone estimations in the luteal phase, and/or endometrial biopsy. Progestogen supplements have been shown to be of limited value in the treatment of this condition and the use of gonadotrophin has not yet been fully assessed.

3. Intrauterine adhesions

   In patients with unexplained infertility and who have questionable findings on hysterosalpingogram, the use of hysteroscopy has demonstrated a higher incidence of intrauterine pathology than in control groups. Pregnancy rates may be improved when these factors have been treated.

4. Asymptomatic infection
Intrauterine T-mycoplasma and chlamydia may cause infertility without obvious macroscopic damage.

5. Psychological factors
Many believe that unexplained infertility is all psychological. This is not true. However, infertility and the investigation and treatment of infertility may itself cause emotional trauma. Many women suffer severely every time a period comes. Most studies, however, cannot find a difference in the basic personalities of infertile and fertile women. Despite this, infertility gives the couple an insoluble problem that strains them physically, emotionally and financially. Suicide is twice as common in childless couples. Despite common belief, adoption does not increase the chance of pregnancy.

Recent advances in the treatment of infertility

1. *In-vitro* fertilization (IVF)
This refers to the process used to conceive a child outside the body. Ova may be picked up from stimulated ovaries either using a laparoscopic technique or transvaginal ultrasound. The technique was developed by Steptoe and Edwards and the first IVF baby was born in the UK in the late 70s. By the end of 1987 6000 babies were born by this technique worldwide.

The technique was developed to overcome infertility in women with damaged tubes, but the indications have broadened to include women with unexplained infertility and men with poor sperm counts.

The success rate is low (about 15%). The miscarriage rate is high, so the take home baby rate may be reduced to 10% per cycle.

2. Gamete intra-Fallopian transfer (GIFT)
This was developed in 1984 in San Antonio, Texas by Dr Ricardo Asch. This technique involves the placement of gametes (eggs and sperm) separately into a catheter followed by injection directly into the Fallopian tubes during laparoscopy. Fertilization occurs in the Fallopian tube, not outside the body as with IVF.

GIFT is not suitable for women with damaged tubes, but has higher success rates than IVF in women with other causes of infertility. The main indications for this technique are couples with unexplained fertility or a severe male factor or women with an immunological infertility.

Genital tract infections and discharge

Michael Webster

12.1 GENERAL INSTRUCTIONAL OBJECTIVE

The students should understand genital tract infections so that they can diagnose, appreciate the management and initiate the treatment of these conditions.

12.2 SPECIFIC BEHAVIOURAL OBJECTIVES

1. Discuss pathological and physiological vaginal discharge.
2. Discuss the aetiological factors involved in common genital tract infection.
3. Discuss the clinical features of genital tract infections.
4. Examine patient(s) and demonstrate an ability to differentiate between normal vaginal secretion and pathological discharge.
5. Examine patient(s) and demonstrate an ability to elicit and recognize signs of endometritis, salpingitis and pelvic peritonitis.
6. Indicate the appropriate investigations that will aid the diagnosis and management of genital tract infection.
7. Discuss the appropriate therapy of genital tract infections.
8. Explain the public health and the possible social implications of genital tract infection.
9. Discuss the sequelae of genital tract infection.

12.3 REASONS FOR LEARNING ABOUT GENITAL TRACT INFECTION

Vaginal discharge is the single most common presenting complaint of patients attending a general gynaecological clinic. It is frequently associated with other symptoms such as pain, vaginal pruritus and dyspareunia, or presents as a complication of contraception. The discharge may be pathological or be excessive 'physiological' discharge. The distinction between the various cases of pathological discharge is important so that appropriate therapy may be commenced. Inappropriate therapy will frequently aggravate the presenting problem or produce further iatrogenic problems. Inappropriate treatment of a physiological discharge may create a pathological discharge.

Genital tract infection, if not diagnosed early and treated appropriately, may have extremely disabling long-term effects on both the patient and her partner because of infertility or recurrent acute exacerbation of a chronic infection, which may eventually result in surgical pelvic clearance to relieve her symptoms.

Thus, although vaginal discharge and pelvic infection are common gynaecological problems and the diagnosis and treatment are straightforward, mismanagement can result in aggravation of the patient's symptoms and the initiation of long-term problems.

12.4 ACHIEVEMENT OF SPECIFIC BEHAVIOURS

Students will take part in tutorial discussion groups and clinicopathological conference on the bacteriology, symptoms and signs of pelvic infection as well as the appropriate methods of confirming the diagnosis and the appropriate treatment for each type of infection. In the clinics and wards, they will be expected to be able to elicit the symptoms and identify the signs of genital tract infection, and to perform appropriate 'office' investigations, take appropriate bacteriological swabs and suggest appropriate therapy.

12.5 VAGINAL DISCHARGE

The vagina of a hormonally active woman is moist, due to secretions from vaginal transudate and cervical mucus, and to a lesser extent from uterine secretion, fallopian tube secretion and Bartholin's gland secretion.

The volume of this secretion that is accepted as normal by individual women covers a wide range. Excessive normal secretion (called leucorrhoea) is usually associated with staining of underclothes and vaginal odour due to the heat denaturation of the proteins in the secretions. The secretions are clear to white and range in consistency

- Ovarian steroids—preg, pill, ectropion, Ovulatory cascade.
↑ Uterine sec^t pre + post mens.
↑ vaginal sec^t sex, irritation.
granuloma
Pelvic congestion.

from the thick mucus prior to ovulation to a thin watery more profuse secretion (the ovulatory cascade).

Increased production of the normal secretions is associated with:

1. Increased production of the ovarian steroids (oestrogens in particular), which occurs:
   (a) At the time of ovulation — ovulatory cascade.
   (b) When oestrogenic oral contraceptives are used.
   (c) In pregnancy.
   (d) With cervical ectopic columnar epithelium (also incorrectly called a cervical erosion), hypertrophy of endocervical columnar glands, and their extension from the cervical canal onto the ectocervix (commonly as a result of increased oestrogenic stimulus).
2. Increased vaginal transudate, which is associated with:
   (a) Sexual excitement.
   (b) Vaginal irritation, such as chemical irritation from inappropriate or too frequent douches or vaginal applications.
3. Uterine secretion, which occurs:
   (a) Prior to menstruation. Secretory changes induced in the endocervical and endometrial glands may give a premenstrual increase in vaginal discharge.
   (b) Following menstruation when the last days of menstrual flow may be prolonged.
4. Pelvic congestion, which may be due to pelvic pathology or be psychosomatic.
5. Granuloma (arising in the suture line at the vaginal vault following a hysterectomy), which can give rise to a profuse discharge. It is best treated by cautery, either chemically or by diathermy.

Management of leucorrhoea

ADEQUATE HISTORY

Make specific enquiries about:

1. Timing of discharge — midcycle or premenstrual exacerbation.
2. Oral contraception — especially oestrogenic type.
3. Use of douches, additions to bath water or deodorizing sprays.
4. Recent medications — especially vaginal applications.
5. Recent pregnancy.

EXAMINATION

Exclude pelvic or vaginal infection (if there is any doubt, take a high vaginal swab and an endocervical swab.) Assess the amount of discharge.

TREATMENT

1. Explain the cause — reassurance that it is not due to an infection may be all that is required.
2. Eliminate any aggravating cause (such as high-dose oestrogenic pill or inappropriate vaginal applications).
3. Give general advice regarding hygiene, limiting local heat to the genital area, taking frequent showers during hot weather, avoiding deodorizing sprays, using cotton underclothes that absorb some of the secretions.
4. Ablative therapy (cryocautery, diathermy, laser) to the cervix to reduce the number of endocervical glands. This may be used in a minority of persistent cases. However, if the original precipitating factor is still present (e.g. oral contraception) relief will be short lived.

Cotton Knickers etc

Pathological discharge

PRESENTATION

This usually presents with other symptoms, such as vaginal/vulval pruritus, dyspareunia or pelvic pain. Many of the infective causes of vaginal discharge produce a classical vaginal reaction; however, more frequently, there is a non-specific discharge and a non-specific vaginal reaction. Experienced gynaecologists can frequently misinterpret the nature of the vaginal discharge.

TRICHOMONAL VAGINITIS

This is caused by a flagellated unicellular organism with four flagella anteriorly and a terminal membranous stylus similar in size to a neutrophil. It is harboured, usually asymptomatically, by the male and is transmitted as a venereal disease. It can also be found in the vagina of asymptomatic patients, and appears to require more than just its presence in order to become established and to cause symptoms.

(Raising the vaginal pH shortly after menstruation may allow the establishment of the infection.)

The discharge is classically frothy and yellow-green in colour, and has a typical odour. The amount of the discharge varies; in actue cases it is usually profuse and commonly associated with pruritus. The vaginal walls and cervix may have an inflamed appearance, with punctate 'strawberry' spots. However, if these signs are absent, the diagnosis can be confirmed by placing a drop of the discharge (diluting it if necessary with saline) on a slide, and examining for motile organisms. These are usually easily distinguished from the only other motile 'organisms' commonly found in the vagina–sperm.

Treatment consists of 200 mg of metronidazole (e.g. Flagyl) orally, three times daily for 7 days. Alternatively, tinidazole (Fasigyn) may be given as a single dose. The male partner should be treated with the same dose, certainly whenever there is a recurrence. It is advisable to treat an asymptomatic woman in whom trichomonas has been found, before it becomes an established infection.

MONILIAL VAGINITIS (THRUSH)

This is caused by the yeast-like fungus *Candida albicans*, which appears microscopically (following Gram staining) as long filaments (mycelia) or as spores. It can be found in the vagina of asymptomatic women. The discharge is classically thick, white and cheesy, and tends to stick to the walls of the vagina, leaving a reddened area when removed. The vagina may be extremely sore, making examination painful. Pruritus is a frequent and often major complaint.

The organism thrives in the presence of carbohydrate, thus it is common during pregnancy or the second half of the menstrual cycle, in diabetes and following broad-spectrum antibiotics, which destroy the normal vaginal flora.

The source of the infection may be the patient's own gastrointestinal tract or, as with trichomonas, it may result from transmission during coitus.

The treatment is to remove any precipitating cause. Local vaginal therapy is the treatment of choice; oral therapy may be used for resistant or recurrent cases.

1. Mycostatin (Nystatin) in the form of pessaries or cream may be used over 14–28 days. The patient should be instructed to place the pessaries or the cream applicator as high as comfortable in the

vagina, so that the whole length of the vagina is exposed to the medication. The treatment should be continued for at least 14 days even if the symptoms have subsided. Oral Nystatin tablets (usually given as one tablet three times a day) will remove monilia at least temporarily from the gastrointestinal tract, and thereby reduce the risk of self-reinfection of the vagina. Oral Nystatin does not treat monilial vaginitis, as it is not absorbed from the bowel.

2. Imidazole drugs appear to be equally effective in shorter courses; for example clotrimazole, econazole or miconazole in cream or pessaries for 3 or 6 days. Clotrimazole may be given as a single-dose pessary (500 mg) which is an advantage when patient compliance is a problem. Vaginal applications may be supplemented with cream for vulvitis. Ketoconazole is the only imidazole drug that is significantly absorbed after oral administration and may be useful for recurrent vaginal candidiasis. FLUCONAZOLE – D. fluc)50

3. Dihydroxyquinoline (Floraquin) pessaries. One twice a day may be used for both monilia and trichomonas.

4. Natamycin (Pimafucin) pessaries can be used for both trichomonal and monilial vaginitis. (However, both Floraquin and Pimafucin are not as effective as the more specific therapy of imidazole drugs for monilia or Flagyl for trichomonas.)

5. Gentian violet has stood the test of time in the treatment of monilial vaginitis. It has the one serious disadvantage in that it is very messy to apply and stains clothing.

When examining a patient with gross monilial vaginitis, it is useful to gently remove as much of the discharge and monilial plaques as possible without distressing the patient. This will aid local medications in curing the vaginitis and relieving the symptoms earlier.

GARDNERELLA VAGINITIS

This is caused by a small, non-motile, gram-variable coccobacillus (*gardnerella vaginalis*). It can be found in the vagina of asymptomatic women. The typical clinical presentation includes a variable amount of discharge that has a fishy or unpleasant vaginal odour and has a homogeneous, thin consistency, which may cause local irritation but not pruritus.

Microscopic examination of a wet preparation mounted on a slide will show large numbers of coccobacilli floating between and attached to vaginal epithelial cells in a stippled manner ('clue cells'). When 10%

10%

potassium hydroxide is added to the wet mount preparation a fishy amine odour is released (sniff test). The combination of the typical clinical findings and a positive sniff test is diagnostic of gardnerella vaginitis, even if clue cells are absent.

Metronidazole is the treatment of choice (700 mg t.i.d. × 7 days). Tetracycline and ampicillin have also been shown to be effective, as has douching therapy with povidone-iodine (Betadine). Investigations have shown that the majority of male partners of infected patients harbour the organism in the urethra. It is therefore recommended that the male sexual partner be treated with metronidazole at the same time.

ATROPHIC VAGINITIS

This is associated with the very thin vaginal epithelium of the postmenopausal woman, which is often easily injured and infected. The responsible organisms are usually non-specific (producing a mixed growth on culture) and of low virulence. The discharge is thin, purulent and often blood stained and the vagina may appear red and have many tiny bleeding points. Vaginal, vulval and perineal soreness are frequently present and may make an adequate examination of the patient difficult.

Treatment consists of oestrogen, either locally in the form of pessaries or cream, or orally. If the uterus is still *in situ*, it is wise to give the oestrogens cyclically with the intermittent exhibition of progestogen to reduce the risk of endometrial hyperplasia.

CHILDHOOD VAGINITIS

This is uncommon and may be associated with a wide range of organisms, which are usually of low virulence. However, *Neisseria gonorrhoeae* and *Trichomonas vaginalis* do occur in children. Whenever a child presents with a vaginal discharge, always suspect a foreign body. + sexual abuse

When examining a young child vaginally, a nasal speculum is a good substitute for a speculum, and a paediatric cystoscope is a useful instrument for removing foreign bodies.

Treatment may also include oral antibiotics, according to sensitivities of the organisms found in a swab from the discharge. In severe cases, 0.2 mg of oestrogen daily, or twice daily, for 7–10 days, may help in improving vaginal resistance to infection.

CHRONIC CERVICITIS

This almost never occurs as a single entity. When there is infection in the tissues of the cervix, there is also more widespread infection of the parametrium, endometrium and/or fallopian tubes. The term 'chronic cervicitis' has been used loosely in many cases to describe ectopic columnar epithelium on the ectocervix. Chronic cervicitis occurs when the stroma of the cervix is involved in a chronic bacterial infection. This may occur when ectopic columnar epithelium becomes infected but more commonly follows a delivery, an abortion or an operation during which the cervix is torn and then becomes infected.

The term 'erosion' is often used to describe any lesion on the cervix that is not normal squamous epithelium. Included under this broad term of erosion may be found such conditions as physiological ectopic columnar epithelium, infected ectopic columnar epithelium, chronic cervicitis, dysplasia of the cervix, neoplasia of the cervix and even true erosions due to loss of epithelium. The term is thus too broad and should not be used when a better description is available.

Ectopic columnar epithelium is a response to oestrogen stimulation, and is thus common during pregnancy and in women using oral contraceptives.

If the discharge is causing distress to the patient, remove the precipitating cause, such as oral contraception, and any factor giving rise to discomfort, such as heat and non-absorbent clothing. Ablative therapy such as cervical cauterization by diathermy, under anaesthesia or cryocautery without anaesthesia may be used when the discharge is particularly troublesome. However, if the precipitating cause is not removed, the discharge will return.

Trachelorrhaphy, or cervical amputation, is usually only performed when the cervix has been lacerated or traumatized.

Diathermy and trachelorrhaphy may give rise to primary or secondary haemorrhage, cervical stenosis or cervical incompetence.

When there is a bacterial chronic cervicitis, the bacteria and their antibiotic sensitivities should be determined by a cervical and high vaginal swab although systemic antibiotics have little effect when used alone, and the main treatment is surgical.

CHEMICAL VAGINITIS/CERVICITIS

Repeated inappropriate therapy of a vaginal discharge can precipitate irritation of the vaginal epithelium, causing discomfort, and lead to destruction of the normal flora. Infection should be excluded by a vaginal swab, the inappropriate therapy withdrawn, and the patient reassured. The problem in self-limiting and, if necessary, a bland cream, for example, Acijel with an appropriate pH may be administered. Severe chemical vaginitis may result from douches with such substances as undiluted Dettol, PHisoHex, lye or Condys crystals. This may be so severe that admission to hospital for pain relief and catheterization may be required.

A foreign body — the commonest being a forgotten tampon in the adult patient, or any variety of objects in the infant or child — may produce an offensive discharge. The only treatment required is removal of the foreign body and occasionally a mild antiseptic douche, such as very dilute aqueous solution of chlorhexidine. Any child with a vaginal discharge should be considered as having a foreign body in the vagina, until proved otherwise by an adequate examination which in some cases will require an anaesthetic.

CHLAMYDIA TRACHOMATIS

Genital tract infection with *Chlamydia trachomatis* (serotypes D–K) is an important and common sexually-transmitted disease. It is the most commonly identified cause of urethitis in young men. In women it has been isolated from multiple sites in the genital tract including the cervix (mucopurulent cervicitis), the urethra (frequency/dysuria syndrome), Bartholin glands (Bartholinitis), the endometrium (endometritis) and the fallopian tubes (salpingitis). In most western communities chlamydial infection is much more common than gonococcal infection.

Infection in women is frequently asymptomatic. Routine screening at family planning and antenatal clinics have shown 5–10% of sexually active women have an unsuspected cervical chlamydial infection. Tubal damage resulting in infertility may result from both acute chlamydial salpingitis or from asymptomatic unrecognized chlamydial infection.

In pregnancy cervical chlamydial infection has been associated with premature delivery, amnionitis and puerperal infection. Chlamydial infection occurs in 60–70% of the neonates born to women with cervical chlamydial infection. Neonatal conjunctivitis occurs in 35–50% of cases and neonatal pneumonia in 10–20% of cases.

Until recently *Chlamydia trachomatis* could only be detected by cell culture techniques that were expensive and not readily available. Direct identification of chlamydia is now possible with immunofluorescent staining using monoclonal antibodies to chlamydia antigen.

Tetracycline and erythromycin are the antibiotic agents most commonly used for treatment of known or suspected chlamydial infection. The current recommendation is doxycycline 200 mg daily for 10 days, abstinence from intercourse during treatment and the concurrent treatment of sexual partners. Erythromycin (500 mg t.i.d. for 10 days) is an alternative for treatment during pregnancy or lactation.

12.6 HERPES GENITALIS

The type II herpes virus is becoming a more frequent infecting agent of the vulva, vagina, perineum and bladder. The symptoms are of severe discomfort in the infected area, which may be associated with urinary retention in severe infections. The retention is due to the severe dysuria when urine comes into contact with the infected area, or may be due to infection in the bladder or urethra. The primary and secondary infections have a similar appearance to the vesicles of a cold sore, which is usually caused by the type I herpes virus.

Herpes infection can be confirmed by viral culture and can be suspected from inclusion bodies in the cells taken from a cervical smear. Venereal spread of the disease is possible and is predisposed to by a moist environment, such as excessive leucorrhoea, or by any decline in general health.

Treatment is difficult. Povidone-iodine and a white light source were thought to be curative, as was idoxuridine (Stoxil). Acyclovir is active against herpes simplex viruses and can be used for acute and recurrent genital infections. To be effective the drug must be given as early as possible in the acute illness. Prophylactic treatment may be given for recurrent severe disease.

Severe episodes may require hospitalization, systemic pain relief, catheterization and treatment of secondary infection.

12.7 HUMAN IMMUNODEFICIENCY VIRUS INFECTION

Human immunodeficiency virus (HIV) infection is a newly-discovered communicable disease that has become pandemic in less than 5 years. HIV is a blood-borne and sexually transmissible organism and was identified as a retrovirus in 1983.

The routes of infection include:

	Infection risk
1. Blood or blood product transfusion	Almost certain
2. Sharing needles	Very high
3. Mother to child	50%
4. Passive (receptive) anal intercourse	Very high
5. Vaginal intercourse (male to female)	High
6. Anal intercourse (active partner)	Medium
7. Vaginal intercourse (female to male)	Medium
8. Oral sex	Low
9. Kissing	Hypothetical only

Following infection an acute mononucleosis-like illness may develop within 6 weeks of exposure to HIV. Some people remain symptomless after primary infection although the majority will develop antibodies to HIV within 6 months of exposure. Once a diagnosis of AIDS has been made the patient should be referred to a specialized AIDS unit. These units take a comprehensive approach to the management of the patient with emphasis on medical and neuropsychiatric assessment, patient counselling and education.

Artificial insemination has been shown to transmit HIV when semen is obtained from infected donors. All donors must now sign a declaration regarding risk factors and semen is accepted only if the donor is HIV seronegative. The semen is stored for 6 months and used only if the donor is found to be seronegative when retested after that time.

In pregnancy where the mother is HIV antibody positive the risk of AIDS in the fetus is approximately 30%. The risk of HIV infection in the infant may be higher than 65%, following intrapartum exposure. Careful supervision is required in pregnancy and the infant should be delivered in a unit capable of providing a high level of perinatal support. Currently, Caesarean section is not indicated. Breast-feeding has been associated with postnatal HIV transmission and its presence in cell free breast milk has been demonstrated.

12.8 PELVIC INFECTIONS

These infections affect the genital organs above the level of the cervix. The infection may extend into the pelvic cavity giving rise to pelvic peritonitis, involve nearby organs or form a pelvic abscess.

Pelvic infections are usually bacterial, the commonest bacteria being anaerobic organisms, chlamydia and gram-negative organisms, especially *Escherichia coli* and *Neisseria gonorrhoeae*. The symptoms vary widely, depending upon the main site of the infection, the extent of the infection and whether it is acute or chronic.

Acute infection

PUERPERAL AND POSTABORTAL INFECTIONS

The placental site and any placental remnants provide good culture media for infection. The most common organisms are anaerobic organisms (bacteroides), *Escherichia coli, Chlamydia trachomatis,* other gram-negative bacilli, clostridium and streptococcus. Invasion of the tissues is rapid, and general systemic symptoms result from the toxaemia. Bacteraemia may also occur and progress to septicaemia with possible death of the patient from septic shock, unless adequate treatment is commenced promptly.

Acute inflammation is found in the endometrium. Acute salpingitis of the interstitium is common, with only minimal involvement of the endosalpinx until late in the disease (unless the gonococcus is involved). A tubo-ovarian abscess may form, and any peritonitis is usually localized to the pouch of Douglas.

Clinically, in well-established infection, the patient looks ill, with a marked pyrexia, tachycardia and perhaps rigors. Pelvic pain and tenderness are present after the infection has spread beyond the endometrium. There is usually a brown or blood-stained offensive heavy lochial loss. The uterus may be soft and larger than expected due to delayed involution, and tender as the infection spreads towards the serosal surface of the uterus.

Signs of peritonitis may be present if the infection has involved the pouch of Douglas, although the lower abdominal rebound tenderness and guarding may not be as marked as expected. (Pouch of Douglas infection produces less marked abdominal signs.) Bowel sounds are usually present.

If septicaemia and endotoxic shock develop, the blood pressure may fall and the pulse becomes weak and difficult to detect. The temperature may become subnormal and the patient's skin is cold and has a cyanosed blotchy appearance. Oliguria or anuria may develop.

The first evidence of pelvic vein thrombophlebitis, induced by the pelvic infection, may be pulmonary embolism. The differential diagnosis must include acute ruptured appendicitis; if there is any doubt, a laparotomy or laparoscopy is indicated.

Treatment

Take steps to identify the infecting organisms by:

1. Taking vaginal and endocervical swabs (for immediate microscopy of a smear from the swab) and culture for organisms (aerobic and anaerobic).
2. Blood for culture is best taken during the upward spikes of the temperature.
3. Midstream urine specimen for possible urinary tract infection.

Broad-spectrum antibiotic therapy should be started as early as possible, in an adequate dose so as to combat possible gram-positive or gram-negative organisms as well as anaerobic organisms. A possible combination is a high-dose penicillin (which may be given intravenously) together with an aminoglycoside, such as streptomycin, kanamycin or gentamicin and metronidazole, for anaerobic cover. These drugs should be continued until the patient has been asymptomatic for 48 hours.

Blood loss is replaced and fluid and electrolyte balance must be carefully controlled. Oliguria or anuria require prompt correction.

If products of conception remain in the uterus, they should be removed carefully after the patient has been resuscitated and an antibiotic cover has been established.

GONOCOCCAL INFECTION

This is one of the commonest venereal diseases, after chlamydia infection. It frequently is not detected in the female by either the patient or doctor, as it is commonly asymptomatic unless it produces an acute pelvic infection. The organism is fragile and will not be detected by normal bacterial swabs or cultures.

Gonorrhoea commonly spreads from the cervix via the endometrium to the endosalpinx, with possible exudation into the pelvic cavity with involvement of the ovary and peritoneum.

As the endosalpinx is the first affected part of the tube, adhesive occlusion of the tube (particularly at the fimbriated end) is common, forming a pyosalpinx.

Clinically, the patient may present with symptoms of urethritis or salpingitis, cervicitis being asymptomatic apart from some discharge. If pelvic infection develops, the vaginal discharge precedes the elevation of the temperature and abdominal pain. There is bilateral pelvic tenderness and severe excitation pain on moving the cervix. Swellings or thickenings of the adnexae may be present but examination usually provokes so much pain that these are difficult to detect. The systemic upset is not marked, despite the pyrexia.

A differential diagnosis must consider ectopic pregnancy, a complicated ovarian cyst, appendicitis and peritonitis. The bilateral nature of the lesion and the history is likely to indicate the diagnosis. If there is doubt, a laparoscopy should be performed. If the diagnosis of salpingitis is confirmed, the opportunity should be taken to obtain a swab of the pus.

Prior to treatment, bacteriological swabs should be taken to confirm the diagnosis. The sites to be swabbed should include endocervix, high vagina, urethra and, depending on history of sexual contact, the pharynx and anus.

An endocervical swab for culture taken with an ordinary cotton-wool swab-stick will probably not produce any growth, for the gonococcal organisms are destroyed quickly when they are allowed to dry. The best method of collecting a specimen for identification of organisms is to use a charcoal-impregnated swab-stick or a calcium alginate (Calgi) swab-stick. These allow the discharge to be absorbed into the swab, keeping them moist at the correct pH. By plating the swabs immediately or transporting them in Stuart's transport media, a high recovery rate for culture is obtained. The organisms are grown on a chocolate-agar medium in a carbon dioxide-enriched atmosphere.

Antibiotics in large doses are indicated and penicillin is the antibiotic of choice. This treatment should be continued for 10 days or until the patient has been afebrile and asymptomatic for at least 48 hours. If the patient is allergic to penicillin, spectinomycin (Trobocin), erythromycin (Erythrocin) or tetracycline (mysteclin, Achromycin) may be used.

Secondary infection by other organisms is not uncommon. When this occurs, a regime similar to that for postabortal pelvic infection is commenced.

Peritonitis should be treated with the patient in a sitting position; with attention to fluids, electrolytes and urinary output. Tubo-ovarian abscess may develop with severe infection and is managed by surgical drainage, usually at laparoscopy.

Chronic pelvic infection

Chronic pelvic infection is an important cause of dysmenorrhoea, dyspareunia, menstrual disturbances and infertility. It usually arises because of inadequate, inappropriate, delayed or too short a course of treatment. The uterus is not usually involved, except in the rare event of pelvic tuberculosis.

CHRONIC SALPINGITIS AND OOPHORITIS

The main changes are associated with occlusion of the fallopian tubes and (with the gonococcus), destruction of the endosalpinx. Distortion of the tubes with peritubal adhesions is also common. If both the fimbrial and isthmic ends of the tubes are blocked, a pyosalpinx may form. Extension of the infection from the tube to the ovary results in chronic inflammatory changes or abscess formation (usually as a tubo-ovarian abscess).

Clinically the patient may complain of dysmenorrhoea, which is characteristically a prolonged pelvic ache. Backache is also common.

Menstrual irregularity, with frequent periods and menorrhagia, is probably related to ovarian involvement in the inflammatory process, and consequent hormonal dysfunction.

A surprising number of patients with chronic inflammatory changes have no symptoms but present with infertility.

SIGNS

It is sometimes possible to detect a mass or bilateral swellings in the pelvis. The uterus is often enlarged and fixed in retroversion, and attempts to antevert it are unsuccessful.

MANAGEMENT

The treatment depends on age, parity, desire for further pregnancies, the nature of the lesions and their extent and response to treatment.

In general the management is conservative, by medical therapy — although surgical treatment is indicated if there is no improvement.

Medical treatment includes correction of anaemia, analgesics, heat and antibiotic therapy. Antibiotics are not as effective in chronic disease as in the acute condition, and there is also the difficulty of obtaining organisms for culture and sensitivity.

Surgery is indicated if:

1. There is no response to intensive therapy and the general health of the patient continues to deteriorate.

2. There are acute exacerbations of chronic inflammatory disease.
3. Local tenderness persists without improvement.
4. Masses in the adnexa or pouch of Douglas increase in size or show no diminution.
5. Menstrual disorders continue and cause incapacity.

Laparotomy should be undertaken during antibiotic therapy and, where possible, material for culture should be obtained at operation. The operation may be a simple salpingostomy or salpingo-oopherectomy, or a complete pelvic clearance may be required.

PELVIC TUBERCULOSIS

This is usually secondary to pulmonary tuberculosis. The fallopian tubes are commonly affected. Many patients are asymptomatic, the diagnosis only being found when specially looked for during investigation of infertility, oligomenorrhoea, vaginal discharge, anaemia, high temperatures or weight loss.

Endometrium obtained at curettage should be examined histologically and sent for guinea-pig inoculation.

Intensive and prolonged anti-tuberculosis therapy is required. The prospects of a successful pregnancy, even after successful treatment, are not great and the risk of an ectopic pregnancy is high.

VENEREAL DISEASE

See trichomonas, gonorrhoea, chlamydia and herpes as described earlier in this chapter. Syphilis should be suspected in any patient in whom gonorrhoea has been diagnosed. Like gonorrhoea, it is commonly asymptomatic in the female, the primary chancre not being observed in the vagina or inner aspects of the vulva.

Treponema pallidum is a slowly multiplying spirochaete, which requires moisture and tissue for survival, transmitted by blood or exudate, entering via lacerations or abrasions in the vagina. The incubation period averages 3 weeks. The primary or chancre stage lasts 1–5 weeks. The typical chancre is a single ulcer (commonly with a rolled edge and a chamois leather-like base), often accompanied by a non-suppurative lymphadenopathy. It is usually painless, except when secondary infection occurs in a vulval chancre. The secondary syphilis stage may last 2–6 weeks and is the most contagious stage. The eruption may take many forms and mimic many types of rashes. The areas commonly affected are the oral cavity ('snail-track' ulcers), palms, soles and genital area. Condylomata lata may develop, and these are accompanied by generalized adenopathy.

There may be a prolonged latent phase following the secondary stage before the tertiary stage develops. The tertiary stage may affect any part of the body, producing neurosyphilis (including GPI), cardiovascular changes and gumma.

Congenital syphilis may only be acquired by the fetus after the 16th week of gestation. If the infection occurs early in the pregnancy, the fetus will usually die *in utero;* if later in pregnancy, the fetus will be born with the stigmata of congenital syphilis; if the infection is acquired late in pregnancy, the stigmata may occur after birth. Congenital syphilis can be prevented by adequate treatment of the mother.

Diagnosis is by adequate investigation of those at risk or at special risk, such as the pregnant patient. There are two basic types of test:

1. Sensitive screening tests, such as the Reiter protein complement fixation (RPCF) test; the Wassermann reaction (WR); the venereal disease research laboratory (VDRL) test; and the Kahn reaction. All these tests give false positive results.
2. In order to confirm the diagnosis, more specific tests such as the *Treponema pallidum* immobilization (TPI) test or the fluorescent treponema antibody test (FTA) should be performed.

The diagnosis can also be confirmed by dark-ground examination of exudate from the chancre to detect the spirochaetes.

Treatment is by penicillin in adequate doses (e.g. Bicillin 2–4 million units intramuscularly on two occasions several days apart, or procaine penicillin 1.2 mega units for 10 days).

Serological tests should be repeated at least 3-monthly for two years to confirm the cure. If there is any doubt about the cure, the CSF should also be examined.

Social implications of pelvic infections

Pelvic infections (especially chlamydia) may cause infertility, and chronic infection gives rise to long-term morbidity.

Venereal diseases (both chlamydia and gonorrhoea) are increasing in frequency in our community. Social groups that form the largest untreated pool of carriers are prostitutes and male homosexuals. The asymptomatic female carrier may only be found by tracing male contacts. Failure of notification of one diagnosed patient may allow a wide spread of the infection. The natural reticence to notify partners must be overcome for public health measures to be effective. Appropriate swabs should be taken of any undiagnosed vaginal discharge or any genital tract infection.

Functional variations of the female genital tract

Rogerio A. Lobo

13.1 GENERAL INSTRUCTIONAL OBJECTIVE

The students should appreciate variations from the normal function of the female reproductive system so they can identify patients who have symptoms of gynaecological disorders without corresponding abnormal physical signs and then initiate management.

13.2 SPECIFIC BEHAVIOURAL OBJECTIVES

1. Discuss the symptoms and signs of normal menstruation.
2. Discuss the investigation of a patient with abnormal uterine bleeding.
3. Discuss the hazards of giving hormonal therapy for abnormal vaginal bleeding before performing adequate examination and investigations.
4. Discuss those factors that may cause abnormal uterine bleeding without demonstrable physical causes.
5. Indicate factors that may cause amenorrhoea without demonstrable physical causes.
6. Discuss the aetiology, clinical features and management of dysmenorrhoea without demonstrable physical causes.
7. Discuss the causes of dyspareunia without demonstrable physical signs.
8. Discuss counselling of patients with dyspareunia without demonstrable physical cause.
9. Discuss the causes and management of pelvic pain without demonstrable physical cause.
10. Discuss the causes and management of leucorrhoea.

11. Elicit, present and discuss the history of a patient with a gynae-cological disorder without demonstrable physical cause.
12. Demonstrate ability to recognize normal physical signs of pelvic examination.
13. Discuss causes and management of postmenopausal problems.
14. Counsel women with postmenopausal problems.

13.3 REASONS FOR LEARNING ABOUT VARIATIONS FROM NORMAL FUNCTION OF THE FEMALE REPRODUCTION SYSTEM

A number of women present to their doctor complaining of symptoms such as pain, irregular bleeding, dyspareunia, vaginal discharge, hot flushes, loss of libido, depression, etc., which appear to have no pathological basis. These symptoms are due to variations from the normal physiological processes and before any form of management can be introduced for these problems, it is essential to understand the basic mechanics that produce the symptoms.

13.4 THE HORMONAL CONTROL OF THE MENSTRUAL CYCLE

Levels of control

An understanding of the hormonal control of the normal menstrual cycle is essential to the rational management of fertility regulation by hormonal techniques and the treatment of disturbances of menstruation and fertility due to ovulatory failure.

In broad outline, the changes in the endometrium that govern the frequency and duration of menstruation are determined by steroid hormones produced by the ovary.

The central control mechanism for menstrual cyclicity resides in the area of the medial basal hypothalamus where gonadotrophin-releasing hormone (GnRH) is secreted in a pulsatile fashion from the area of the arcuate nucleus. GnRH is secreted episodically with pulses actually occurring every 90 minutes. Only when GnRH is produced in this pulsatile manner will luteinizing hormone (LH) be delivered into the peripheral circulation. Multiple complex neuronal contributions around the area of the arcuate nucleus are responsible for the tonic control of the pulsatile GnRH secretion. These neuronal centres have specific neurotransmitters which are in turn modulated by higher supratentorial centres which are vulnerable to environmental and emotional inhibitory influences. GnRH is delivered through the portal system to the pituitary where LH and follicle-stimulating hormone (FSH) are produced and released. In the area of the third ventricle there are ependymal neuronal structures called tanycytes which also interact with the cerebrospinal fluid and therefore constitute an additional release mechanism for GnRH. Measurements of peripheral LH may be used to detect pulses which reflect the episodic release of GnRH. In women with disorders of the hypothalamic–pituitary–ovarian axis, there may be either exaggerated LH pulses as in polycystic ovary (PCO) syndrome or decreased pulses in the case of hypothalamic amenorrhoea.

The effects of GnRH on the pituitary are influenced by GnRH priming as well as by the pituitary context of LH and FSH. This in turn is also influenced by the oestrogen status of the patient. At the time of ovulation, when oestrogen levels are high, LH is secreted with increased amplitude. Sex steroids also influence gonadotrophin secretion. Oestrogen and progesterone both have negative and positive effects on the hypothalamic–pituitary axis. During the early follicular phase, when oestrogen is low, negative feedback does not occur, resulting in increased LH and FSH discharge. The FSH, in particular, primes follicular development and the production of oestrogen. With adequate pulsatile gonadotrophin release, follicular growth ensues and oestrogen rises in the circulation. When the dominant follicle reaches 18 mm or more in size and oestradiol levels reach 150 pg/ml for 36 hours or more, the positive influence or positive feedback of oestrogen on the pituitary as well as the hypothalamus comes about. This results in a surge of LH from the pituitary but there is probably an associated increase in GnRH from the hypothalamus as well. While the former is more important for follicular rupture and ovulation, the GnRH effect from the hypothalamus helps the amplitude of this response. Following ovulation, a corpus luteum is formed which secretes progesterone primarily in response to a slower pulsatile activity of LH. Progesterone levels in the luteal phase should be > 10 ng/ml at a peak of corpus luteum development (on day 21 of a 28-day menstrual cycle). Progesterone appears to inhibit the pulsatile release of GnRH and also inhibits further development of follicles within the ovary, thus preventing superovulation.

While GnRH is the releasing factor responsible for gonadotrophin secretion there are other hypothalamic factors which release other hormones from the pituitary. Thyrotrophin-releasing hormone (TRH) is responsible for the secretion of thyroid-stimulating hormone (TSH) which in turn releases thyroid hormone. In addition, there is growth hormone-releasing hormone (GHRH) and corticotrophin-releasing factor (CRF) which releases ACTH as well as other peptides from the anterior pituitary gland. The only major anterior pituitary hormone which does not have an identified specific releasing factor is prolactin (PRL). PRL is released from the anterior pituitary but is primarily under a tonic inhibitory control. This PRL inhibitory factor has been thought to be dopamine, which is clearly inhibitory, but there are possibly other inhibitory control mechanisms in addition. TRH is known to be at least one factor which directly stimulates PRL release from the pituitary gland.

From the posterior pituitary oxytocin and vasopressin are secreted. These hormones are thought to play a minor role in the reproductive axis but can accentuate the effects of CRF on the ACTH axis. They also have a role in memory and may be linked with PRL secretion.

An important interaction of the CRF–ACTH axis with reproduction occurs with the advent of stressful stimuli and events. With stress, CRF increases. This in turn not only stimulates ACTH and cortisol but also elicits the release of opioid peptides, the precursor molecule of which is pro-opiomelanocortin (POMC). POMC in turn is selectively cleaved not only to ACTH, but to β-endorphin and other opioid peptides. β-Endorphin has been shown to directly inhibit GnRH and therefore may play a significant role in the reproductive axis. There is evidence that increased opioid peptide secretion can occur in some states of amenorrhoea resulting from chronic stress, as well as in hyperprolactinemia. Although PRL can directly inhibit the reproductive axis at the level of the hypothalamus, pituitary or ovary, one of the possible mechanisms at the level of the hypothalamus may be via β-endorphin release.

Specific tests for hormonal evaluation of the hypothalamic–pituitary axis

GnRH can be used exogenously to stimulate the release of LH and FSH and is being used therapeutically for the induction of ovulation. If the GnRH molecule is substituted in certain positions, such as in the 6th and 10th positions, a long-acting agonist of GnRH will be produced. GnRH agonists, because of their prolonged affinity for the GnRH receptor, causes down-regulation of gonadotroph cells which eventually results in amenorrhoea and a form of medical castration.

This process has been used therapeutically for treatment of precocious puberty and endometriosis as well as uterine fibroids and other conditions such as cancer.

GnRH can be used in a stimulation test to determine the integrity of pituitary and LH and FSH release. A 100 µg bolus of GnRH can be given intravenously which will elicit a maximum response of LH by 20–30 minutes and one of FSH between 45 and 60 minutes. While it is extremely rare to have a true deficiency of the pituitary, this can certainly occur in cases related to postpartum hemorrhage (Sheehan's syndrome) as well as in cases of pituitary tumours. Most often the cause of amenorrhoea is due to hypothalamic inactivity where endogenous GnRH release, which is necessary to prime the pituitary, has not occurred. In this instance, a normal response with GnRH may not be elicited, although the pituitary is normal, and priming of the pituitary is required. Daily intramuscular injections of GnRH (100 µg) are given for approximately 4–5 days after which a routine GnRH test is administered as described above. When this is carried out, a normal response is usually elicited.

TRH can be used to stimulate the secretion of PRL as well as to evoke responses in TSH. In general, a 200% increase or a tripling of the baseline level of PRL is considered a normal response. TSH responses should be at least $7\,\mu U$ at 30 minutes. Exaggerated responses ($> 28\ \mu U/ml$) suggest hypothyroidism and blunted or absent responses suggest hyperthyroidism.

ACTH can be used to stimulate cortisol and adrenal androgens from the adrenal but is rarely needed to test for deficiency states. A better test for the integrity of the hypothalamic–pituitary–adrenal axis is the insulin tolerance test or the use of metyrapone. This is used when there is a question of panhypopituitarism, for example in Sheehan's syndrome. An insulin tolerance test results in the release of stress-related hormones such as ACTH, growth hormone and PRL. Details of this testing can be found in any textbook on this matter.

Knowledge of the oestrogen status of a given patient is extremely important in the evaluation of amenorrhoea. This shows whether she is merely anovulatory or has a more serious defect in the reproductive axis. This may be accomplished by either measuring an oestrogen level (in this instance a specific oestradiol assay is important) or by administering a progestin. It requires approximately 40 pg/ml of oestradiol to have positive withdrawal bleeding in response to progestin. This level of oestrogen is similar to that of the early phase of the menstrual cycle. The level of oestradiol may be presumed to be above

40 pg/ml if there is withdrawal bleeding after administering a progestin which confirms the anovulatory state. Progesterone in oil, 100–150 mg, may be administered intramuscularly. Bleeding usually ensues within a week and this can be anything from a brownish discharge to frank bleeding. Alternatively, various progestins can be administered orally for 5–7 days. This is accomplished with either medroxyprogesterone acetate in doses from 10 to 30 mg or with norethindrone from 5 to 10 mg daily. Details of testing for states of oestrogen deficiency and the evaluation of patients lacking a response to intramuscular progesterone can be found under the section on amenorrhoea.

13.5 DYSFUNCTIONAL UTERINE BLEEDING (DUB)

Physiology of normal menstrual shedding

In response to oestrogen, the endometrial tissue builds up from the functional basal layer to cause a proliferation of glandular tissue and stroma. This normally occurs until midcycle, around day 14, when ovulation ensues. Following the rise in progesterone which is secreted by the corpus luteum, an organization of the endometrium occurs. In the presence of progesterone, oestrogen growth of the endometrium is arrested abruptly because of the anti-oestrogenic effect of progesterone. Following this, an organization of the endometrium occurs where the endometrium is functionally held together because of the production of mucopolysaccharides which function as a ground support.

Progesterone also influences the endometrium in that the glands undergo secretory transformation. In the presence of adequate progesterone stimulation during the luteal phase, when endometrial shedding occurs, an organized slough occurs down to the level of the decidua basalis. Menstrual bleeding is arrested by the two mechanisms: the first is platelet plug formation and the second is due to prostaglandin stimulation of uterine contractions ($PGF_{2\alpha}$).

Key concepts in understanding the pathophysiology of DUB are:

1. Oestrogen causes growth of the endometrium.
2. Progestin results in support.
3. Platelet plug formation is the first line of defence for cessation of shedding.
4. Prostaglandin interaction is important for uterine haemostasis.

Definitions of dysfunctional uterine bleeding

1. Menorrhagia — Excessive bleeding at regular intervals (generally > 80 ml per month).
2. Hypermenorrhoea — Prolonged bleeding at regular intervals (1 and 2 are sometimes used interchangeably).
3. Metrorrhagia — Variable amounts of bleeding at abnormal and frequent intervals.
4. Menometrorrhagia — Excessive bleeding, often prolonged, at abnormal and frequent intervals.
5. Polymenorrhoea — Bleeding at regular intervals less than <21 days.
6. Oligomenorrhoea — Bleeding at irregular intervals of greater than 35 days.
7. Hypomenorrhoea — Decrease in amount and duration of menses.

DUB is an exclusionary diagnosis. It refers to conditions where all anatomical and exogenous causes of bleeding have been ruled out in a non-pregnant reproductive-age woman. This also excludes women with bleeding disorders, medical endocrinopathies and all postmenopausal women. A common misconception is that a woman on birth control pills may have DUB. However, a woman on exogenous sex steroids may bleed because of the hormonal effect of those steroids on her endometrium, but not because of her endogenous state.

The greatest prevalence of DUB occurs in the perimenarchial period and in the perimenopausal woman. The primary problem which occurs in the adolescent is that her hypothalamic–pituitary axis has not yet reached maturity. There is an absent positive feedback of oestradiol on GnRH–LH release which results in anovulation. The oestrogen stimulation of the endometrium with an abrupt fall in oestrogen levels occurring in the absence of ovulation leads to heavy bleeding episodes.

The most important factor to rule out in teenagers who present with heavy bleeding is the occurrence of a blood dyscrasia (not DUB) causing bleeding. In acute adolescent menorrhagia, this can occur in up to 20% of cases and may represent the initial presentation of the bleeding disorder. Most of these are platelet disorders.

The perimenopausal woman is relatively oestrogen deficient. FSH levels rise in the circulation even before the last menstrual period. The relative deficiency of oestrogen coupled with the progressive dissociation between the hypothalamic–pituitary axis and the ovary results in an erratic response of the endometrium and irregular bleeding. While anovulation usually occurs, ovulatory dysfunction can also result.

Mechanisms of dysfunctional uterine bleeding

While progesterone withdrawal is the normal mechanism which results in menstruation, the most common cause of bleeding in DUB is due to a build-up of endometrium in the absence of progesterone (anovulation). This results in breakthrough bleeding when the height of the endometrium can no longer be supported in the absence of progesterone.

Any acute cessation of oestrogen (oestrogen withdrawal) can result in breakdown of the endometrium and bleeding. This occurs in teenagers when, in the absence of positive feedback and an LH surge, the follicle stops its development and oestrogen levels fall.

Clinical management

It is imperative to know whether ovulatory or anovulatory bleeding is occurring. After adequate history and physical examination, which is important to rule out the most obvious medical and anatomical conditions, pregnancy should be ruled out in reproductive-age women. It is also important to have some objective monitor of the amount of bleeding (e.g. haematocrit). After this, if bleeding has been a significant problem, an endometrial biopsy (not a dilatation and curettage [D & C]) will provide valuable information in that the histological nature of the bleeding endometrium can be evaulated.

Most causes of DUB are due to anovulation. This may become obvious in history taking or will be noted by the finding of a proliferative endometrium on biopsy. Occasionally, an endometrial biopsy will reveal a secretory endometrium. This can be a cause of DUB if the progestin support has been inadequate or if there is a subtle anatomical defect not detected on physical examination (endometrial polyp, submucous fibroid, adenomyosis, etc.).

Treatment

Treatment of DUB may be divided into acute and long-term phases.

ACUTE PHASE

If heavy bleeding occurs particularly in conjunction with a low haematocrit and it is necessary to stop bleeding acutely, a regimen with oestrogen is needed. Oestrogen causes growth of the endometrium. Thus, regardless, of the cause of bleeding, a proliferative growth of the endometrium can be achieved over denuded bleeding endometrial surfaces. This process, however, takes time and a minimum of 4–6 hours is needed for the oestrogen effect to be observed. In very high doses, oestrogens may stabilize platelet function as well through unknown mechanisms. High-dose oestrogens can be administered parenterally (25 mg Premarin IV q 4 hours) or orally 2.5 mg q.i.d. If bleeding does not stop within 2 days, a curettage should be considered. Once bleeding stops, the oral dose should be continued for at least another 7 days with the addition of a progestin (e.g. Provera 10 mg) to help slough the endometrium at the end of the week. During this time, iron therapy is recommended. An alternative method is to give oral contraceptive pills four times a day. The high-dose oestrogen in the pill helps to control bleeding while the progestin helps to organize the endometrium. After 4 pills a day of an oral contraceptive containing 50 µg of ethinyloestradiol and a progestin for a week, withdrawal bleeding occurs. However, this withdrawal bleeding usually ceases because the endometrium has been influenced by the progestin. It is absolutely essential to add a progestin for at least a week to any acute regimen which is designed to stop bleeding.

LONG-TERM MANAGEMENT

This may be divided into patients who are anovulatory or ovulatory.

Anovulatory DUB

Anovulatory patients are the majority of patients. The adolescent bleeder who has DUB (platelet and other bleeding disorders ruled out) only needs progestin until her hypothalamic–pituitary axis matures. Provera may be prescribed at a dose of 10 mg q.i.d. for 10 days each month for 3 months.

The reproductive-age woman may be treated in a similar fashion or be given oral contraceptives. She may receive clomiphene if she wishes to conceive.

The perimenopausal woman may also receive Provera but is better served with sequential treatment with oestrogen and progestin (as for menopausal patients) because of oestrogen deficiency and her relative lack of progestin receptors.

Ovulatory DUB

In the woman with a secretory endometrium, an anatomical lesion should be ruled out. A hysterosalpingogram will reveal a filling defect which may explain the bleeding. If there is no anatomical lesion, therapy should be directed at suppressing the endometrium. This is accomplished by oral contraceptives or a progestin for 21 days each month (e.g. Provera 10 mg). At the time of bleeding, an antiprostaglandin will reduce blood loss further. This latter effect is primarily due to the suppression of prostacyclin which opposes the pro-aggregatory effects of platelets and has been found to be excessively produced in patients with DUB. There is some evidence that low doses of danazol (200 mg/day) may be effective in women who are difficult to treat.

Most recently, laser ablation of the endometrium has been advocated but is an alternative only to be considered if future fertility is not desired. Hysterectomy may be another therapy if all else fails, or if other indications exist.

THE ROLE OF DILATATION AND CURETTAGE

A dilatation and curettage need not be routine for DUB. It should be recommended for:

1. Women with hypovolaemia and haemodynamic compromise. A D and C will control bleeding much faster than using high-dose oestrogens.
2. Women over the age of 40 or those who have significant medical illness.
3. Failed medical management (e.g. after a trial with high-dose oestrogens and progestins).

13.6 DYSMENORRHOEA

Pain just before and during menstruation may be the result of exaggeration of the normal physiological changes that occur at this time, or be the consequence of pathological changes within the reproductive organs.

Physiological changes (first-day dysmenorrhoea)

After menstruation and before ovulation, the myometrium of the non-pregnant human uterus is exposed to the action of oestradiol. The action of this hormone on the smooth muscle of the uterus is to produce contractions of high frequency but low amplitude. After ovulation, the progesterone secreted by the corpus luteum modifies myometrial activity by reducing the frequency of contractions but increasing the amplitude. After withdrawal of progesterone at the end of the menstrual cycle, the endometrium undergoes disorganization and fragmentation whereby prostaglandins are liberated. The prostaglandins produce large uterine contractions on the first day of menstruation. These contractions are not unlike the contractions which occur during labour and give rise to pain and stimulation of the sympathetic nervous system. Prostaglandins reaching the alimentary tract may produce nausea and occasionally diarrhoea. After the first of day of menstruation, the uterine contractions gradually diminish.

Foreign bodies within the uterine cavity (e.g. intrauterine device) can stimulate contractions. Intrauterine devices may produce 'cramps' and heavy menstrual flow (menorrhagia), accentuating the discomfort experienced during menstruation. The principal prostaglandin liberated which is responsible for uterine contractions and pain is $PGF_{2\alpha}$.

Clinical features of primary dysmenorrhoea

Age. When menstruation first commences, bleeding is often painless because of anovulatory cycles and the lack of liberation of $PGF_{2\alpha}$. Some girls, however, experience painful periods from the initiation of menarche.

Parity. After the first confinement, dysmenorrhoea is often less severe owing to the softening of the cervix and its response to uterine contractions.

Pain. The distribution of pain is suprapubic, extending into both iliac fossae and down the inner and front aspect of the thighs. It is referred to the T10 to L1 dermatomes. The pain is maximal at the commencement of the menstrual flow and is milder on the second day.

Frequency. About 40% of normal young women experience some discomfort with their periods, but 7% between the ages of 17 and 24 seek medical advice because of the severity of the dysmenorrhoea. About half of those who seek medical advice are unable to carry on with their work or social activities on the first day of menstruation and have to lie down for part of the day.

Secondary dysmenorrhoea

The discussion above pertains to primary dysmenorrhoea. If dysmenorrhoea appears for the first time later in life, it is considered 'secondary' and usually signifies an organic aetiology. The history of secondary dysmenorrhoea alerts the clinician to pathological states. Careful history and physical examination are necessary to rule out pathological conditions. This may be supplemented by X-ray studies and/or direct visualization at laparoscopy. Pelvic infection, adhesions, ovarian masses or tubal pathology, endometriosis and adenomyosis are some of the more common causes of secondary dysmenorrhoea. If any of these diseases is present, therapy is directed specifically at the disorder.

Treatment

Antiprostaglandins are the primary therapy for dysmenorrhoea. Newer agents like ibuprofen, mefenamic acid and others are more effective than aspirin. These agents are capable of inhibiting or relieving dysmenorrhoea in over 75% of women. If the synthetase inhibitors are ineffective, then hormonal therapy may be used.

Oral contraceptives may be effective by suppressing endometrial growth and suppressing $PGF_{2\alpha}$ production.

SURGICAL APPROACHES

These approaches are not usually advocated but may be used as adjuncts or may be considered if other therapy is ineffective.

DILATATION OF THE CERVIX

Mechanical dilatation of the cervix produces partial relief of dysmenorrhoea in about one-third of women. However, with forceful dilatation of the cervix there is the risk of an incompetent internal os in future pregnancies.

PRESACRAL NEURECTOMY

The sensory fibres from the uterus travel back to the spinal cord through the presacral nerves and over the surfaces of contiguous large vessels. Dysmenorrhoea may be relieved by cutting these sensory fibres. However, this involves a laparotomy, and the results are not always completely satisfactory. Its major role is as an adjunctive procedure to conservative pelvic surgery, such as in the treatment of endometriosis.

13.7 THE PREMENSTRUAL SYNDROME (PMS)

Some women become miserable and unhappy the week before the onset of their periods and many are 'off colour' or depressed for 2–3 days premenstrually. Other women only complain of carbo-hydrate intolerance and others may have breast tenderness and/or significant fluid retention. In general, somatic complaints should be separated from the mood disorders of anxiety and depression. Those who experience headaches just before or during menses sometimes develop a migraine-type affliction associated with nausea and vomiting. Acne often becomes more prominent premenstrually. These effects, with the exception of migraine, are thought to be the result of progesterone produced during the second half of the cycle.

PMS is a heterogeneous group of disorders which results in sig-nificant disability in many women. It is imperative to document the disorder by having patients fill out daily symptom cards for 1 or 2 cycles. If symptom scores in the luteal or premenstrual phase exceed those of the follicular phase then true PMS may be operative. By documenting symptomatology throughout the menstrual cycle, signi-ficant psychopathology may also emerge. Evaluation in conjunction with a psychologist or psychiatrist is recommended.

There is no accepted aetiological basis for PMS and there are probably several factors involved in this heterogeneous syndrome. A relative progesterone lack and/or an acute brain opioid withdrawal phenomenon are two of the most popular theories.

Treatment

Therapy is best directed at the particular complaint. Mastodynia is effectively treated with bromocriptine or danazol. Fluid retention is best alleviated by spironolactone of another diuretic. Depression and mood disturbances respond well to placebo. High-dose progesterone suppositories have been advocated by many but the responses are similar to responses obtained with placebo. Alprazolam for anxiety and depression has been found to be more effective than placebo for treating some women. Progesterone has been used as an adjunct in the second half of the cycle but the response is not encouraging. However, suppression of the complete menstrual cycle by a GnRH agonist has been successful. Occasionally the use of continuous progestins or oral contraception has relieved symptoms.

13.8 PELVIC PAIN

Pelvic pain not associated with menstruation is a common complaint and can be an extremely difficult problem to diagnose and treat. In the absence of positive findings on physical examination, subtle abnormalities or functional, psychological disorders are likely.

Exclusion of urinary, gastrointestinal and musculoskeletal abnormalities, which may be the cause of pain, is important in evaluating the patient. This can be accomplished by appropriate X-ray and other diagnostic tests as indicated.

Abnormalities of the reproductive organs including pelvic adhesive disease, chronic salpingitis and other tubal pathology, endometriosis and adenomyosis are all possible diagnoses. An entity called pelvic congestion which is associated with dilated tortuous ovarian veins has been described, but if existent, is an inconsistent and rare finding. If history and physical examination are negative, a diagnostic laparoscopy is still necessary to rule out organic pathology. After this, if needed, psychological evaluation may be appropriate. Many women who complain of pain are sufficiently reassured after a negative laparoscopy and cease to have major complaints thereafter.

13.9 AMENORRHOEA AND ANOVULATION

Definitions

Primary amenorrhoea may be diagnosed if menstruation has not occurred by the age of sixteen or if there has been no breast development by the age of fourteen and a half.

Secondary amenorrhoea is generally defined as the absence of cyclic menses for 6 months. Some clinicians prefer a 3-month time interval for the absence of menses and others use the absence of menses for 1 year in women who are oligomenorrhoeic.

Primary amenorrhoea

Primary amenorrhoea may be simply categorized based upon the presence or absence of the breast and uterus. Breast development signifies appropriate oestrogen production. If breast tissue is absent and the uterus is present by examination or ultrasound, the differential diagnosis is between gonadal dysgenesis and hypothalamic–pituitary failure or hypogonadotrophic hypogonadism. A karyotype helps make this distinction and is particularly valuable in the absence of classic phenotypic features of Turner's syndrome. A skull X-ray or computerized axial tomography (CT) scan is essential to rule out a central nervous system (CNS) lesion if the karyotype is normal.

If breast tissue is present and the uterus is absent, the differential diagnosis is between testicular feminization (TF) and congenital absence of a uterus. A normal female testosterone level rules out TF while a level in the male range can be confirmed by the finding of a male karyotype, 46,XY. Congenital absence of the uterus, which is more common than TF, may be confirmed by a biphasic basal body temperature or weekly progesterone levels signifying normal ovulatory ovarian function in the absence of uterine tissue. A laparoscopy is not necessary. In these two disorders, the 'vagina' ends blindly and may require either dilatation therapy or a vaginoplasty.

If both breast and uterus are absent, then a rare abnormality exists and a karyotype is required. This usually occurs in patients who have a 46,XY karyotype and have a defect in steroidogenesis or have a situation where the testes were lost at some point in development. These patients usually require referral for a complete diagnosis.

If both breast and uterus are present, then the patient needs to be evaluated for some arrest in development which precludes normal menstruation. This includes a PRL-secreting adenoma or another CNS lesion. Alternatively, an outflow abnormality of the uterus may exist which was caused by infection such as pelvic tuberculosis. In the absence of an outflow tract abnormality, these patients are evaluated as are all patients with secondary amenorrhoea (described below).

TREATMENT OF PRIMARY AMENORRHOEA

Gonadal dysgenesis is treated with oestrogen replacement. If a Y line exists in the karyotype, the streaks need to be removed to prevent the development of a neoplasm. CNS lesions in patients with hypogonadotrophic hypogonadism are treated as required from a neurosurgical standpoint.

TF is treated with oestrogen replacement. Gonadectomy (of testes) is required by the time of maturity to avoid a neoplasm. There is controversy if this should be carried out in childhood or after adequate breast development by age 18. Congenital absence is treated with reassurance and screening for associated skeletal and renal abnormalities. A vaginoplasty may be required, or dilator therapy and intercourse in patients with TF and congenital absence of the uterus.

Patients with both breast and uterus present ultimately require treatment after a firm diagnosis is made.

Secondary amenorrhoea

Outflow abnormalities of the uterus have to be ruled out here. The history of prior instrumentation of the uterus, of any kind, is an important clue. The uterus may be sounded or a hysterosalpingogram should be ordered. Hormonal induction of menses with both oestrogen and progestin is an unreliable diagnostic test.

If outflow abnormalities have been ruled out, the oestrogen status of the patient needs to be established by a progestin challenge test. Progesterone in oil, 150 mg intramuscularly, will induce bleeding in women with an adequate oestrogen status. This signifies a problem of anovulation due to a myriad of CNS causes (e.g. stress, exercise, psychological disturbances, etc.). At this juncture, gonadotrophin assays are important as is PRL. Hyperprolactinaemia may be a cause of secondary amenorrhoea and anovulation even in the absence of galactorrhoea. If LH is high, it suggests the diagnosis of PCO even in the absence of hirsutism. If LH is normal or low, a hypothalamic dysfunction responsible for anovulation is operative.

If the progestin challenge test is negative, oestrogen deficiency may be assumed in the absence of an outflow tract abnormality. Gonadotrophin measurements are necessary here. If FSH levels are normal or low, a central disturbance of the hypothalmic–pituitary axis is present and a CAT scan is required as well as a more indepth evaluation of pituitary function including measurements of thyroid status (free thyroxine index rather than TSH). If FSH levels are high, the diagnosis is premature ovarian failure. This is diagnosed in women who have amenorrhoea prior to the age of 40. Karyotypic abnormalities are common in women under age 25 and women in this age group should have karyotype carried out. Although there are many possible aetiologies for premature ovarian failure, we do not advocate laparoscopy or ovarian biopsy. It is important to rule out polyglandular autoimmunity in this group. Tests for hypothyroidism, antimicrosomal and antinuclear antibodies, calcium, phosphorus and urinary-free cortisol are some of the tests which should be considered.

TREATMENT OF SECONDARY AMENORRHOEA

If patients respond to progestin challenge, anovulation is either treated with induction of ovulation or intermittent progestin withdrawal. In PCO, hyperandrogenism is best suppressed as described below.

Hypo-oestrogenism in patients with secondary amenorrhoea is treated with oestrogen replacement in the same way as postmenopausal women. If a woman with hypothalamic failure wishes to conceive, she can be treated with either human menopausal gonadotrophins or pulsatile GnRH.

13.10 HYPERPROLACTINAEMIA

Prolactin is a hormone which is influenced by stress events as well as oestrogen and certain drugs. Its control is primarily inhibitory.

Galactorrhoea is the most common physical finding in hyperprolactinaemia, yet galactorrhoea may occur with a normal PRL level and rarely PRL may be elevated when galactorrhoea has not been elicited. Drug ingestion (e.g. tranquillizers) is a common cause of galactorrhoea and hyperprolactinaemia and careful history taking is required. Hypothyroidism may be present in up to 5% of patients with galactorrhoea and hyperprolactinemia and thyroid function testing (TSH) is important to include in patient evaluation.

Hyperprolactinaemia may result in amenorrhoea or luteal deficiency but can be associated with normal menses. PRL inhibits the hypothalamic–pituitary axis and may potentially affect ovarian function directly as well. Menstrual disturbances, infertility and galactorrhoea are the major indications for measurement of PRL.

If PRL is > 20 ng/ml during the day, unassociated with stress or food intake (which causes a transient rise), further evaluation is necessary. A TSH assay is a sensitive test for hypothyroidism. Patients with consistently elevated PRL levels > 60 ng/ml should have a CT scan or magnetic resonance imaging (MRI) of the pituitary to rule out an adenoma. Patients with levels slightly above 20 ng/ml and who have regular menses can be followed. If the PRL level is < 60 ng/ml but is consistently > 20 ng/ml and the patient has anovulation, a CT scan or MRI is indicated.

Most abnormalities of the pituitary are PRL-secreting microadenomas (< 1 cm), although occasionally macroadenomas will be detected. With larger tumours, visual field evaluation and more complete endocrinological and neurological assessment are necessary. A microadenoma may not require treatment unless oestogen deficiency exists or pregnancy is desired. Knowledge of the oestrogen status in hyerprolactinaemia patients is essential and may be assessed by progestin challenge and/or an oestradiol assay. Amenorrhoea and oestrogen deficiency in hyperprolactinaemia are also associated with significant osteoporosis.

Treatment of hyperprolactinaemia

After ruling out drug exposure and hypothyroidism, indications for treatment of hyperprolactinaemia are:

1. Macroadenomas
2. Oestrogen deficiency
3. Infertility

Other patients may be followed clinically and with PRL assays at 6-month intervals.

In all patients bromocriptine is used to suppress PRL. A starting dose of 2.5 mg daily is increased up to 10 mg or more in order to suppress PRL levels to normal or until symptoms and signs disappear. Side effects of dizziness, nausea, hypotension and nasal congestion may be significant and bromocriptine should be administered with caution in small incremental doses. Normal oestrogen status and ovulatory function are important endpoints of therapy.

In patients with macroadenomas, depending on the response to bromocriptine, neurosurgery may be advocated as an additional measure. Once bromocriptine is stopped, rapid regrowth can occur. In patients with microadenomas, repeat pituitary scans are only requested every 2–3 years or after a pregnancy has occurred. Although there is no consensus, we do not advocate the use of bromocriptine in pregnancy for microadenomas unless symptoms occur. For patients with macroadenomas, the maintenance dose of bromocriptine during pregnancy may be prudent.

13.11 HYPERANDROGENISM/HIRSUITISM/ POLYCYSTIC OVARY SYNDROME

Excessive androgen secretion in women may lead to anovulation as well as acne and hirsutism. Androgen may be secreted in excess by the ovaries, adrenals or peripheral tissues, including skin. The best blood marker of each of these three compartments is:

1. Testosterone (T) for the ovary (reflecting about two-thirds of circulating T).
2. Dehydroepiandrosterone sulphate (DHEA-S) for the adrenal (90% an adrenal product).
3. 3 α-Androstanediol glucuronide for the peripheral compartment.

When a patient presents with clinical signs of androgen excess, the following differential diagnosis should be considered:

1. Iatrogenic or drug-related hirsutism.
2. Abnormal gonadal or sexual development.
3. Idiopathic (familial) hirsutism.
4. Polycystic ovary syndrome.
5. Stromal hyperthecosis.
6. Androgen-producing ovarian tumours.
7. Cushing's syndrome.
8. Adult manifestation of congenital adrenal hyperplasia.
9. Androgen-producing adrenal tumours.

Clinical evaluation should be directed at establishing the most likely diagnosis by history and physical examination and then by determining the source(s) of excessive androgen production. A serum T level two and a half times above the upper limit of the laboratory suggests an ovarian neoplasm. DHEA-S levels above 8 µg/ml suggests an adrenal neoplasm.

Only the most common conditions will be included here. The most likely diagnoses in hirsute women are 'idiopathic' or constitutional hirsutism and PCO. 'Idiopathic' hirsutism appears to be a genetically endowed, familial problem of skin sensitivity in most cases and may be reflected in elevated levels of peripherally-derived androgens like 3 α-androstanediol glucuronide. It may be diagnosed in ovulatory women with near-normal levels of T and DHEA-S. While free T levels may be slightly elevated, this does not explain the source or severity of hirsutism.

PCO is a heterogeneous group of disorders characterized by peri-menarchial onset of chronic anovulation and hyperandrogenism, whether or not hirsutism is present. Patients are often obese and typically have enlarged cystic ovaries. However, the latter finding is not an absolute requirement. The adrenals and ovaries may both be sources of increased androgen production and patients are hyper-oestrogenic as well (increased oestrone and free oestradiol) leading to problems of dysfunctional bleeding and endometrial hyperplasia. PRL levels may be slightly elevated. The cardinal biochemical feature of PCO is inappropriate gonadotrophin secretion with high serum LH levels (> 21 mIU/ml) and FSH levels which are low or normal resulting in a ratio of LH : FSH which is elevated. This finding occurs in three-quarters of the patients with PCO.

Tumours of the adrenal or ovary are suggested by their rapid clinical course, abnormal findings if present on physical examination, and elevated levels of T and/or DHEA-S. Specific imaging techniques are often required (ultrasound, CT) and, rarely, selective venous catheterization studies will be helpful.

Adult onset of mild, attenuated congenital adrenal hyperplasia resulting from a deficiency of 21-hydroxylase, or, rarely, 11-hydroxylase can be found in approximately 5% of hirsute women. The vast majority of cases are due to a mild 21-hydroxylase deficiency which is not associated with salt wasting. These diagnoses should be kept in mind when evaluating young hirsute patients who have high levels of androgens, who may be shorter, have a strong family history of hirsutism and who may have hypertension (patients with 11-hydroxylase deficiency). The specific measurements of 17-hydroxyprogesterone before and/or after ACTH stimulation will establish the diagnosis.

Treatment

The favoured treatment is based upon the source of hyperandrogenism. Clearly, operative therapy is indicated for neoplasms but should not be considered in PCO. Oral contraceptives primarily inhibit ovarian androgens, increase binding globulin and thereby lower free T levels dramatically. Oral contraceptives also inhibit adrenal androgens to a minor degree (30%). Prednisone or dexamethasone in low doses 2.5 or 0.25 mg, respectively) suppress moderate elevations in adrenal androgens without major effects on cortisol secretion. Close monitoring is necessary for signs of hypercortisolism and excessive pituitary–adrenal suppression.

Cyproterone acetate and spironolactone are the best agents for peripheral androgen disorders like 'idiopathic' hirsutism. If hirsutism is mild, the combination pill with ethinyloestradiol 50 µg and a progestin may be used while larger doses of cyproterone are usually required for more severe cases. Spironolactone 100–200 mg is effective in 70% of patients with the complaint of hirsutism. With these agents, healthy patients have few side effects, and specifically, hyperkalaemia is rarely encountered with spironolactone. Combinations of oral contraceptives, dexamethasone and spironolactone may also be used effectively.

13.12 MENOPAUSE

The average age of the menopause is 51.4 years. Hormonal changes of the menopause are listed in Table 13.1. Clearly as much as a third of a woman's life is spent in a state of hormonal deficiency. In this context, as women live longer, the quality of that time is extremely important. Except for the rare individual, virtually all women are candidates for oestrogen replacement, whether or not they suffer from vasomotor instability. Table 13.2 lists the major body systems benefited by oestrogens. Only 75% of women entering the menopause complain of hot flushes or vasomotor instability. However, to exclude the other 25% of the postmenopausal population from receiving oestrogen would be erroneous for the reasons outlined below.

Psychological function and mood are improved with oestrogen. However, improvement in depression for example, only occurs within the normal range. Oestrogen has no place in the management of psychotic depression. Nevertheless, anxiety decreases and the sense of well-being, short-term memory and insomnia may be improved in symptomatic women. While these changes may largely be due to decreases in vasomotor instability, even in asymptomatic women, psychological profiles have been shown to improve.

It has been clearly established that oestrogen can prevent the development of postmenopausal osteoporosis, even though the mechanism for this benefit has not been established. Calcium supplementation, although important because of the relative deficient dietary intake of calcium, has been shown not to be of benefit when used as sole therapy. To sufficiently replace calcium, a total daily intake of 1500 mg of elemental calcium is required. There is insufficient data on other

Table 13.1 Hormonal changes of menopause

FSH elevated +++	Oestradiol$_2$ decreased ++
LH elevated ++	Oestrone$_1$ decreased +
	Testosterone decreased +
PRL normal or decreased	Androstenedione decreased +
ACTH normal	DHEA-S decreased +
TSH normal	Cortisol normal
	FTI normal

Table 13.2   Body systems benefited by oestrogen

1. Vasomotor symptoms
2. Psychological symptoms/mood
3. Connective tissue and bone homoeostasis
4. Genitourinary atrophy
5. Cardiovascular

regimens, including 1,25-dihydroxyvitamin D, calcitonin and fluoride, for their recommendation for the prevention of osteoporosis. The effective preventive dose for decreasing bone resorption for all women is the equivalent of 0.625 mg of conjugated equine oestrogens (CEE, Premarin). Other natural oestrogen compounds may be equally beneficial. There is some evidence that the addition of a progestin imparts an additional benefit by stimulating bone formation.

Collagen content in skin, bone and the pelvic diaphragm decrease with oestrogen deficiency but also as a function of age. There is evidence that replacement therapy alleviates many of these problems and is beneficial, to some extent, for the wrinkling of skin and stress urinary incontinence. Very small doses of local oestrogen application (0.3 mg CEE) aid greatly in improving the vaginal epithelium and for problems of atrophy, senile vaginitis and dyspareunia. Much larger doses ($\sim$ 1.25 mg CEE) are required orally for this purpose.

Contrary to earlier belief, natural oestrogen replacement (as opposed to synthetic compounds used in birth control pills) is beneficial for the cardiovascular system and appears to be cardioprotective. The incidence of cardiovascular disease (which increases in women after the menopause) is reduced by at least 50% in those women receiving oestrogen. Furthermore the chance of dying upon sustaining a myocardial infarction is reduced by 50–60% in those women receiving oestrogen. Natural oestrogen replacement has no major effect on blood pressure, carbohydrate tolerance or coagulation factors. Indeed, hypertension, which occurs rarely with oestrogen replacement, has to be viewed as an idiosyncratic reaction. The more natural oestrogens such as oestrone sulphate and oestradiol have been shown to actually decrease blood pressure in normo- and hypertensive women in prospective studies.

The purported mechanism for the cardioprotective effect of oestrogen replacement is related to lipid metabolism. Oestrogen imparts a beneficial lipoprotein profile by increasing high-density lipoprotein$_2$–cholesterol with its apolipoprotein A$_1$ and by lowering low-density lipoprotein-cholesterol. However, there are probably other cardiopro-tective properties of oestrogen as well which need to be elucidated.

In women with a uterus, progestins need to be prescribed to prevent endometrial hyperplasia. It has been established that lower doses of progestins are sufficient as long as progestin therapy is maintained for 12 days. Because progestins tend to oppose the beneficial effects of oestrogen on lipoprotein subfractions, lowering the dose to 2.5 or 5 mg of medroxyprogesterone acetate (Provera) or 0.35–1 mg of nor-ethindrone/norethisterone (micronor, Norlutin) is important as long as therapy continues for 12 days. Usually 5 mg of Provera or 0.7 mg of norethindrone/norethisterone are needed. In women without a uterus, there is no proven benefit of adding a progestin although this is often recommended by those who believe progestins also reduce the risk of breast cancer.

There is no evidence at present that oestrogen replacement in-creases the risk of breast neoplasia. However, oestrogen is contraindica-ted in women with breast carcinoma. The only other contraindications are invasive undifferentiated uterine cancer, severe thromboembolic disease and severe liver disease. To a certain extent, the latter two contraindications may be dealt with on a selective basis by using a parenteral form of oestrogen or a progestin-only preparation.

Estraderm (0.05 and 0.1 mg) is a transdermal therapy which avoids potentially harmful hepatic first passage effects. This also occurs with use of the subcutaneous oestradiol pellet (Progynon 25 mg), oestrogel (a cream) or injectable oestrogens. Estraderm, oestrogel or the pellet may be considered according to the patient's preference or for those women who dislike the oral route and/or who have hepatic-related problems such as the idiosyncratic reactions of hypertension and thrombophlebitis. Injectable oestrogens tend to result in pharmaco-logical dosing and should be avoided. Parenteral oestrogens, however, have the disadvantage of not altering lipoprotein fractions as favourably as with the oral route.

Progestins alone may be of some benefit for the alleviation of vasomotor symptoms and maintenance of bone mass. Oral Provera 10–20 mg/day is required or 150 mg Depo Provera intramuscularly every 3 months has been used effectively. These methods are less preferable primarily because of their potential negative impact on the cardiovascular system.

The most popular regimens for replacement therapy are found in Table 13.3. Cyclic therapy using one of the natural oestrogens may be used for 25 days each month or used continuously if symptoms

Table 13.3 Replacement regimens

Cyclic
  Oestrogens
  Conjugated equine oestrogens — Calendar days 1–25
  (Premarin) 0.625 mg (or every day)

                                      or

  Oestrone sulphate
  (Ogen) 0.625–1.25 mg

                                      or

  Micronized oestradiol
  (Estrace) 1 mg

                                      or

  Oestradiol valerate
  (Progynova) 1–2 mg
Progestins
  Medroxyprogesterone acetate — Days 14–25
  (Provera) 5–10 mg (or 12 days each month)

                                      or

  Norethindrone (NET) 1 mg
  Norethisterone
Continuous combined
  Premarin 0.625 or
  Ogen 1.25 mg or
  Estrace 1 mg plus Provera 5–10 mg or
  NET 0.3–1 mg
Options: Every day or 5 days each week (Monday to Friday)

occur at the end of a cycle. The dose should be increased only for symptomatic complaints (Ogen or Estrace may be slightly less potent). Synthetic oestrogens (e.g., Estinyl, Estigyn) should be avoided unless very small doses are used because of their marked hepatic stimulatory effects. Twelve days of progestins should be used at the end of the 25-day regimen. If bleeding occurs before day 10 of progestin therapy, the dose of progestin should be increased. Normal withdrawal bleeding should ensue with this regimen and should not warrant the use of routine endometrial biopsies.

In women wishing to achieve amenenorrhoea, various continuous combined regimens have been used (Table 13.3). Early experience with these regimens suggests that bleeding control is difficult and although endometrial atrophy usually occurs, continuous spotting and bleeding for several months may be disheartening. Several changes in the oestrogen/progestin combinations may be required to achieve amenorrhoea.

Prolapse and urinary incontinence

Barry G. Wren

14.1 GENERAL INSTRUCTIONAL OBJECTIVE

The students should understand the nature and significance of utero-vaginal prolapse and urinary incontinence so that they can diagnose these conditions and appreciate the management of such patients.

14.2 SPECIFIC BEHAVIOURAL OBJECTIVES

1. Discuss the applied anatomy of the uterus, vagina and supporting structures.
2. Discuss the aetiological factors of utero-vaginal prolapse.
3. Explain the meaning of urethrocoele, cystocoele, enterocoele, rectocoele and the degree of uterine prolapse.
4. Demonstrate an ability to examine a woman with utero-vaginal prolapse and relate the history to the physical findings.
5. List the types of management of utero-vaginal prolapse.
6. Discuss urinary continence in the female.
7. List and define the types of urinary incontinence.
8. Discuss the aetiological factors of each type of urinary incontinence.
9. Demonstrate an ability to diagnose the type of urinary incontinence by taking a history and performing an adequate physical examination.

14.3 REASONS FOR LEARNING ABOUT PROLAPSE AND URINARY INCONTINENCE

Women who have had children, or who have passed through the climacteric, may often present to their doctor with complaints that suggest the bladder, uterus or rectum is involved in a prolapse. It is important to be able to take a history, examine and correctly diagnose these conditions, to then initiate management, or to refer to an appropriate person who can manage the problem.

As a large number of women will present with symptoms referable to the bladder and vagina, it is necessary to understand the anatomical, physiological and clinical significance of these structures.

14.4 ANATOMY AND PHYSIOLOGY

The uterus is normally supported in the midpelvic plane by the two fascial thickenings known as the transverse cervical ligaments (Fig. 14.1). This dense fascial tissue begins on either side of the cervix, the lower portion of the uterus and the upper third of the vagina, and runs laterally to insert in a broad area over the lateral wall of the true pelvis.

The transverse cervical ligaments are given added support by the smaller pubo-cervical ligaments and by the utero-sacral ligaments behind.

The round ligaments *do not* support the uterus. They may assist in anteverting the fundus, but do not carry any weight. The broad ligaments (Fig. 14.2) are a thin filmy collection of fascia above the transverse cervical ligaments, and are enclosed by peritoneum anteriorly and posteriorly. Like the round ligaments, they give no support to the uterus.

The perineal body, the levator ani muscle and the mucles surround-

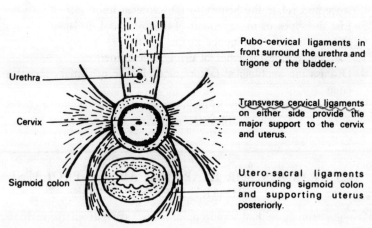

Pubo-cervical ligaments in front surround the urethra and trigone of the bladder.

Urethra

Transverse cervical ligaments on either side provide the major support to the cervix and uterus.

Cervix

Sigmoid colon

Utero-sacral ligaments surrounding sigmoid colon and supporting uterus posteriorly.

Fig. 14.1 Ligamentous supports of the cervix and uterus.

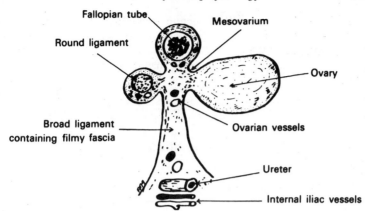

Fig. 14.2 Anatomy of broad ligaments.

ing the vaginal introitus do not support the uterus, but play their part in determining the size of the vaginal introitus.

The bladder and the urethra are supported by fascial tissue surrounding the urethra, bladder trigone and vagina. This tissue inserts into the back of the symphysis pubis and the lower pelvic floor muscles. The fascial supports may become thickened in places to resemble ligaments and are often given names such as the pubo-urethral ligament or suspensory ligament of the bladder, trigone or urethra.

Like all sexual tissue, the fascial planes are dependent on oestrogen to maintain a good tone and to continue to provide support to organs such as the urethra, bladder, cervix, uterus and rectum. When oestrogen is withdrawn from these tissues, not only does the epithelium become atrophic, but so does the surrounding support tissue. This general weakening of the pelvic supports eventually predisposes to stretching and finally prolapse.

Normally the bladder is a very distensible organ, with a thickened and relatively fixed base called the trigone. The trigone lies almost directly over the cervix and the upper third of the vagina, and is thus supported by the fascia. Urinary continence is achieved by a sphincter-like action of the proximal spiral muscle bundles which surround the urethra in its whole length as well as by the maintenance of an angle between the urethra and the bladder.

Any intra-abdominal pressure on the bladder thus will not produce loss of urine if the angle is maintained. However, when the angle is progressively lost until a 'funnel' is produced, stress incontinence may result.

A bladder that has prolapsed, producing a large cystocoele, may not be associated with stress incontinence if the urethral position and the vesico-urethral angle are maintained. However, a much smaller cystocoele associated with a urethocoele may demonstrate severe stress incontinence.

14.5 INCONTINENCE

Stress incontinence

Stress incontinence is that condition occurring when urine is lost with some degree of raised intra-abdominal pressure. This increase in pressure is transmitted to the bladder and if the sphincter closure pressure is exceeded by the intravesical pressure then urine is lost. A large number of women suffer from minor degrees of stress incontinence when 'caught unawares' (coughing, sneezing, laughing, etc.) but if it becomes embarassingly frequent, then it should be investigated and treated.

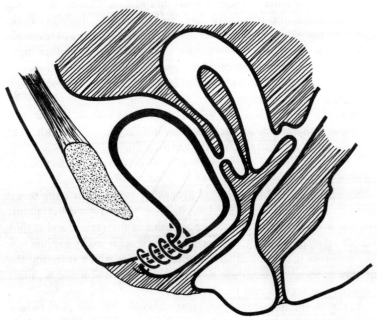

Fig. 14.3 Spiral muscle surrounding sphincter and urethra controls the closure of the urethra.

Also *TRUE INCONTINENCE — constant, due to vesico-vaginal fistula.

*Neurogenic bladder

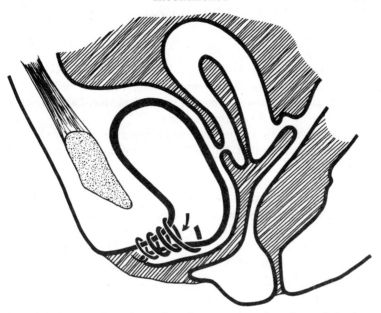

Fig. 14.4 Weakened spiral muscle with cystocoele and urethrocoele leads to stress and urgency incontinence.

Urge incontinence

Urge incontinence occurs when there is an uncontrollable desire to micturate. This usually takes place when urine enters the fore part of the proximal urethra. Urine in the proximal urethra initiates a reflex, mediated through the sacral plexus, which results in detrusor muscle contraction and a marked desire to empty the bladder.

Both urge and stress incontinence may be present in the same patient and are both associated with weakness of the spiral muscle bundles which surround the urethra (Figs 14.3, 14.4).

Irritable or unstable bladder

Irritable or unstable bladder occurs in those women who have an increased detrusor muscle activity either due to intravesical irritation (bladder infection), extravesical irritation (tumours, pregnancy, etc.) or due to nerve excitation (psychological or induced).

Investigations

It is important that whenever a woman presents with symptoms or signs of stress incontinence, urge incontinence or an unstable bladder, she should be investigated before therapy is undertaken. A urodynamic study is most important. During this procedure, the intravesical pressure, vesical volume and the detrusor tone are measured as well as the closure pressure of the urethral sphincter.

Cystoscopy can disclose evidence of inflammation or other changes to the bladder epithelium. Finally, a cystographic study can disclose descent of the bladder base, loss of the urethral sphincter tone and dilatation of the urethra.

Any evidence of irritable bladder with associated sphincter incontinence should be treated with anticholinergic drugs such as probanthine and a central nervous system anxiolytic agent such as imipramine. Excellent results without recourse to surgery may be obtained by judicious use of such drugs.

14.6 PROLAPSE

Classification

BLADDER PROLAPSE

The bladder may prolapse as a cystocoele and bulge down from the anterior wall of the vagina, eventually producing a mass protruding through the introitus. If it remains within the vagina, the cystocoele is regarded as a stage I cystocoele; if a portion protrudes through the introitus, this is a stage II cystocoele; and if all the bladder has prolapsed, this is a stage III cystocoele, which is usually associated with a complete uterine prolapse (procidentia).

Often the cystocoele is also associated with a urethral prolapse. This is known as a cysto-urethrocoele, which is associated with stress incontinence.

UTERINE PROLAPSE

When the uterus has prolapsed but the cervix is still within the vaginal introitus, this is termed a stage I uterine prolapse (Figs 14.5–14.7). When the cervix protrudes through the introitus, this is a stage II prolapse; and when the fundus of the uterus has also come outside the vagina, this is a stage III prolapse or procidentia.

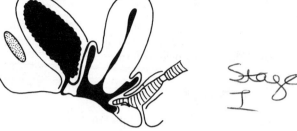

Fig. 14.5 Prolapse. Demonstrating early descent of the uterus, but no associated bladder movement. The urethro-vesical angle is still intact and no stress incontinence occurs.

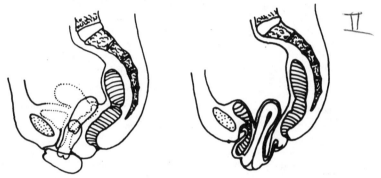

Fig. 14.6 Illustrating the stages in descent and prolapse of the uterus. Shows how as the uterus prolapses, the bladder is dragged out as well to produce a cystocoele.

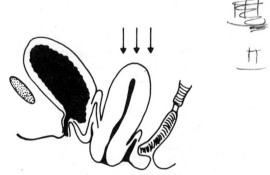

Fig. 14.7 Prolapse of the uterus outside the vagina. Increased intra-abdominal pressure has forced the uterus outside the vagina, dragging the bladder with the anterior wall of the uterus. A cystocoele has developed, but there is no associated stress incontinence because the urethro-vesical angle remains intact.

RECTOCOELE

When the fascia between the rectum and vagina has been torn or stretched, the rectum tends to bulge forward during defaecation, allowing a rectocoele to form.

ENTEROCOELE

In the pouch of Douglas behind the cervix and between the two utero-sacral ligaments, there is a weak area of the posterior vaginal fornix that consists of vaginal epithelium, thin fascia and peritoneum only. Although the space is small, increased intra-abdominal pressure may force loops of bowel against this weak point and produce a hernia into the posterior aspect of the vagina.

Causes of prolapse

There are three major factors associated with the development of a prolapse of the genital organs:

1. Childbirth.
2. Withdrawal of oestrogens.
3. Increase in intra-abdominal pressure.

Chirdbirth is an antecedent cause of prolapse in the majority of cases. This is probably due to several factors. During pregnancy the pelvic tissues become engorged, hypertrophied, softened and elastic, allowing much flexible movement and stretching of tissue that would otherwise tear or overstretch. However, despite this attempt to prepare

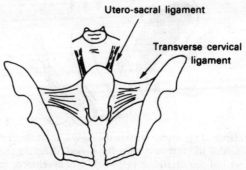

Fig. 14.8 Diagram to illustrate the ligamentous supports of the uterus.

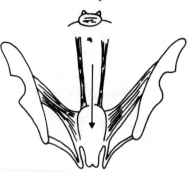

Fig. 14.9 Diagram to illustrate how the utero-sacral ligaments and the transverse cervical ligaments become stretched during prolapse of the uterus. Not only does this cause a dragging pain, but the uterus begins to descend through the vagina.

the genital tract for an easy delivery, there are many times when the delivery does disrupt the fascial supports. This is more likely to occur during a prolonged labour due to disproportion when maternal expulsive efforts or forceps application attempt to deliver the fetus through an incompletely dilated cervix, where rotation and delivery of the head cause torsion of the vagina or when fundal pressure is exerted on the uterus to expel the placenta. All these manoeuvres or activities can produce tearing and disruption or overstretching of the fascial ligamentous supports of the uterus, vagina, bladder or rectum.

Following a delivery, the elastic tissue returns to normal — but if the tissue is weakened by atrophy (oestrogen lack) or by increased intra-abdominal pressure (fat, coughing, ascites, etc.), then the fascial supports give way and allow the bladder, uterus or rectum to prolapse (Figs. 14.8, 14.9).

Symptoms and signs

The symptoms and signs depend to a large extent on the organs involved, but commonly there is:

1. A feeling of a lump or mass within the vagina. This is often expressed as a feeling of fullness and is due to the cervix and uterus prolapsing down the vagina to the introitus.
2. A low backache or bilateral lower abdominal dragging pain. This is due to the pelvic organs dragging down on the usually non-supportive tissue and ligaments, such as utero-sacral ligaments, round ligaments and the broad ligaments.

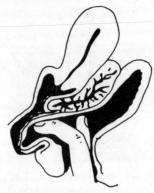

Fig. 14.10 Demonstrating how to differentiate between a rectocoele and an enterocoele employing rectal examination.

3. Symptoms of stress incontinence.
4. Repeated attacks of dysuria, urinary frequency and urgency due to the distortion of the trigone and urethro-vesical angle.
5. Urinary infection due to organisms invading the retained pool of urine.
6. Difficulty in emptying the bowel — often the rectocoele must be pushed back to allow evacuation.
7. Lax vagina, with little or no sensation during intercourse.
8. A discharge or bleeding caused by ulceration of dependent portions of the prolapse (decubitus ulcers).
9. A lump between the thighs, which may be felt when a complete procidentia develops.

Management

When a prolapse has been diagnosed, the management usually lies within the province of the gynaecologist. The basic steps in management are:

1. Reduce excess weight.
2. Treat a cough or respiratory infection.
3. Administer oestrogen to improve the vaginal epithelium and the pelvic fascia. It normally takes 6–12 weeks before there is sufficient improvement in postmenopausal women to allow a surgical approach.

4. Operate to restore normal anatomical planes and anatomy. The operations commonly employed are:

   (a) Manchester repair. The bladder is exposed and fascia united firmly under the bladder neck and trigone. The cervix is amputated, the transverse cervical ligaments shortened and finally the rectocoele is cured as the perineum is restored to normal.

   (b) Vaginal hysterectomy and repair. The Manchester repair technique is used, together with removal of the uterus from below.

   (c) Marshal–Marchetti–Krantz and other operations for stress incontinence. The fascial supports of the urethra and bladder are sewn to the back of the symphysis pubis.

   (d) Sling operation. A sling is passed under the bladder neck and attached to the rectus sheath behind the symphysis pubis to treat stress incontinence.

Postoperative care of vaginal operations

Because patients cannot pass urine through the oedematous inflamed urethra for several days, a suprapubic catheter should be inserted so as to allow complete drainage of the bladder until it begins to function normally. During this phase of suprapubic drainage, care must be taken that the bladder urine remains sterile: careful drainage techniques, appropriate chemotherapy and sometimes bladder irrigations with antiseptic solution are required.

Benign and malignant tumours of the female genital tract

Barry G. Wren

15.1 GENERAL INSTRUCTIONAL OBJECTIVE

The students should understand the nature of benign and malignant lesions of the female reproductive system and the significance of the pre-malignant conditions of that area so that they can identify those patients requiring further investigation and can appreciate their management.

15.2 SPECIFIC BEHAVIOURAL OBJECTIVES

1. Indicate possible aetiological factors involved in malignancy of the reproductive systems.
2. Describe the macroscopic features of benign and malignant neoplasms of the female reproductive system.
3. Describe the common pre-malignant lesions of the reproductive system and discuss their significance.
4. Discuss the clinical features and complications of the common benign lesions of the female reproductive system, such as endometriosis, adenomyosis, fibromyoma, ovarian tumours, uterine polyps, Bartholin's cysts and cervical lesions.
5. Discuss the clinical features and complications of common malignant lesions of the female reproductive system, such as ovarian carcinoma, adenocarcinoma of corpus, squamous-cell carcinoma of cervix, squamous-cell carcinoma of vulva.
6. Discuss the clinical differences between benign and malignant lesions of the female reproductive system.

 7. Identify by history and examination a patient with a malignant or pre-malignant lesion and record the findings.
 8. Take a cervical smear and indicate a knowledge of other techniques available to make a diagnosis of malignant and pre-malignant lesions of the female reproductive system.
 9. Describe the symptoms and signs that would arouse suspicion of the presence of a malignant neoplasm of the female reproductive system.
10. Outline the possible management of benign, malignant and pre-malignant lesions of the female reproductive system.
11. Discuss counselling of a patient with a benign, malignant or pre-malignant lesion of the reproductive system.
12. Discuss the clinical behaviour and prognosis of common malignant neoplasms of the female reproductive system.
13. Discuss the clinical behaviour of common benign neoplasms.

15.3 REASONS FOR LEARNING ABOUT BENIGN AND MALIGNANT TUMOURS IN THE GENITAL TRACT

Women attending a doctor or a clinic may present with symptoms or signs that may be due to a benign or malignant lesion. It is important that not only should doctors understand the basic disease process, but they should also be aware of how it may present, what steps should be taken to diagnose the problem and how it may be managed. Failure to diagnose and initiate management may lead to a delay that will increase morbidity or mortality. Doctors should be able to differentiate most benign from most malignant diseases and when the latter is suspected, they should be able to direct the patient to the most appropriate institution for early treatment.

The details of management are not necessary, but a broad concept of what is involved is essential so that counselling and post-treatment advice can be properly directed. The symptoms or signs may lead to an early and accurate diagnosis of the underlying disease; and failure to detect such a disease may lead to an erroneous management plan.

Patients attending the gynaecological clinic and those admitted for surgery will often be found to have some form of genital tract tumour. Most of these patients will have benign tumours, such as ovarian cysts, fibromyomata, adenomyosis, endometriosis, polyps or Bartholin's cysts. Benign lesions of the cervix, such as ectopic columnar epithelium and polyps, must be differentiated from cancer of the cervix — abnormal uterine bleeding due to fibromyomata, polyps or dysfunctional uterine haemorrhage will often mimic carcinoma of the endometrium, and tumours in the pelvis due to benign follicular cysts or endometriosis may be confused with malignant ovaries.

15.4 TYPES OF TUMOURS OF THE GENITAL TRACT

The common benign tumours of the genital tract are:

1. Physiological ovarian cysts, such as follicular and luteal cysts.
2. Dermoid cysts.
3. Mucinous and serous cystadenomas of the ovary.
4. Fibromyomas of uterus and ovaries.
5. Adenomyosis of the uterus.
6. Endometriosis of the pelvis.
7. Endometrial and endocervical mucous polyps.
8. Ectopic columnar epithelium of the cervix.
9. Bartholin's cysts and abscesses.

The common malignant tumours are:

1. Mucinous and serous cystadenocarcinomas of the ovary.
2. Carcinoma of the endometrium.
3. Carcinoma of the cervix.
4. Sarcoma of the uterus.

15.5 PHYSIOLOGICAL OVARIAN CYSTS

The ovary is composed of stroma in which rest the primordial germ cells, both of which are derived from the common mesenchymal cells of the primitive gonad. As development occurs, the stromal or mesenchymal cells that surround each primordial germ cell differentiate into granulosa cells and theca cells.

Under the influence of follicular-stimulating hormone from the anterior pituitary, one (or more) germ cell and the surrounding granulosa cells begin to grow and form a follicular cyst. The granulosa cells normally produce oestradiol, which reaches a peak of production about the 12th to 14th day and stimulates the production of releasing factor from the hypothalamus. This in turn causes the pituitary to release luteinizing hormone in large quantities and thus precipitates the rupture of a follicle. The resultant ovulation leaves a corpus luteum, which continues to produce oestrogen and progesterone for a further 5–8 days, followed by a gradual decrease in levels (leading to menstruation) unless pregnancy eventuates.

If the delicate balance of hormonal levels is disturbed in any way a number of dysfunctional actions may occur. If the developing Graafian follicle produces low levels of oestrogens, then the induction of a surge of luteinizing hormone fails to occur and ovulation may not eventuate. In this case follicular-stimulating hormone continues to be produced (as well as low levels of luteinizing hormone) and the follicle continues to grow. Normally a follicle reaches about 2 cm in size prior to ovulation, but it may grow to the size of a golf ball (4 cm) or occasionally even larger under the continued influence of follicular-stimulating hormone. The patient will present with a history of amenorrhoea (due to sustained levels of oestrogen), followed by irregular bleeds for some weeks afterwards. Because of the prolonged influence of oestrogen, the endometrium is hypertrophied, may become cystic or even polypoidal, and will eventually produce heavy blood loss (metropathia haemorrhagica). On examination, the uterus is usually not enlarged, the cervix is closed and a round mobile mass can be palpated in the region of the ovary. It is sometimes difficult to differentiate such cases from an ectopic pregnancy or even a normal early pregnancy, so when doubt exists, order a pregnancy test. Most cases of dysfunctional uterine haemorrhage due to anovulation occur in women aged over 35, or in girls who have not yet established their cycle. In all these cases there is no need to operate on the ovarian cyst as it will usually spontaneously regress.

The cyst should be observed for one month, and only if it is more that 5 cm in diameter or persistent for more than one month should a surgical approach be made. An oophorectomy is not required, the cyst can be simply punctured or shelled out of the ovary. The follicular cyst is usually easily identified, as it is 1–5 cm in diameter, thin-walled and filled with clear fluid. The only symptom directly referable to the cyst is haemorrhage or torsion of the cyst, which gives an ache or pain referred to the iliac fossa, or the medial side of the thigh.

Other physiological cysts are corpus luteum cysts, which produce progesterone, and the polycystic ovaries associated with the increased production of luteinizing hormone.

Physiological ovarian cysts of follicular origin are so common that they probably account for 80–90% of all identified tumours of the ovary; they are typically less that 5 cm in diameter, and usually regress spontaneously over a period of one month.

15.6 BENIGN OVARIAN TUMOURS

Mucinous ovarian tumours

Benign mucinous cystadenomas account for 10% of non-physiological ovarian tumours. They are usually multilocular cysts with a smooth, thickened white wall and usually a semi-solid mass present in one region. Occasionally these cysts are bilateral. They may grow to a huge size, filling the whole abdomen and producing marked pressure effects. The cyst is lined by a tall columnar epithelium, which produces a glycoprotein secretion resembling mucin. If the cyst is accidentally ruptured at removal or ruptures spontaneously, the epithelial cells of the cyst may seed onto the peritoneum and produce a myxoma peritonei. This leads to the abdominal cavity becoming filled with mucin — eventually leading to marked bowel problems and death.

About 5–10% of mucinous cystadenomas are found to be malignant at removal.

Serous cystadenomas of the ovary

These cysts account for 35–40% of ovarian tumours. They are usually thin-walled, unilocular cysts with many intracystic papillae. About 30% are found to be bilateral. They usually are not very large — only 5–10 cm in diameter. The secretions that fill the thin-walled cyst are generally clear or straw coloured. The lining epithelium is columnar and is said to resemble the epithelium of the endosalpinx. About 30% of these cysts are thought to undergo malignant change.

Other benign ovarian tumours

Fibromas and luteomas of the ovary are solid tumours, which are less common. They are derived from ovarian stroma and depending on the amount of active tissue within each type of tumour, may secrete excessively large or very small amounts of oestrogen.

Dermoid cysts make up about 25% of all ovarian tumours and are often found to be the cause of cystic enlargement of an ovary. The benign teratomas contain skin, hair, sebaceous glands, teeth and bone. Because of the sebaceous glands, they contain thick, greasy, yellow secretions, which have a very distinct appearance and are highly irritant to the peritoneum.

[handwritten margin notes: heavy – fall into Pouch of Douglas ∴ 10 cm max ∅]

15.7 OVARIAN MALIGNANCY

Any tumour may present as a malignancy and it is often difficult to determine whether the lesion is a primary malignancy or whether there is a change from a benign epithelial stage. However, it is generally conceded that both events may occur.

The common malignant ovarian tumours are serous cystadenocarcinomas, mucinous cystadenocarcinomas, secondary ovarian carcinoma (from bowel, lung or breast — Krukenberg tumours) and sarcoma. Granulosa-cell tumours produce oestrogen and therefore may be associated with endometrial hyperplasia, atypical hyperplasia or even an increased incidence of carcinoma of the endometrium.

Malignant tumours of the ovary usually have a very poor prognosis because they are not detected until very late in the course of the disease.

Clinical features of ovarian tumours

Ovarian tumours are notoriously difficult to diagnose early in their course, and they are usually detected when a patient presents for a routine check-up. However, they do have some symptoms and signs that are important indications of a potential tumour.

Symptoms and signs (Table 15.1)

1. Vaginal bleeding. Postmenopausal women often have an episode of postmenopausal bleeding when an ovarian tumour is present. This bleeding occurs from the endometrium, which may become proliferative under the influence of oestrogen. The oestrogen is derived from ovarian stromal cells (surrounding any tumour of the ovary) that differentiate to produce theca-like cells, which have the potential to produce oestrogen. Premenopausal women may present with irregular vaginal bleeding from the same source.
2. Ascites. A number of tumours of the ovary produce an increase in irritation of the peritoneum (fibromas, carcinomas), and thus produce an increase in ascitic fluid. A peculiar combination of fibromyoma of the ovary, ascites and hydrothorax is known as Meigs' syndrome.
3. Pain. If a cyst undergoes torsion or a vessel bleeds into the cyst, then moderate to severe pain may be experienced. Generally the

Table 15.1 Differentiation between malignant and benign ovarian tumours

	Benign	Malignant
Consistency	Usually smooth walled and cystic	Solid, nodular or part solid/part cystic, with irregular papillae
Fixation	Usually freely mobile	May be fixed, with extension or adhesions
Number of tumours	Only 15% are bilateral	75% are bilateral
Ascites	Usually not a significant amount	Often very copious, with blood staining
Presence of vessels on tumour	No significant increase	Large dilated vessels coursing over the surface, leads to frequent haemorrhage and blood-stained ascites

pain from an ovarian tumour is referred to the iliac fossa and the inner aspect of the thigh.

4. Abdominal swelling, nausea, vomiting and cachexia. These are found when the tumour produces metastases to the bowel, the diaphragm or the omentum.

5. Urinary frequency. This is a common symptom when the tumour is large enough to encroach on the capacity of the bladder.

6. A palpable mass within the pelvis or arising from the pelvis into the abdominal cavity.

7. An ovarian mass is always dull to percussion in the middle and resonant in the flanks. This sign helps to differentiate an ovarian cyst containing fluid, from ascites in the abdomen.

8. An ovarian tumour within the pelvis will generally not move when the cervix is moved up and down. This sign helps to differentiate fibromyomas of the uterus (which are attached to the uterus) from solid ovarian tumours.

Management of ovarian tumours

In the reproductive phase, women presenting with an ovarian tumour that is less than 5 cm in diameter should have the mass rechecked after one month. Physiological tumours usually regress during this time. If the mass persists, is greater than 5 cm in size or is found in postmenopausal women, then a laparotomy should be performed to remove the tumour.

If the tumour appears to be clinically benign, it should be shelled out of the ovary in reproductive women. In postmenopausal women, both ovaries should be removed.

If the tumour appears to be malignant then a frozen section histopathological examination should be carried out as an emergency procedure. If malignancy is confirmed then a bilateral salpingo-oophorectomy and hysterectomy should be performed as well as exploration of the upper abdomen. Any secondary deposits should be removed together with omentum and a peritoneal debulking operation. Surgery should be followed by a course of chemotherapy — presently a combination of chlorambucil and cis-platinum for 6 cycles gives the best response. The overall survival rate for ovarian malignancy is only 30% — most patients die following bowel obstruction, ureteric involvement and cachexia.

15.8 UTERINE TUMOURS

Fibromyoma

Fibromyomas, as the name suggests, are tumours composed of muscle and fibrous connective tissue. They are the most common type of genital tract tumour, and in about 99% of cases are associated with the uterus.

They are usually hard, spherical masses that may range in size from a few millimetres up to 30 cm in diameter. They are surrounded by a pseudocapsule, consisting of compressed myometrial tissue, in which run the blood vessels that supply the tumour.

It is rare to find a fibromyoma in women aged under 30; and most are detected in women aged over 35 — about one-third of all women over this age will be found to have a fibromyoma. However, in the majority of cases the tumours are relatively small and do not cause any symptoms, so no treatment is required.

The symptoms depend on the site and the six of the tumour. The three common sites for uterine fibromyoma are (Fig. 15.1):

1. Subserous. The tumour has grown and extruded to the serous surface of the uterus, forming a sessile or a pedunculated tumour covered by peritoneum.
2. Intramural. The tumour is found within the uterine musculature and apart from enlarging the uterus, produces only a localized thickening in the wall.

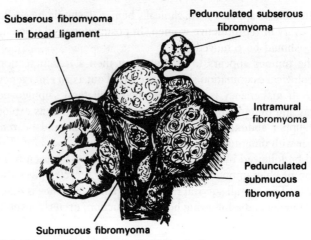

Subserous fibromyoma in broad ligament

Pedunculated subserous fibromyoma

Intramural fibromyoma

Pedunculated submucous fibromyoma

Submucous fibromyoma

Fig. 15.1 Fibromyoma of the uterus. (After Jeffcoate.)

3. Submucous. The tumour has grown into the cavity of the uterus, the surface being covered by endometrium.

SUBSEROUS FIBROMYOMA

These tumours may produce symptoms related to their size, pressure on surrounding organs or due to degeneration. They may reach the size of a football, producing a distended abdomen, bowel symptoms, heavy dragging ache and marked urinary frequency. Other patients have no symptoms, even when the subserous tumour is so large as to be visibly obvious. However, a general principle to be followed is that subserous fibromyomas should be removed if they are so large that they rise out of the pelvis (equivalent to about 14 weeks' gestation) or if they produce pressure symptoms. The commonest pressure symptoms are related to urinary frequency (due to irritation of the trigone or encroachment on the capacity of the bladder) and obstruction to venous return of blood from the lower limbs. This last symptom will only occur with large fibromyomas that fill the pelvis and compress the pelvic veins and the inferior vena cava.

INTRAMURAL FIBROMYOMA

Like the subserous tumours, these may reach a large size, making the uterus itself increase in size, and increase the length and surface area of the uterine cavity. This increased endometrial surface area leads to an increase in blood loss with each menstrual flow, often causing anaemia over a prolonged period of time. Other symptoms may be due to pressure on pelvic organs (urinary frequency) and a dull dragging ache in the pelvis during each menses. This dull dragging ache or pain is due to the increase in pelvic and uterine congestion related to menstruation, and the associated oedema of the myometrial tissue.

SUBMUCOUS FIBROMYOMA

These tumours produce two very specific symptoms:

1. An increase in menstrual flow, due to: *MENORRHAGIA — Regular*
   (a) Increase in surface area.
   (b) Increase in vascularity of the degenerating endometrium covering the fibromyoma.
   (c) Presence of endometrial polyps at the junction of the fibromyoma with the normal uterine cavity.
   (d) Occasional degeneration of the lower pole of a polypoid submucous fibromyoma.
2. Colicky uterine pain, due to the efforts of the uterus to expel the submucous fibromyoma. The fibromyoma may act as a foreign body (like an IUD), and the uterus actively tries to pass the tumour. The cervix will then dilate and the fibromyoma may present into the vagina as a red, bleeding or degenerating tumour.

Fibromyomas that produce menstrual problems are mainly submucous and intramural tumours. They rarely cause intermenstrual or irregular bleeding, and the symptom complained of most commonly is heavy regular periods. Subserous fibromyomas never cause menorrhagia, but as fibromyomas are often multiple it is common to find an enlarged irregular uterus with tumours at all three sites (see Fig. 15.1).

Fibromyomas may undergo hyaline, cystic or fatty degeneration due to interference with the blood supply to the tumours. Red degeneration is a rare complication associated with pregnancy — the fibromyoma becomes necrotic and haemorrhagic, causing acute pain and discomfort. Other complications associated with pregnancy are:

1. Incarceration of a retroverted gravid uterus, causing urinary retention and abortion.
2. Obstruction to labour when a fibroid involves the cervix or lower uterine body.

3. Torsion of a pedunculated subserous fibroid.

Submucous fibroids may produce infertility, but intramural and subserous fibromyomas usually do not interfere with conception.

MANAGEMENT

Fibromyomas that are found during a routine examination and have given no symptoms should not be treated unless they are larger than a 14-week pregnancy.

Fibromyomas that cause symptoms should be removed by myomectomy when the woman is aged under 35, and by hysterectomy when the women is older. However, individual variations to this will arise due to the desire for further pregnancies, size of family, request for symptomatic relief and occasionally when sterilization is a concomitant request.

Whatever method of management is used, prior diagnostic curettage should be performed so that submucous fibromyomas, polyps or endometrial neoplasia can be excluded.

15.9 ADENOMYOSIS

Adenomyosis is a peculiar disease of the uterus, caused when the basal layer of endometrial cells grows into the myometrium, producing crypts and glandular invasion of the muscle. Each crypt or gland is connected to the uterine cavity from which it has arisen, and the endometrium that is shed eventually finds its way into the endometrial cavity of the uterus.

This condition produces a range of symptoms and signs, varying from none to extreme discomfort. About 10% of all women who have a hysterectomy are found to have evidence of adenomyosis on pathological examination, but only about one-third of these women will have complained of symptoms referable to the disease.

Most women with symptoms of adenomyosis are aged over 35, have a history of normal fertility and pregnancies, and present with dysmenorrhoea. The dysmenorrhoea is heavy, dragging and congestive, beginning on the first day of each period, reaching a peak of discomfort on day 2 or 3, and gradually subsiding as the menses cease. Because there is a menstrual loss into each crypt and gland in the myometrium, these glands become distended during menses and produce tension on the surrounding myometrial cells. The blood within each crypt finds its way slowly to the endometrial cavity, so that patients with adenomyosis will have a prolonged menses that is only occasionally heavy.

The signs that may indicate adenomyosis are:

1. Slight enlargement of the uterus. (It is unusual for adenomyosis to cause uterine enlargement beyond the size of an 8-week pregnancy.)
2. Generally uniform firm uterine shape and consistency. (Occasionally there may be a single focus of adenomyosis, which can resemble an intramural fibromyoma.)
3. Tenderness of the uterus when it is squeezed, particularly during a period. (The uterus is generally a non-tender organ.)

Pathologically, the uterus has a whorled, striated appearance with much fibromyomatous material surrounding blood-filled clefts. It can be distinguished from fibromyomas in that there is no 'capsule' of compressed myometrium. Most areas of adenomyosis can be found close to or connected to the uterine cavity, and very few areas are detected near the serosal surface.

Management

Symptomatic adenomyosis does not respond well to hormonal therapy, as the offending cells are derived from the basal layers of the endometrium. However, younger women may be treated with a course of progesterone (e.g. 5 mg norethisterone daily) for 3–6 months. If there is no improvement at the end of this course, then hysterectomy is indicated.

15.10 ENDOMETRIOSIS

Endometriosis is often confused with adenomyosis, but is similar only in that both originate from the same cellular layer.

There have been several hypotheses put forward to account for the development of endometriotic cysts, and it is likely that all may be involved. However, the most popular and plausible hypothesis is that put forward by Sampson. He suggests that endometrial cells spill out through the tubes onto the ovaries and peritoneum of the pouch of Douglas, and implant in these sites to form cysts containing endometrial fluid. The cause of spill of endometriotic cells is not confirmed, but involves several physiological principles:

1. There is an increase in uterine contractions (due to prostaglandins) when secretory endometrium is undergoing menstrual breakdown.
2. Nulliparous women usually have a tightly closed internal cervical sphincter, which may remain contracted during a menses.
3. Menstrual flow may exceed the capacity of the uterine cavity, and the excess may flow into the tubes.
4. Tetanic spasmodic uterine contractions may force menstrual blood out through the tubes to spill onto the peritoneal cavity.

Supportive evidence for these concepts is to be found in the following:

1. Most patients are aged between 25 and 35 when the signs are first detected.
2. Most patients give a history of first-day, spasmodic dysmenorrhoea during the first five to ten years of menstrual life.
3. There is a high incidence of endometriosis among women with cryptomenorrhoea.
4. Early pregnancy, which leads to dilatation of the cervical sphincter, usually relieves the dysmenorrhoea and the subsequent development of endometriosis.
5. Women who have their families early in their reproductive life have less evidence of endometriosis.
6. Women with a history of spasmodic dysmenorrhoea and subsequent infertility are often found to have endometriosis and extensive adhesions in the pelvis.
7. The common sites for endometriosis are the ovary (70%) uterosacral ligaments (30%) and the pouch of Douglas (20%).

Symptoms

Endometriosis produces a multitude of symptoms, but the most extensive of disease processes may be found at laparotomy with virtually no symptoms.

1. Dysmenorrhoea is a common associated factor. Initially patients often give a history of spasmodic, first-day cramp or colic (due to the increased uterine muscle activity), but after 5–10 years (when the endometriotic cells implant and begin to grow into cysts) the pattern of period pain changes. The dysmenorrhoea begins several days before each period, is congestive in nature and reaches a peak

Luteinized unruptured follicle

towards the middle or end of each cycle, subsiding gradually over several postmenstrual days.

2. Dyspareunia is also a common symptom. This occurs due to the penis pressing on and moving the cysts and the associated adhesions.

3. Infertility occurs due to fibrosis and adhesions around the ovary. There is no tubal obstruction, but the tube and ovary may be so involved in adhesions that the ova cannot freely enter the fimbrial end of the tube. *ALSO LUF syndrome*

4. Abdominal pain and discomfort, particularly on defaecation and micturition are common.

There is only occasionally a disturbance in menstrual function and flow, which is probably due to coincidental ovarian or uterine pathology.

Pathologically the tumours are blood-filled 'chocolate cysts' whose walls are composed of flattened endometriotic cells. The cyst itself is surrounded by dense, fibrotic material and adhesions, which may simulate infection, neoplasia, myoma, diverticulitis, hernia or any other abdominal tumour or obstruction.

Diagnosis

Endometriosis should be suspected whenever a patient presents with one or more of the above symptoms. The diagnosis is usually confirmed by pelvic findings of nodules or small tumours in the pouch of Douglas, the utero-sacral ligaments, the recto-vaginal septum or on the ovaries. Often the uterus is retroverted, fixed and very tender to move. Any history or physical findings suggestive of endometriosis should be followed up with a laparoscopy or laparotomy to confirm the diagnosis.

Management

Initially the management should be conservative, with an attempt to treat the disease with hormones. Progestogens (which act as an anti-oestrogen) prevent further growth of endometrium and produce hypoplasia of the glands. If continued for 6 months or more, any small lesions in the pelvis may regress and disappear. The use of progestogens is successful in 25% of cases where the lesions are very small. The androgenic progestogen (Danazol/Danacrine) has marked anti-oestrogenic activity on endometrial cells and has been found to be most useful in the treatment of endometriosis.

Larger endometriotic deposits, involving a dense capsular fibrosis, will not regress in spite of prolonged progestogen therapy. The offending tissue should be removed surgically. The larger cysts can be cut out, whilst the smaller lesions can be cauterized. However, in spite of all measures taken, the endometriosis, fibrosis and accompanying symptoms often persist, and will remain a cause for discomfort until after the menopause.

15.11 CARCINOMA OF THE ENDOMETRIUM

Carcinoma of the endometrium commonly affects postmenopausal women, the average age of presentation being in the early 60s.

The endometrium may show all the features of neoplastic atypy, ranging from atypical hyperplasia, well-differentiated change to poorly-differentiated adenocarcinoma — and the gross features may vary from papillary overgrowth to necrotic ulceration. Squamous metaplasia may occur with well-differentiated adenocarcinomas, and this condition is termed adeno-acanthoma.

Aetiology

Although the cause for carcinoma of the uterus is not known, a number of associated factors have been noted:

1. Late menopause. Women who menstruate beyond the age of 50 have a higher incidence of carcinoma of the endometrium than women who reach the menopause earlier. Prolonged exhibition of hormones, especially oestrogen, may play a part.
2. Relative infertility. Women who have a long history of infertility have a higher incidence of neoplasia. Again, anovulation and unopposed oestrogen are thought to be factors.
3. Dysfunctional uterine haemorrhage due to oestrogen influence or anovulation is also implicated. The action of unopposed oestrogen is to produce endometrial and cystic hyperplasia. Occasionally the cells and glands are associated with stromal hyperplasia and atypical hyperplasias, which are thought to be pre-malignant conditions.
4. Feminizing tumours of the ovary such as granulosa and theca-cell tumours are associated with a higher incidence of carcinoma of the endometrium.

5. Recent evidence suggests that exogenous oestrogen given for post-menopausal symptoms is also associated with an increased (2–3 times greater) incidence of neoplasia of the uterus.

Other factors such as race, parity, diabetes and pregnancy have been implicated in the past, but recent studies have suggested that these factors are not important.

Clinically, carcinoma of the uterus presents with abnormal uterine bleeding. Any irregularity of menstrual function, intermenstrual or postmenopausal bleeding should be investigated by a full curettage. Some women ignore the slight haemoserous discharge, which may present for some months, and only attend when frank blood is visible. Any amount of bleeding should be regarded as potentially derived from a malignant site.

The uterus may enlarge or become softer, but only when the tumour is growing and is more extensive. Occasionally the endocervical canal may become occluded and haematometra (or even pyometra) may result. Extension to the bladder or to the peritoneal surface suggest a poor prognosis.

Metastases occur primarily to the pelvic lymph nodes, the para-aortic nodes and occasionally to the inguinal nodes or there may be widespread haematogenous dissemination. Direct spread to other pelvic organs or trans-peritoneal migration to abdominal cavity sites is very common in the late stages of the disease.

Pain is a late symptom in the disease, as is bowel involvement.

Staging of carcinoma of the endometrium (Fig. 15.2)

Stage 1: Carcinoma confined to the uterus.
Stage 2: Carcinoma involving the uterus and cervix.

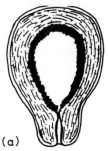 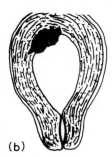

(a)   (b)

Fig. 15.2 Carcinoma of endometrium. (a) Diffuse involvement of uterine cavity; (b) Localized tumour involving myometrium.

Stage 3: Carcinoma extending outside the uterus but not outside the pelvis.

Stage 4: Carcinoma extending outside the pelvis or involving the bladder or rectum.

Diagnosis

The diagnosis is made by examining tissue obtained by curettage for evidence of histological neoplasia, and the staging of the disease is made by clinical examination and chest X-ray (cystoscopy and proctoscopy, if advanced).

Management

The basic management depends on several factors:

1. Age. No bar to surgery if medically fit.
2. Stage of the disease. Early diagnosis and early staging allow more curative management to be undertaken.
3. Availability of appropriate therapy.

Stage 1. The ideal management of Stage 1 carcinoma of the uterus is to perform a total abdominal hysterectomy with bilateral salpingo-oophorectomy. Whilst performing this surgery, gland biopsy and peritoneal tissue should be obtained to determine if any extension has occurred. If the post-operative histopathological examination demonstrates any evidence of tumour in the lymph glands, the peritoneum, or there has been myometrial invasion deeper than one-third, then post-operative radiotherapy should be administered.

Stage 2. Stage 2 tumours are usually given a course of preoperative irradiation before attempting a hysterectomy and bilateral salpingo-oophorectomy with removal of as much pelvix tissue as is possible.

Stages 3 and 4. Stage and 3 and 4 tumours are usually treated with radiotherapy and palliative surgery only. If following a combined radiotherapeutic and surgical approach, there is evidence of extension of the disease then the use of progesterone (medroxyprogesterone — Provera 100–200 mg t.i.d.) may cause reversion of the neoplastic changes in some women.

Prognosis

Stage 1 tumours treated adequately have a 5-year cure rate of 80% while Stage 2 tumours have a 5-year cure rate of about 65%. Stage 3 and 4 tumours of the endometrium have a generally poor prognosis with a cure rate of 15–25%.

15.12 TUMOURS OF THE CERVIX

The most common benign lesion of the cervix is ectopic columnar epithelium. Normally the endocervix is lined by mucus-secreting columnar epithelium, which is under the influence of oestrogen. The ectocervix is covered by flat squamous epithelium, which normally is of a mid-pink colour, and is smooth and regular. Under the influence of oestrogen (during menarche, pregnancy, the taking of certain oral contraceptives, exogenous oestrogen, endogenous oestrogen-producing tumours), the endocervical glands proliferate and grow onto the ectocervix. This outgrowth of columnar epithelium produces a velvety red or orange, roughed epithelium which secretes a profuse clear mucus discharge. Occasionally the mucus epithelium may become infected with coliform bacilli, trichomonas or other pathogens and then a yellow or brownish mucus discharge is evident. Because columnar epithelium is usually only one or two cell layers thick, it is easily broken down and eroded, leading to bleeding and a pus-like discharge.

The ectopic columnar epithelium is continually undergoing metaplastic change to squamous epithelium, during which neoplasia may be found. Regular Papanicolaou smears should be performed on women who have evidence of ectopic columnar epithelium. Ectopic columnar epithelium is in fact not an 'erosion' although it is often discussed in this context when describing cervical lesions. (A true erosion occurs when the whole of the epithelium is lost, leaving a 'raw' area of granulating or stromal tissue.)

Ectopic columnar epithelium, particularly following a pregnancy, may become involved in a chronic infective state and lead to chronic cervicitis. More commonly, however, the cervix is mildly inflamed or not even infected. For simple ectopic columnar epithelium, the surface epithelium should be burnt using a flat cautery point, allowing normal squamous epithelium to grow back after 3–4 weeks. Where chronic cervicitis is present, a deeper stromal cautery may be required.

When metaplasia to squamous epithelium occurs naturally, a number of glands and crypts will be buried under the surface and so lead to occluded glands. These eventually become round, firm, discrete cysts known as Nabothian follicles. They are seen around the external os of a cervix that has undergone metaplastic change to squamous epithelium — they are benign and require no treatment.

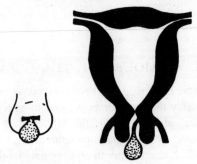

Fig. 15.3 Demonstrating how an endocervical polyp presents at the cervical os.

Polyps

Occasionally, under the influence of oestrogen, the endometrial or endocervical glands hypertrophy until the tissue is thick and polypoidal. These polyps usually develop stalks and protrude out through the cervical os (Fig. 15.3). The majority are less than 0.5 cm in size, but some may grow to 5 cm in diameter. They usually cause abnormal bleeding (e.g. menorrhagia, intermenstrual bleeding or postcoital bleeding) or are occasionally associated with colicky abdominal pain (as the uterus attempts to expel the polyp).

The treatment is simply to twist the polyp or cauterize its base. The polyp must be examined histologically, as about 1–3% have evidence of neoplastic change in the base.

15.13 CARCINOMA OF THE CERVIX

This is the second most common cancer affecting females, accounting for almost 10% of neoplasia of women.

The most common age for detection of carcinoma of the cervix is 45–55, when most other abnormal bleeding symptoms are also commonly found. It is important to be aware of the symptoms and signs of carcinoma of the cervix so that the disease may be diagnosed early and appropriate management initiated.

Factors associated with carcinoma of the cervix

1. The commonest associated factor with the development of carcinoma of the cervix appears to be the papillomavirus. There are

41 known strains of wart virus but only 4 or 5 are thought to have a malignant influence on cervical cells (strains 16 and 18 are particularly virulent).

2. Intercourse. Women who have intercourse with multiple partners have a higher incidence of neoplasia than women who have infrequent or no intercourse. It is believed that sperm, semen, bacterial or viral infection may all predispose to change within the metaplastic cell. It has also been shown that prostitutes have over 100 times greater risk of developing carcinoma of the cervix than do nuns.

3. Childbirth appears to increase the risk of carcinoma about 5–10 times.

4. Other viral infections such as herpes genitalis may be associated with an increased incidence of abnormal change in the cervix.

5. Early age at first and subsequent intercourse increases the risk.

It was once thought that circumcision of the male partner reduced the incidence of carcinoma of the cervix. However, the evidence for this suggestion was the low incidence of carcinoma among orthodox Jewesses, who rarely have intercourse when 'unclean' (i.e. when menstruating, bleeding for the 12–16 weeks postpartum, or having profuse vaginal discharge). But during these times ectopic columnar epithelium is undergoing metaplasia to squamous epithelium, so by avoiding intercourse during these periods, the incidence of carcinoma of the cervix is reduced. The incidence among liberal Jewesses, who do not necessarily refrain from intercourse at these times, is the same as that among Gentile women.

The actual causative agent for carcinoma of the cervix is still unknown. However, large population studies of women in various age groups suggests that there may be a latent phase of 5–10 years, during which cervical epithelium is undergoing a change to dysplasias, carcinoma-in-situ, and finally to invasive carcinoma. If a Papanicolaou smear is taken regularly from the total squamocolumnar junction, then these changes can be identified by detecting abnormal cells with large irregular pyknotic nuclei, or even mitotic divisions, and unusual cell shape.

An abnormal smear result may be found in a slide prepared from the cells taken from a clinically normal cervix. This common finding occurs because the initial cellular changes are intra-epithelial and therefore the early disturbance of the normal surface is macroscopically not visable.

Clinical symptoms and signs

1. Carcinoma-*in-situ*, because it is still intra-epithelial, usually has no presenting symptomatology. The use of the Hinselman colposcope allows magnification of the cervix and therefore easier visualization of abnormal epithelium. When the site is painted with Schiller's iodine, the margins of abnormal epithelium can be seen to stand out. (Glycogen-containing squamous epithelial cells normally take up iodine and stain a mahogany-brown colour, whereas neoplastic or mucus-secreting cells remain non-staining.) When an abnormal smear is reported in the absence of a visible cervical lesion, then a colposcopy, selective biopsy and cautery (or laser) should be performed. A cone biopsy should be performed if there is no colposcopic evidence of abnormality of the ectocervix.

2. Invasive carcinoma may present with symptoms, such as intermenstrual bleeding, postcoital bleeding, postmenopausal bleeding, brown or haemoserous discharge or occasionally (in extensive cases) bladder or bowel symptoms. However, early invasive carcinoma or carcinoma of the endocervix may be detected only at a routine check-up, when a Papanicolaou smear suggests an abnormality and a subsequent cone biopsy proves early invasion to be present. The signs of the disease are a reflection of the stage of the tumour.

   (a) Visually, there may be an exfoliating growth, an ulcer or an intraepithelial spread of the cancer over the cervix and the vagina. Bleeding is a common accompaniment, and any trauma produces a steady ooze or frank haemorrhage.

   (b) Digital vaginal examination usually discloses a firm, often friable mass or ulcer which may extend onto the vaginal epithelium, laterally into the paracervical tissue, to the side walls and pelvic nodes or to the bladder or the rectum.

   (c) Occasionally there may be spread to pelvic glands, liver, scalene node or other sites.

   (d) Rectal examination may disclose parametrial thickening and extension to the pelvic walls or the lymph nodes.

Pathology

Carcinoma of the cervix is usually of the squamous type, although 20% of tumours are derived from columnar epithelium and have the usual characteristics of an adenocarcinoma.

The tumours may vary from well-differentiated squamous-cell carcinomas to poorly differentiated anaplastic lesions; the response to treatment and the survival rate depending not only on the stage of the tumour but on the degree of cell differentiation.

They usually spread by direct invasion to surrounding tissue — by lymphatic spread and occasionally by the haematogenous route. Direct invasion of the paracervical tissues, parametrium, uterus and vagina is the commonest extension — spread to the pelvic lymph nodes (obturator, internal, external, common iliac and pre-sacral nodes) is frequent but the bladder and rectum are rarely involved.

Staging of carcinoma of the cervix

Stage 0: Carcinoma cells are found within the cervical epithelium, but no invasion of the underlying tissue has taken place.

Stage 1: The cancer is strictly confined to the cervix.

Stage 2: The carcinoma has extended beyond the cervix, but has not reached the pelvic walls or lymph nodes. If may extend to the upper two-thirds of the vagina, to the paracervical tissues or to the uterus.

Stage 3: The carcinoma has extended to the pelvic side-walls or has involved the lower third of the vagina.

Stage 4: The carcinoma has involved the bladder, the rectum or spread to tissue outside the pelvis.

All staging is performed clinically, and before the results of investigations or treatment are available.

Diagnosis

When the history, physical examination or Papanicolaou smear suggest that a carcinoma of the cervix may be present, the definitive pathological diagnosis depends on the results of a biopsy taken from the cervix.

An abnormal smear in the presence of a cervical lesion indicates that a punch (or knife biopsy) should be taken from the edge of the lesion. However, when the same smear results are obtained from a relatively normal-looking cervix, then a colposcopy and biopsy should be performed to make certain that all the squamo-columnar junction is examined. If the squamo-columnar junction is not readily visualized or if no abnormal lesion is seen, then a cone biopsy should be performed if the Papanicolaou smear is persistently suspicious.

In both cases, curettage should also be performed to eliminate the

possibility that the abnormal Papanicolaou smear is derived from adenocarcinoma of the endocervix or uterus.

Management

For squamous-cell carcinoma of the cervix, the management depends
entirely on the stage of the tumour.
Stage 0. If Schiller's iodine and a colposcope are available so that the
abnormal area is easily identified, then (multiple) punch biopsies from
the most obvious abnormal areas followed by extensive radical diathermy is the method of choice in management.

However, if the cervix appears to be clinically normal to inspection
after an abnormal Papanicolaou smear, then a cone biopsy should be
performed. If the histopathology suggests complete excision, then
follow-up smears should be taken every 6 months for two years, with a
yearly smear after that time.

An incomplete excision requires either a second cone biopsy or a
hysterectomy. Vaginal vault cytology should be performed regularly to
check that recurrence has not taken place.
Stage 1. These are treated by one of the following methods:

1. Radical hysterectomy with gland dissection and a generous cuff of
   the vagina.
2. Combined external irradiation or intracavitary radium followed by
   extended surgery.
3. Using external and internal irradiation only to treat the cancer.

In the best of hands all techniques appear to give about an 80%
5-year survival rate.
Stages 2 and 3. These are usually treated by external irradiation followed by intracavitary radium. The survival rate varies from 40 to 60%
depending on the stage of the tumour.
Stage 4. These are also treated by intracavitary and external irradiation. Survival rates are low and depend on whether only the bladder
and rectal mucosa and involved.

Adenocarcinoma of the cervix is usually treated surgically, as the
tumour cells respond poorly to radiotherapy. However, recent figures
suggest that a combined approach gives best results.

15.14 VAGINA

There are very few pathological lesions that affect the vagina, because
it is very resistant to any epithelial change. However, benign cysts may
be found:

1. A cystocoele or urethrocoele is relatively common in multiparous women. This lesion is invariably in the midline anteriorly and is easily diagnosed. This is discussed in Chapter 14 under the title 'prolapse'.

2. Inclusion cysts may occur near the vaginal introitus following episiotomies and surgery on the vagina. They cause no problems and do not require treatment.

3. Gartner's duct cysts may be seen in the antero-lateral area of the vagina, and are the result of cystic dilatation of the vestigial mesonephric duct (Wolffian duct). They are generally asymptomatic and require no treatment unless very large and distorting the vagina or urethra. They are thin-walled, translucent, greyish, soft cystic swellings which should not be opened until after an IVP excludes any urinary tract connection.

4. Periurethral cysts may enlarge and protrude from the anterior wall of the vagina, simulating a urethrocoele. However, they are usually firm and cystic. They should not be incised as it may lead to a urinary fistula.

Carcinoma of the vagina

This is relatively rare and is usually of the squamous-cell type. The treatment is generally by needles or plaques of radium implanted directly over the tumour.

15.15 VULVA

Infective lesions of the vulva may include:

1. Bartholin's abscess.
2. Lymphogranuloma inguinale.
3. Granuloma venereum.
4. Vulval warts.

Bartholin's abscess

This usually presents with an acute, tender, painful swelling in the posterior third of the labia. The duct may become obstructed following inflammatory invasion by bacteria (usually coliform or *Neisseria gonorrhoeae*), and the gland then is infected.

It is an acute condition requiring emergency admission and treatment. Although the abscess tends to 'point' outside the vagina, the surgical drainage of a Bartholin's abscess should be into the vagina

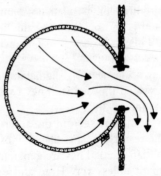

Fig. 15.4 Bartholin's abscess — demonstrating drainage by incision and marsupialization.

itself. The operation to drain a Bartholin's abscess is called 'marsupialization' (Fig. 15.4). The technique is to incise into the abscess and then sew the margins of the incision so that the abscess wall is allowed to unite to the vaginal epithelium, to form a pouch. In this manner the abscess continues to drain into the vagina and when it resumes functioning, the Bartholin's gland secretions empty into the vagina.

Vulval warts

These are usually due to viral infection and can be transmitted venereally. All warts in the vaginal/vulval area appear to increase rapidly in size and extent in moist conditions or during pregnancy so that when other vaginal discharges are present, the warts (condylomata acuminata) appear to flourish profusely. They are often painful, irritating or itchy and are best treated by cautery or painting with 25% podophyllum in tincture of benzoin.

Urethral carbuncle

This is usually due to prolapse or overgrowth of the urethral mucosa. A small inflamed polypoid-like lesion is seen at the urethral introitus. It can be treated with cautery or excision if symptoms warrant its removal.

Vulval malignancy and dermatoses

A number of vulval lesions present with symptoms and some with signs. All of these conditions require careful investigation, as some are due to pre-malignant or malignant conditions and some are benign dermatoses.

The commonest presenting symptom is an itch or an irritation, whilst bleeding, ulceration, papules or warts may be manifestations of vulval lesions.

Hypertrophic dystrophy

This is a chronic inflammation of the subdermis, which leads to ischaemia, increase in keratinization and hypertrophic changes in the epithelium. There is a typical appearance of white plaques and patches in the epithelium, and often the intradermal cells may resemble cancer. It is thought that hypertrophic dystrophy may lead to squamous-cell carcinoma of the vulva.

If a malignant change does not occur, the hypertrophic dystrophy eventually leads to atrophy and fibrosis. This causes the vaginal introitus to shrink, leading to stenosis, 'hooding' of the clitoris and urethra, and eventually to almost complete closure of the vagina.

Hypertrophic dystrophy should be treated with oral oestrogen (in postmenopausal women), together with a local cortisone ointment. If any areas appear suspicious, a biopsy of the site should be performed to exclude a malignant change.

Kraurosis vulvae

This is a condition often mistaken for hypertrophic dystrophy, as it also causes stenosis of the vulva with atrophic changes. However, although the epithelium is pale, there are no plaques. The condition is not pre-malignant. Like hypertrophic dystrophy it occurs following the menopause and will often respond to oestrogen therapy and local creams.

Dermatoses

Women who suffer from chronic dermatological conditions such as psoriasis, intertrigo, fungal infections, vitiligo, etc., may manifest the disease in the vulval and pubic areas. Close inspection is required to diagnose a dermatological cause.

Malignant vulval lesions

The commonest vulval malignancy is squamous-cell carcinoma. This condition is unusual before the age of 65, and usually presents itself as

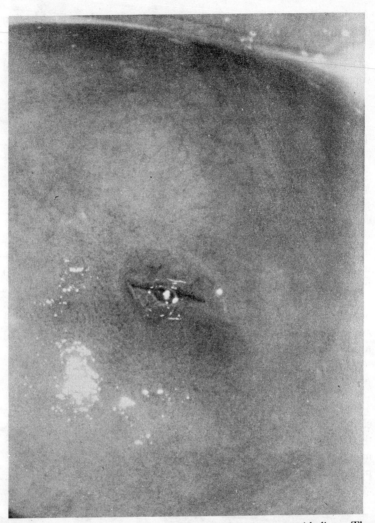

Plate 1 The ectocervix is covered by original squamous epithelium. The external os is in the centre of the colpophotograph. The white areas are due to light reflection. (Plates 1–7 are from Coppleson, Pixley and Reid (1978) *Colposcopy*, 2 edn, Charles C. Thomas, Springfield MA.)

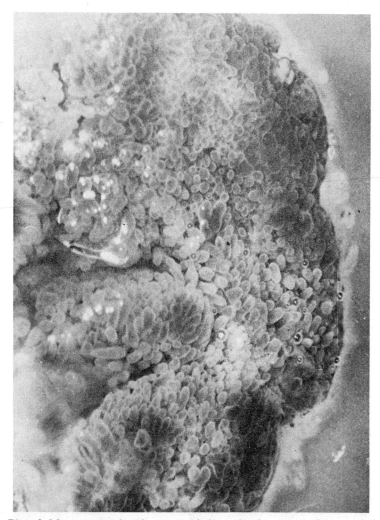

Plate 2 More commonly columnar epithelium also forms part of the cervical covering and here displays the characteristic grape-like or villous colposcopic appearance, which in pregnancy is even more conspicuous. The external os is seen in the centre on the left. Columnar epithelium is laid down on the ectocervix either during embryogenesis or by eversion in the first pregnancy. It appears red to the naked eye and is commonly referred to, incorrectly, as cervical erosion.

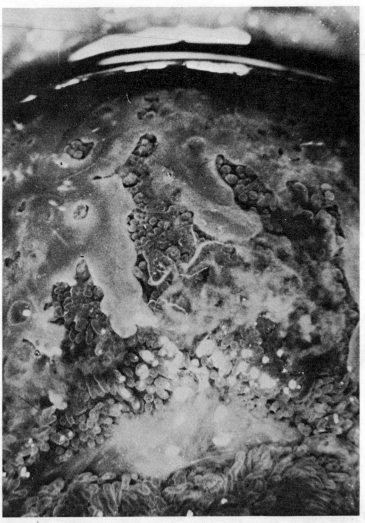

Plate 3 Typical transformation zone. Due to the acid pH in the vagina, the exposed columnar epithelium undergoes metaplasia. Mature normal metaplastic squamous epithelium is seen to form fingerlike processes replacing the columnar epithelium which is still visible as islands in the metaplastic epithelium and near the cervical os below. A plug of white mucus is present at the os.

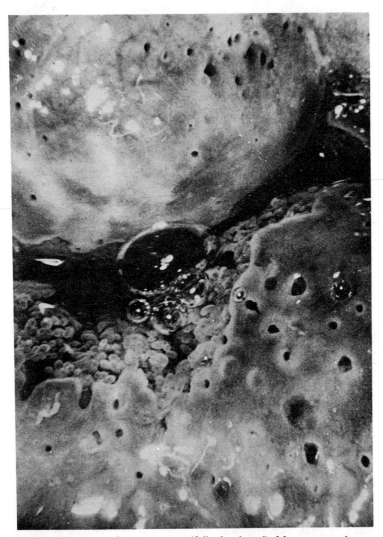

Plate 4 Typical transformation zone (fully developed). Mature normal meta-plastic epithelium has completely replaced the columnar epithelium previously present on the ectocervix. Several gland openings, representing the remnants of the pre-existing glands in the columnar epithelium can be seen. Where these glands are occluded by the metaplastic epithelium, retention cysts (Nabothian follicles) result. This change is irreversible and this woman is now almost free of risk of developing squamous cancer of the cervix.

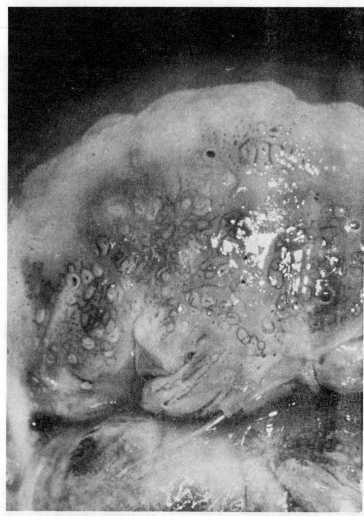

Plate 5 Atypical transformation zone. The columnar epithelium on the ectocervix has been completely replaced by the less common atypical metaplastic squamous epithelium. White epithelium and mosaic structure, the characteristic colposcopic attributes of dysplasia and carcinoma *in situ* are seen. The atypical transformation zone is 'the field of neoplastic potentials'.

an ulcerated, bleeding lesion. It is slow growing but extremely difficult to cure successfully. Most patients are old, frail and unable to tolerate the major surgical attack necessary to remove the tumour and the affected glands. Even when surgery is undertaken, there is a high recurrence rate. Most women with carcinoma of the vulva will be alive after five years, but many of them will have a recurrence of the condition.

Other malignancies of the vulva include:

1. Melanoma, which is potentially very serious.
2. Basal-cell carcinoma.
3. Intra-epithelial carcinoma (Bowen's disease, Paget's disease).

Human sexuality

Rosalind Robertson

16.1 GENERAL INSTRUCTIONAL OBJECTIVE

The students should understand the psychology and physiology of human sexuality and the principles of available therapy for patients with sexual problems so that they can initiate appropriate management.

16.2 SPECIFIC BEHAVIOURAL OBJECTIVES

1. Describe the physiological changes that occur in the human sexual response cycle.
2. Describe deviations from the normal anatomy that cause physical sexual problems.
3. Discuss factors that may modify the human sexual response cycle:
   (a) Physical
   (b) Psychological
   (c) Social
   (d) Cultural
4. Discuss factors that influence libido and sexual arousal in the individual and partners:
   (a) Physiological disturbances (illness, fatigue, depression, anxiety).
   (b) Personality differences.
   (c) Attitudinal differences.
   (d) Hormonal influences (both exogenous and endogenous).
   (e) Sexual techniques.
   (f) Effects of drugs and alcohol.
5. Discuss how a couple's general relationship influences their sexual behaviour.
6. Discuss factors affecting satisfactory intercourse, e.g. impotence, premature ejaculation, loss of libido, vaginismus.

7. Discuss the physical and emotional factors affecting the achievement of orgasm.
8. Discuss the principles of psychosexual counselling.
9. Elicit, present and discuss the history of a patient with a psychosexual problem.

16.3 REASONS FOR LEARNING ABOUT HUMAN SEXUALITY

Every medical practitioner at some stage will be confronted by a patient who complains directly of a sexual problem, or who presents a problem that on deeper enquiry will be found to be due to some psychosexual cause. These multiple presentations may be as varied as depression, pelvic pain, loss of libido or vaginismus. Women may complain of absence of orgasm or headaches due to marital conflict. Most often, the patient and her partner require a full investigation and counselling to allow them to understand their mutual problems, although occasionally therapy directed to one partner only may help resolve the issue. The medical practitioner must have the knowledge and skill to recognize the presentation, explore its cause and direct the couple to the correct mode of management. It is important to be sympathetic and appear to have the time to listen to any problems.

16.4 HUMAN SEXUALITY

Sexual drive or libido is generated in the brain and can occur without requiring any stimulus outside the body. However, sexual drive is capable of being affected by the emotional state, past experiences, environment and by many influences external to the body. Every person has a sexual urge or libido and the level of the response to this basic urge depends on many factors. These can be grouped into two separate but inter-related parts:

1. The Biological. The brain contains centres that enhance or stimulate sexual drive. In this regard, sexual drive is regulated like other biological drives such as thirst and hunger. The centre located in the brain stimulates or depresses the physical reflex in the sacral portion of the spinal cord. When erogenous zones are stimulated impulses are transmitted to the sacral portion of the spinal cord. Return impulses then stimulate the blood vessels in the genital region, so that engorgement occurs.
2. The Psychological. This is a reflection of the need or motivation to

engage in sexual activity at a given time. Psychological need for sex is a complex issue, as emotional state, environment and experiences, play an important role.

16.5 THE SEXUAL RESPONSE CYCLE

The response cycle consists of four phases. The duration of each of the phases varies greatly with the individual and the circumstances. The only major difference in the physiological response between the two sexes is the presence of a refractory period when the male is unable to respond to a second stimulation until a certain period of time has elapsed. For this reason the male is usually unable to have repeated orgasms over a short space of time. This refractory period may well be due to inhibitory impulses from the ejaculatory reflex centred in the lumbar portion of the spinal cord.

VASOCONGESTION AND MYOTONIA

Vasocongestion and myotonia are the two underlying mechanisms in both sexes which lead to the various organ responses. Vasocongestion is the engorgement of blood vessels in superficial and deep tissues, but especially in the genital organs. It begins at the start of sexual excitement and precedes myotonia, the second response. Myotonia is increased muscle tension. Myotonia affects both smooth and skeletal muscles, and occurs both voluntarily and involuntarily. With continual stimulation, muscle tensions build up to a certain point and then a reflex stretch mechanism causes the muscles to contract vigorously. The result of these contractions is a release of muscular spasm and a decrease of vasocongestion. At the time these contractions are occurring, the individual experiences the peak of physical pleasure known as orgasm.

1. The excitement phase

In all individuals there is a base level of sexual drive, which is variable. Starting from this, within 10–30 seconds of the beginning of any effective mechanical or psychological sexual stimulation, there is marked vasocongestion. This produces vaginal lubrication in the female and erection of the penis in the male. At the same time in the female there is lengthening and distension of the inner two-thirds of the vagina. As the plateau phase is approached the uterus is elevated and the inner part of the vagina distends. The blood vessels in the labia minora and

EXCITEMENT
PLATEAU
ORGASMIC
RESOLUTION

Clitoral shaft also undergo vasocongestion and the nipples become erect. This phase is variable in duration and dependent on the form of stimulation.

2. The plateau phase

The outer third of the vagina becomes markedly engorged, so that the vaginal opening decreases by at least one-third. The clitoris retracts under the clitoral hood, almost inaccessible to direct stimulation but still responding to pressure from traction of the clitoral hood. The engorged labia minora undergo a vivid colour change, from pink to bright red in nulliparous women and red to deep wine colour in parous women.

3. The orgasmic phase

This usually lasts 5–10 seconds, and begins with contractions in the outer third of the vagina. Uterine contractions may also begin at this time. At the same time, respiration, heart rate and blood pressure have all increased. During orgasm, there is a release of muscular spasm and engorgement of blood vessels, and a peak of physical pleasure.

4. The resolution phase

During this time, in the female, the plateau and orgasmic phases may be reactivated by adequate stimuli. Following orgasm, the clitoris that has been retracted returns to its normal position within 5–10 seconds. The contraction in the outer third of the vagina ceases and slowly all the organs return to their previously unstimulated state. Unlike the female who maintains higher levels of stimulative susceptibility during the immediate postorgasmic period, the male has a unique refractory period, where sexual tension is reduced to low excitement phase levels. Due to the postorgasmic loss of stimulation response, the male viscera tend to lose superficial and deep vasocongestion more rapidly than the female.

16.6 FACTORS AFFECTING HUMAN SEXUALITY

Various factors affect basic sexual drive and the subsequent sexual response cycle. They are discussed here as two separate but inter-related parts — physical factors and the affect of psychological factors.

Physical factors

1. PHYSICAL TOUCH

Touch is the only type of stimulation to which the body can respond reflexly and independently of higher psychic centres. If a man is unconscious or has a spinal cord injury preventing impulses to and from the brain, an erection can still be obtained by stimulation of the genitals or inner parts of the thigh. This is a reflex from nerve endings to the cord, with resultant vasocongestion and myotonia. The reflex is centred in the sacral portion of the cord. The degree of response depends upon the intensity of the mechanical stimulus and the area of stimulation. Although touch receptors are the same in all areas of the body, they are much more concentrated in those parts that are commonly called the "erogenous zones" (e.g. breasts, inner parts of the thigh, genitals, etc.). Many women who are orgasmic are only able to respond to the point of orgasm by direct manipulation (manual or oral) of the clitoral region.

2. ORGANIC FACTORS

Ageing is a good example. A man usually achieves peak sexual drive at about the age of 19–20 and this slowly decreases, but sexual drive is still present in old age.

In the female this drive tends to reach its maximum somewhat later and then slowly decreases.

3. HORMONES

Hormones play a significant role in the development and maintenance of our sexuality. Oestrogen decreases sexual drive in the male, but testosterone has been reported to increase drive in a female by increasing the clitoral response mechanisms. Progesterone in high dosages tends to decrease libido in the female, as may oestrogen. This is probably related to increasing levels of sex hormone binding globulin.

4. PATHOLOGICAL

Pain, fatigue, chronic debilitating diseases, and neurological diseases.

5. *DRUGS*

Particularly:

- Anticholinergics
- Anorexiants
- Anti-epileptics
- Some cardiovascular drugs
- Some CNS depressants
- Psychotropic drugs (antidepressants, neuroleptics).

Psychological factors

Psychological factors are primarily related to our education and past experiences. There is no doubt that one of the stronger factors in sustaining sexual desire is satisfaction from previous relationships and experiences.

However, other important factors can lead to a depression of sexual response, such as fear. This may be fear of discovery, fear of pregnancy, fear of contracting a sexually transmitted disease, injury, heart attack, or fear of failure, guilt or shame.

Self-esteem and perceived body image are also important factors. If lack of self-esteem or poor body image is an issue, then there may be marked depression in the ability to respond sexually.

The way in which individuals regard themselves as sexual persons also has an important effect on the ability to abandon themselves and enjoy sexual activity.

Development of sexual attitudes during childhood and adolescence can vary greatly depending on the cultural and individual environment and influence sexuality.

General attitudes of the community are also of importance and can affect response.

Interpersonal problems which might be encountered as a cause for sexual problems include:

1. Failure to communicate.
2. Failure to arouse emotionally.
3. Poor sexual technique or boredom with the technique.
4. Poor sex education and lack of sexual experience.
5. Aversion and dislike of partner.
6. Fear of interruption by children or relatives, etc.
7. Fear of pregnancy.
8. Financial pressures.

9. Cultural, social and religious differences.
10. Sexual aversions and perversions.

16.7 SEXUAL COUNSELLING

Sexual counselling involves both therapists and clients in a detailed exploration of the problems causing the sexual inadequacy and then the therapist using a reflective approach, allowing the client to understand the factors which have caused the problem.

Counselling requires skill and patience on the part of the therapist and motivation and involvement by the couple. Used in conjunction with behaviour modification, excellent results may be achieved in the majority of motivated couples. Both counselling and behaviour modification by themselves have high failure rates.

How to counsel

1. Counselling is best done by having both members of the client partnership attend for all visits, creating the understanding that all problems are shared problems.
2. Make sure that you have allowed sufficient time to listen to the problem and have both partners express their interpretation of the problem. It is difficult to conduct any counselling session in less than 1 hour.
3. Make the session a relaxed, non-threatening experience — the more relaxed you appear to be, the more productive the session will be.
4. Do not interrupt to clarify, but allow both parties equal time to present their differing viewpoints.
5. Do not take sides or favour one point of view, even though you may feel strongly that one or the other person is incorrect or being imposed upon.
6. Provide a setting in which the couple learn by self-discovery and awareness, rather than by you being too directive in your approach.
7. Encourage the couple to take an active role in the solutions to their problems. Stress the need for their participation and motivation in problem solving. If they are not sufficiently motivated to work together, their problems will be difficult to solve.
8. Always give client couples a task to complete before they return for their next visit. These tasks may relate to communication

activities (verbal, non-verbal and sexual) or to behavioural modification exercises.
9. Always begin each new session by asking about the homework which has been set at the previous counselling session.

16.8 HUMAN SEXUAL PROBLEMS

Common male problems

1. Premature ejaculation. Ejaculation occurring so quickly (less than 30 seconds after beginning intercourse) that a normal female is unable to obtain sexual satisfaction.
2. Erectile impotence. This may be total or simply related to a particular situation.
3. Retarded or absent ejaculation.
4. Loss of libido.

Common female problems

1. Loss of libido.
2. Orgasmic dysfunction.
3. Vaginismus. Involuntary vaginal muscular spasm, leading to failure of penetration and localized pain.
4. Dyspareunia or painful intercourse.

Management

The aims of the initial consultation are:

1. Establishment of rapport with patient and partner preferably (the relationship must allow interchange between patient and doctor and be non-directive in approach).
2. Taking a sexual problem history, including:
   (a) Description of current problem.
   (b) Onset and course of problem.
   (c) Patient's perception of cause and maintenance of problem.
   (d) Past treatment and outcome (professional and self-treatment) and why the patient feels it did not work.
   (e) Expectation and goals of treatment.
3. Relieve immediate anxiety by reassurance and limited relevant information.

4. Decide if referral to sex therapist is necessary. (Grounds for referral may be insufficient time or resources, poor relationship with patient, or the case being too complicated.)

In almost all cases, the basic problem is compounded by anxiety, either related to inadequate sexual knowledge or to fear of failure. Often all that is necessary is reassurance and limited related information, showing that myths regarding sex (e.g. penis size, coincidental orgasm, etc.) are incorrect, and explaining that any sexual behaviour which is perhaps producing guilt is also practised by others and may be continued without misgivings.

In conducting sex therapy the overall aims should encompass:

1. Overcoming performance pressure.
2. Allowing the couple to learn what kind of stimulation is pleasant and arousing.
3. Building up communication between the partners.

The classic example of this approach is the sensate focus programme, which is a graded approach to intercourse involving all the above concepts. It usually consists of three separate stages. The first is each partner exploring and stimulating the other partner's non-genital regions, and communicating their feelings. Once complete relaxation and confidence is obtained by both partners they move to the second stage, genital stimulation, and finally the third stage, intercourse.

A co-operative partner is required for this or similar programmes. The patient must have some assertive skill, and both participants must feel comfortable with their own body. This type of programme is of great help in loss or lack of sexual interest and limited or no sexual response. It may also be used as an adjunct in the management of the other common problems listed.

Other simple programmes use desensitization in addition to sensate focus. For example, the squeeze technique is used in the treatment of premature ejaculation, and progressive vaginal dilatation for vaginismus. The squeeze technique also requires co-operative partners, and is based on the fact that squeezing for 10–15 seconds just below the head of the penis prior to ejaculation removes the desire to ejaculate. Progessive vaginal dilatation is usually carried out initially by the patient alone, or with the help of her doctor. It is a graded approach using dilators (fingers or glass) of increasing size. Encouraging the patient to use tampons during her menstrual period is also useful.

16.9 SEXUALITY IN PREGNANCY

Pregnancy produces a further set of problems which might cause conflict and increased interpersonal disruption. These can be listed under the following headings:

1. Nausea, vomiting and tiredness.
2. Change in mental attitude to sexual intercourse.
3. Fear of hurting 'the baby'.
4. Feeling cumbersome.
5. Repugnance of the whole sexual act.
6. Feeling fat and ugly.
7. Difficulty in maintaining a suitable position for intercourse.
8. Worry and anxiety about managing a new infant in the house — will they be able to cope.
9. Is the baby normal?

It must of course be remembered that pregnancy may also enhance a close sexual relationship for the following reasons:

1. Sharing the feelings of producing a new life.
2. Enhancing a close interpersonal relationship.
3. Enhancing the physical appearance of women.
4. Increasing the sexual response mechanism.

Advice on sexual activity in pregnancy and the puerperium

It is quite normal for couples to have sexual intercourse during pregnancy and you should advise that there is no contraindication to intercourse throughout pregnancy except if any of the following problems have occurred:

1. Antepartum haemorrhage.
2. Premature rupture of membranes.
3. History of premature labour or of premature rupture of membranes.
4. Vaginal infections such as trichomonas, monilia or venereal disease.
5. If the obstetrician specifically forbids intercourse for a specific reason.

In the puerperium, intercourse may be resumed when:

1. Vaginal cuts or lacerations have healed — usually 3–4 weeks.
2. Blood-stained discharge has ceased — usually 2–3 weeks.

Index